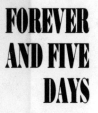

FOREVER
AND FIVE
DAYS

FOREVER AND FIVE DAYS

Lowell Cauffiel

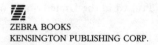

ZEBRA BOOKS
KENSINGTON PUBLISHING CORP.

ZEBRA BOOKS

are published by

Kensington Publishing Corp.
475 Park Avenue South
New York, NY 10016

Library of Congress Catalog Card Number: 91-76056

First printing: March, 1992

Printed in the United States of America

ISBN 0-8217-3710-4

For Deborah

Acknowledgements

Non fiction is not possible without a collective effort by many people. Some of their names already appear in the main text. Others do not, but were equally important in the development, research and writing of *Forever and Five Days*.

I would like to thank reporter Jan Weist, my research assistant in Grand Rapids, for her work with victims; Jeanne McAllister for her timely transcripts; Paul Dinas my editor at Zebra for his belief in this book; attorneys Michael Novak and T. Patrick Freydl for their ongoing expertise, and my agent Russell Galen and the folks with Scott Meredith for their continuing support.

Furthermore, this book could not have been researched without the cooperation of Warden Joan Yukins and Deputy Assistant Warden Dr. George Calvert at the Huron Valley Women's Facility; the psychological insight of Dr. Michael Abramsky; the medical consultations of Dr. Herbert Malinoff, M.D.; the input of Cindy Lent at the FBI's Behavioral Science Unit, and the help of Pat Zacharias and Anita Mack at the Detroit News and Chris Kucharski at the Detroit Free Press.

Above all, I would like to thank my daughter Jessica and son John for their love and patience. And finally, there's no greater gratitude than the kind I've discovered in the company of Bill's crew, both the Tuesday night group and the Chelsea regulars: Eugene, Guss, Dan, John and all the rest.

Author's Note

Forever and Five Days is a work of fact. It is not a "fictionalized" version of the Alpine Manor murder case. The narrative is based on more than twenty-five thousand pages of documents and hundreds of hours of taped interviews conducted by myself, or an assistant, with more than thirty key characters. They include conversations with Catherine May Wood and many interviews over the course of a year with Gwendolyn Gail Graham. Miss Graham also underwent psychological testing and evaluation by Dr. Michael Abramsky, a forensic psychologist I consulted. Other documentation includes police and court transcripts, patients' medical records, Alpine Manor work files, computerization of calendar data and other proven sources and methods of journalistic research. Everything was cross-checked wherever possible. Some individuals requested anonymity, and their fictitious names appear in italics on the first reference. To protect their privacy and dignity, some patients at Alpine Manor not involved in the murder case are called by their first names only.

Love does not rejoice in what is wrong but rejoices with the truth.
—1 CORINTHIANS, Chapter 13.

Prologue:

Wednesday, November 30, 1989

The blows of the sledgehammers rang out in the building, shaking loose the remnants of earth still clinging to the vault. It was no easy task, breaking the seal of the burial chamber that held the casket of the woman.

The interior of the utility garage at the Rosedale Park Memorial Cemetery was frigid and full of shadows in the last minutes of the afternoon. It smelled of earth and fertilizer and motor oil. But mostly, it was cold. An undertaker, a cemetery manager, a vault company representative and two detectives from a suburban Grand Rapids police department shuffled and stamped, waiting for the grisly work to be done.

The air seemed colder inside than out, where earlier the plot under a maple tree had been roped off by yellow crime scene tape. The sun was setting as a backhoe devoured the first layers of earth in the section called Garden of the Gospels. By the time the excavating machine was finished, the scene was illuminated by the harsh, blue glow of television lights beamed in from beyond the yellow tape. The halogen spots turned the pupils of the gravediggers into pencil points, blinding them to the contents of the cavity. When they jumped in with their shovels, they felt like they were about to dig in a bottomless pit. Finally, large flakes of new snow softly pelted the vault as it was chained, lifted to a flatbed truck and shuttled away to the garage.

Some reporters and photographers were waiting outside in the dark, while the workers in the garage went about their work. The news media had showed up at the cemetery after learning of the court order to exhume for autopsy the body of the sixty-year-old woman. She had been embalmed, blessed and buried nearly two years ago. The mere fact she was being dug up was news.

Already they had fragments of a more astounding story. There had been tips that police were investigating deaths in a nursing home called Alpine Manor. Routinely, the facility in the suburb of Walker averaged about forty deaths a year.

"It's not unusual for people to die in a nursing home," a spokesman for the facility had said, trying to calm concerns. "They are all expected to die, sooner or later, of natural causes."

However, they were not expected to die of suffocation. Police were looking at the possibility that patients had been smothered. The homicides, the story went, were the handiwork of employees. One victim had been an Alzheimer's patient. Another had been suffering from gangrene of the leg. One news source claimed to have talked to a witness of the killings. The source wasn't sure if the deaths were to put patients "out of their misery" or just a way of "getting kicks."

Later, the identities of eight possible victims were reported. The number alone shocked the quiet, middle-American city, home of the presidential museum of its favorite son, Gerald Ford. The number of homicides in the city of Grand Rapids for all of 1989 stood at only six. Soon, reports would also surface that the killings were part of some kind of love bond, an unholy cement in a union of lust and death.

Grand Rapids had always been immune to such stories. The city by the Grand River was designated an "All-American City" four times by the National Municipal League. A local minister once dubbed it the "Christian Capital of the World." Beer and wine were available on Sunday, but first you had to find a grocer open on the Sabbath. Civic brochures promoted the ratio of one church for every thousand people. The city was the home of the Christian Reformed Church, the American outpost of Dutch Calvinism. The western side of Michigan was the state's Bible Belt.

Inside the utility garage, the detectives directing the men with the sledgehammers were obsessed with a more earthly pursuit. The investigative process had proven as difficult as the burial seal. Questionable witnesses, elusive facts and hidden agendas had dominated the inquiry. Perhaps the truth was inside the vault.

Finally, gravediggers pried open the long concrete container with crowbars. As they wrestled the heavy top from the vault, the atmosphere of the garage quickly changed. They couldn't get the casket into the medical examiner's van soon enough. With a blast of exhaust, the van left behind the pungent, fleshy smell of death.

Not a half hour later, the casket itself was opened in the autopsy room of a Grand Rapids hospital. Inside the woman of sixty was dressed in a pink jacket and skirt, white ruffled blouse, brassiere, panty hose, a slip and shoes. Her blond hair was highlighted with natural gray. It was still shaped from her final hairdressing.

There was, however, a problem. Some in attendance at the post-mortem examination suspected as much when the vault seal was broken. Also, someone had heard something sloshing in the casket when it was carried into the hospital's autopsy room. The woman's final resting place had not been immune to disturbance. In the twenty-two months of her interment, water had somehow invaded the casket. Extensive mold in a surreal shade of blue-green clung to the woman's face, the back of her neck and portions of her extremities.

At 7:00 P.M., the search for answers began with the stainless cut of a pathologist's knife.

PART ONE

1986

Chapter 1

"I enjoyed taking care of those old people."

—Cathy Wood, December 29, 1989.

For five days she inhaled pure oxygen, as antibiotics fought the infection that tried to steal away her breath. They wanted her comfortable; that was their overwhelming concern. She should have oxygen. She should have antibiotics, if those helped. They didn't want any elaborate life-support systems. Ma would not have wanted her life perpetuated by a mechanical device, they all agreed. That's where the Chambers family would draw the line.

None would be drawn today.

"She's strong as an ox, that Hollander," Ed Chambers said.

Pop's right, Jan thought. Her age, and her constitution—her stalwart Dutch blood, "damned Hollanders," Pop always said—had pulled her through again.

"You know, I'm feeling like she can conquer anything," Jan said.

This she really wished.

Jan searched her mother's face. Her cheeks were narrow without her dentures, but not gaunt. Her forehead was square and high, her nose upturned and well-proportioned. Her hair was the color of faded straw. That and her blue eyes affirmed her ancestral claim to the family names of De Boer and Van Der Sac. Jan spoke quietly.

"Soon you'll be leaving. Soon you'll be outta the hospital, Mom."

Jan looked again, not for color, but brightness, the gleam of recognition. Sometimes Jan could see that in her eyes.

For months, charts like the one hanging at the foot of the hospital bed had differed only in the handwriting and perception of the nurses making the notes. Jan could recite the entries: "Marguerite Chambers. Age, 60. Alzheimer's Disease. Incontinent of bowel and bladder. Involuntary movement of arms. Does not communicate."

Or, sometimes it read, "Unaware of her surroundings."

Or, "Does not communicate except for added activity and facial expressions."

The shape of her mother's body was a constant. Jan usually found her bent forward and inward on her back, or fetal, on her side. Her clenched hands were positioned just below her chin. Together both limbs moved rhythmically as if she were suspended forever in some kind of earnest prayer.

It was the seventh day of April. Tomorrow, Marguerite Chambers would be leaving the hospital. Her daughter Jan Hunderman, however, knew she would not be going home.

Outside St. Mary's Medical Center, balmy winds from the southwest blew across the city of Grand Rapids. Abnormally high temperatures in the seventies provided a peculiar contrast with the urban landscape. Trees everywhere were still leafless from the Michigan winter. Survivors of the Dutch elm disease in the nearby Heritage Hill historic district swayed like stranded stick figures, trying to signal someone in the cloudless sky. Life swelled in new buds, but their old age and their stature, placed this evidence well above the perception of most everyone on the street.

A few blocks north, on the concrete terrain around Grand Rapids Junior College, street life was different. The blast of warm air from the south had brought out young people in force. Bicyclists dodged traffic down the Ransom Avenue hill. Coats littered steps and retaining walls. Students perched anywhere they could find a spot. Some skipped classes. Others read texts, but did so in the sun.

Jan Hunderman had seen Michigan's perennial struggle between winter and spring play out fourteen times since her mother's decline began. She would never forget the first hint. Those monogrammed dinner napkins, in 1972. They announced "Jan & Gary," her wedding.

"Mom forgot to bring them," she told a friend. "But when she raced back to the house to get them, she forgot why she'd gone there in the first place."

"Dumb Hollander," Pop had said.

Everyone laughed. The early symptoms were easy to overlook, easy to fix to some other cause.

Marguerite Chambers might have been able to hide them longer if it had not been for her job. She repaired and calibrated flight instruments, working thirty years at Lear Siegler. Ed Chambers had been arguing the causes of workers since he became president of his UAW local. When it came to his wife's forgetfulness, however, he had to side with management.

"They told me that perhaps it's best they put her on sick leave until you find out what's wrong with her," Pop said.

After a series of examinations in Grand Rapids, the family took her to the Mayo Clinic, then were told about the progressive dementia called Alzheimer's Disease. At the time, Marguerite was only forty-eight. Ed was fifty-one. Jan was turning twenty-one, and her two younger brothers were still in high school. Together, they all watched their mother go back. It was like watching someone's mind age in reverse.

Marguerite had always been active, leading 4-H groups, water-skiing up at the family cottage. She had been a dancer, with an energetic set of dancer's legs.

This was different. The polka and waltz gave way to the jerk and the monkey. She wore loud clothes and tight pants. She became pouty, self-absorbed, then defiant.

"Holy smokes, my mom's turned into a teenager again," Jan told her friends.

In time, as her memory loss became more severe, Ed Chambers took away the car keys. She was parking the family car right in the middle of Alpine Avenue, then locking it up before heading into the stores to shop.

In time, she began asking for help with basic tasks. She asked permission. Scrabble, her longtime favorite game, became difficult, then impossible. Her verbal vocabulary deteriorated as well. She would point at the Scrabble board up at the cottage.

"You wanna play?" Jan asked.

She nodded. They started, then she would simply forget what to do with the letters. Jan usually ended up playing both hands. Her mother got frustrated with that.

"Oh darn," she said.

Often she looked bemused, as though she didn't understand why it was all happening. That was the worse part, Jan thought.

Eight years into the disease, Jan's mother was speaking in fragments: "I wanna." "Come." "This way," and the like. Eventually there were only syllables, repeated as though she had developed a stutter.

The family could sense her frustration and anger.

"If you don't keep a good eye on her," he said, "that Hollander will sneak up on you and beat the hell out of you."

Pop tried to put a humorous spin on things. But Jan could see these kind of things hurt him as well.

Marguerite stayed close in her last months at home. She'd lived on the same parcel of land all her life. So had her ancestors, back when that part of the suburb of Walker was laced with Dutch farms. Ed and Marguerite Chambers' first home was the old farmhouse where Jan's grandmother was raised. Later, they split off a lot from the old De Boer family farm to build their own home and sold the rest off.

During her mother's last summer in Walker, Jan remembered, she had often beckoned Pop outside. He sat on the porch while she waded through wild grass bleached by the late summer sun. There was a field, and across it, a nursery. She always headed for the greenhouses. She gazed through the smears of paint on the windows at the baby plants. She wandered among the saplings lashed to sticks in the nursery yard.

Pop always let her linger for a while, then cupped his hands and called:

"Maaaaaargieeeeee. Maaaaaargieeeeee."

In the last days of August, the screaming began. She screamed spontaneously, cued by no apparent person or event. She sounded as if she were scared, or hurt maybe. Three times neighbors called the police.

Jan's father had retired early to care for her. He was feeding her, leading her like a toddler to the bathroom. Jan visited her mom after work, giving her baths, putting her on the toilet.

The doctor prescribed a sedative for her outbursts. Jan's father called soon after the first dose. His voice was shaking.

"Jan, Ma can't walk!"

Jan sped over to the house. They had to come up with a plan. Her father couldn't carry her to the bathroom. Everyone was doing what they could, but everyone also had to work. She needed twenty-four-hour nursing care in her own home. No one could afford that.

Jan and her father took her to the Kent Oaks Psychiatric Unit, part of the state system. The facility agreed to admit her while the Chambers found a private nursing home.

The memory of their last moments in the admitting room could still send Jan into tears.

Her mother was frightened, confused. Her eyes darted around the room.

"No, Janie," she kept repeating. "No, no, Janie."

When Jan and her father returned to visit the next day, hospital officials said Marguerite Chambers had been transferred to Kalmazoo State Hospital, another mental facility. She was taken there in the back of a police car on the return leg of a transfer of the criminally insane. A month later, the family was advised to commit her.

Jan shuddered when she thought of the hour trips to Kalamazoo, south on U.S. 131 through open flatlands of soy and corn. The asylum sat on top of a hill. Its architectural focus was a twelve-story water tower with a solid brick parapet topped by merlons and crenels. It looked like a chess rook. It looked like the setting for a horror film.

Marguerite was kept on the third floor, behind a series of locked doors. The ward was large and open, full of windows with security screens and bars. Walkways were defined only by a pair of yellow lines on the linoleum floor.

"It smells like peanut butter in here," Ed Junior, Jan's brother, sometimes said.

"To me, it smelled like something died," Jan said later.

One side of the ward had twenty beds, partitioned by curtains. Patients shared dressers. They shuffled about, or sat in wheelchairs. Some mumbled ongoing commentaries of their own particular delirium. Others just glared and shouted angrily at Jan and others when they passed.

Jan usually found her mother sitting among them. She was dressed in pajamas, her hair pulled back in two pigtails. Her vocabulary, by that juncture, had been reduced to one repetitive utterance.

"Hi Mom," Jan would say.

"Nt. Nt. Nt."

Jan knew what she was trying to say: "Shit, shit, shit." It was one of her last words.

It could have been worse, Jan told herself. There was the other half of the ward, the side where she never went. There were ten beds there. They were caged. In fact, they looked like giant baby cribs of steel.

Please God, Jan prayed, I don't ever want to see my mother on the other side.

For two years the Chambers name had sat on waiting lists at several nursing homes. When Ed's eye doctor became involved in the hunt, a bed was made available within days. The facility was called Alpine Manor, a nursing home in Walker, only three blocks from Ed Chambers' home. Two nurse's aides there were former high school classmates of Jan's. She felt even more reassured after talking with the nursing director.

"We'll take good care of your mother," she said. "We don't want you to worry anymore."

The contrast between the state hospital and Alpine Manor was stunning. Rooms were carpeted and clean. Some patients talked nonsense, but few screamed. They sought conversation. There was a reassuring order to the place. Nurse's aides wore pastel colors. Nurses dressed impeccably in white.

Marguerite's room was neat, orderly. There was an intercom and call button. There was a big picture window overlooking a court-yard. There were curtains, not bars.

"Make sure you visit a lot, because the patients who get visitors never get ignored," a friend who worked there advised.

And they did. Ed came every day. Jan and other relatives came at night. Some days she would have up to three visits.

That's the way it had been for three years now, until the most recent complication. When her mother's condition worsened, the whole family prepared for her death. They gathered at her bedside for the death watch. Twice now they had gathered, but Jan's mother had other plans.

"Tomorrow, Mom, you'll be heading back to Alpine Manor."

Her mother's body remained kinetic in the hospital bed. It's been a long time since she's mumbled even a syllable, Jan thought. If she could sit, then walk, what then? Where would she go? And what would she think when she got there?

They knew so little. Jan wondered if she was like a patient with a head injury, the kind that recovered to report people, places and conversations back when everyone thought they were unconscious.

Jan never doubted her mother still knew her, but with Pop, her reaction was profound. Her clenched hand would pop up like a jack in a box when his voice sounded as he strolled through the door. Her eyes wide, she shook her hand repeatedly. When he grabbed it, and squeezed, she calmed.

He often held her that way, slowly positioning her arm back near her breast.

"Dumb Hollander," Pop sometimes said.

Their eyes did all the rest.

The next day, the ambulance left the circular driveway and merged into traffic on Jefferson Street, its engine churning to pull the hundreds of pounds of mobile medical technology that surrounded its cargo.

Inside, Marguerite Chambers was wrapped in a white blanket and strapped onto a portable stretcher. A clear plastic tube like those found in an aquarium snaked up her chest and entered her right nostril. It penetrated her nasal cavity, straddled her pharynx and descended downward into the darkness of her esophagus.

It was another kind of bodily intruder that had put her in the hospital five days earlier. Most likely, she inhaled it with a droplet of liquid supper. Bacteria required only an opportunity. The mode of entry could vary. The strain's ancient resolve to invade and multiply was constant. The result was a fever, a cough and a form of internal suffocation antique medical texts called "the old man's friend"—a condition known as bacterial pneumonia.

As the ambulance left St. Mary's Medical Center, Marguerite Chambers was playing out a medical scenario all too common among the aged. Pneumonia afflicts two million Americans yearly, but kills less than one in ten. Many contract it in nursing homes, but it's no longer treated as a welcome companion. The old nickname was applied before the age of antibiotics. Then, the illness was a quick and relatively easy exit for the elderly, often preventing a longer ravaging by other, slower-acting diseases.

For Marguerite, a drug called Keflex had taken all that was amiable out of the old man's friend. It was her second successful bout with the illness in three years. Now she was headed back to Alpine Manor, discharged from the hospital at 10:00 A.M.

Once on U.S. 131, the ambulance headed north on the freeway that followed the Grand River. The unit passed bridges at West Fulton and Pearl Streets, then elevated with the freeway to reveal a postcard view of the downtown skyline on the Grand's east bank. It cruised by the sparkling tower of the Amway Grand Plaza and the triangular architecture of the Gerald R. Ford Museum.

Beyond the old ironworks, the Grand River hit the white water for which the city was named. Nearly a hundred years ago, it was the site of the nation's largest logjam. There were too many big trees, and not enough water to handle the lure of profits in Grand Rapids sawmills, back when every old tree in Michigan fell to the saw and axe.

Marguerite could not see these sights, and it was impossible to know if she retained any memory of them. Her brain weighed no more than eight hundred grams, three-fourths the weight of a normal person of sixty. Alzheimer's had wasted the rest.

Four miles north of downtown the ambulance left the freeway, headed north on Alpine Avenue and turned onto Four Mile Road. The patient's rib cage pressed against the stretcher straps as cervical collars hanging from the ceiling swayed with the turns.

The ambulance stopped at the front door of Alpine Manor. Attendants carried the stretcher inside, then transferred Marguerite Chambers into a freshly made bed. She was back in her old room on a nurse's station called Abbey Lane. But as she lay there, everything was not the same.

The variation was the plastic tube in her nose. It carried a tan liquid called Enrich. The solution resembled baby formula, though Marguerite never would get a taste. The nasogastric tube, or NG tube, delivered the solution directly to the stomach. Marguerite's physician had ordered her to be tube-fed.

This was not a welcome development. Marguerite kept reaching for the tube, finally disconnecting it at a coupling. In such instances, nursing home procedure called for "safety devices," otherwise known as restraints. A nurse locked Marguerite's right wrist in a thick cuff made of strong felt. This was then cinched with a strong strap, which in turn was wrapped around the right bed rail. This procedure was repeated for her left wrist. Two more were applied to her ankles.

Staked out by these soft shackles, Marguerite Chambers indeed would be fed. A pair of adult diapers handled the rest. As the NG tube pumped in its sweet supper at a rate of 75 cc per hour, fluorescent panels glowed like tiny warped windows of light in Marguerite's glassy eyes. Sometimes she looked as if she were crying.

As a matter of fact, however, that was impossible to tell.

Medical science was supplying most of Marguerite's teardrops. The nursing staff administered a prescription every hour or so to keep her pupils from drying.

They called it Artificial Tears.

Chapter 2

Ken almost caught the ball. He was poised to grab the foul fly as it hurtled downward toward their seats behind the bull pen at Tiger Stadium. Then, it drifted into the upper deck.

"Damn," he said, turning to Cathy.

His wife was cowering in her seat, her eyebrows raised. She was peaking at him behind the little body of their daughter Jamie, age thirteen months. Cathy had held up their only child as a shield from the foul fly.

"Nice maternal instincts, Cath," he said.

When Ken thought about Cathy and motherhood, he always thought about that outing to Detroit. Somewhere during the three-hour ride back to Grand Rapids he eventually chuckled about it. Back then, Ken could dismiss such behavior to his wife's age and inexperience. She was only nineteen.

In time he came to view the incident differently. Now, five years later, mother and daughter had a running feud.

"Jamie's trying to undermine my authority," Cathy said.

His wife was standing in the living room, her hands folded in front of her, as though she were making an official announcement.

Her body was motionless, but her face quite animated. It was a mode he knew all too well. Cathy's quiet rage, he called it.

She tilted her head to one side.

"You're not punishing Jamie, and she's doing these things purposely to upset me."

Her voice was soft, but had a controlled, sighing quality. She tilted her head the other way, and glared.

"Ken. *She* thinks *she's* the boss."

Ken looked at Cathy, then Jamie. The immense size contrast prompted him to shake his head. He pleaded.

"Cath, she's *only* six years old, for Chrissakes. She's only asking questions."

Normal questions, he thought, for someone her age. Most stemmed from simple curiosity. And yes, sometimes Jamie was defiant. He knew that. Sometimes kids *are* defiant. They're just kids, testing the limits.

Cathy, however, approached motherhood as an epic battle of dominance and submission. There was conflict every day. Jamie was being disobedient. Jamie was making her nervous. Jamie wouldn't settle down. Jamie showed her no respect. Ken couldn't understand why Cathy should be so threatened.

This could make their small one-story home on Effie Place very cramped. The house had one bedroom, a living room, a kitchen, a half bath upstairs and a shower in the basement. Three of them shared the northeast Grand Rapids home. They should have been able to afford a larger house. Ken worked production at General Motors, but they spent unwisely early in their marriage. They rented the little house on Effie for two hundred dollars a month from Cathy's mother. He would have liked another landlord.

The last thing Ken needed now was this battle between mother and daughter. As the debate continued, it was becoming increasingly clear to him that Cathy wanted him to do all the trench fighting.

"Ken, make sure Jamie knows I'm the boss."

"No, Cath. She's defiant because you let her. She is not defiant with me because I won't let her. But, I can't do that for you."

Cathy, in fact, was the one who could be downright childish. He remembered the time she demanded that Jamie be disciplined for some transgression real or imagined. The three of them were in the living room.

"I told you your father would punish you," she snapped.

Ken was facing Jamie. Cathy was behind his back. Jamie became almost hysterical.

"Dad, are you going to spank me? Are you going to spank me?"

He couldn't understand why she was so horrified. He hadn't raised a hand. Later, he found out Cathy, from her position behind him, was taunting Jamie. She was making I-told-you-so faces, pointing her finger and giggling at Jamie.

Cathy just had no skills or common sense when it came to parenting, Ken finally decided. She seemed incapable of providing hands-on comfort. If Jamie was flu-ridden, mother kept her distance from daughter. She would absorb herself in a book in her big easy chair in the living room.

"Just go to sleep," she would say coldly. "Just go to sleep."

On the other hand, Cathy did have many qualities Ken admired. She could size up people instantly. She was intuitive. She anticipated people's behavior and often seemed several exchanges ahead of everyone during a conversation. Her mind was exceptionally quick, and she kept it stimulated daily with books. He couldn't remember the last time he had read a novel cover to cover. She had hundreds in the basement.

Cathy also was exceptional at stroking people's egos. It was one of her real talents, even with Jamie. She put her in cute outfits and posed her, snapping photo after photo on outings. She made sure Jamie heard her bragging how cute she was in front of friends. She praised her when she made her happy. Jamie fetched books and soda pops and bags of chips. She called Jamie "Baby Cakes" and "Burger."

"Oh, Burger you make Mommy so happy."

She called Ken her "sweet man." Sometimes he was her "sexy man." He liked that. She made her voice so delicate when she whispered, so precise, so refined. Sometimes she whispered when he called during nine o'clock break. Usually, she was reading. Sometimes she cooed.

"Oooooo, Ken, this book's really romantic. Sexy man, I can't wait till you get *off.*"

Sometimes, she liked to draw out the last word of a sentence, savoring every vowel and consonant.

When this started a couple of years back, Ken always drove straight home. However, then he discerned a pattern. When she whispered erotic innuendos on the phone, he could count on finding her asleep in bed. When there was none of this, he invariably found her up, watching David Letterman or her nose in another book.

Cathy knows how to stroke someone, Ken thought. She's just no good at any of the hands-on stuff.

He could say the same for her housekeeping. Some disorder was acceptable in any lived-in American household, Ken reasoned. But unless he tackled the housework daily, their little home became a claustrophobic cavern with mounting stalagmites of dirty dishes and litter. He could have attributed this to her schedule, but her bad habits began long before she had one.

Often, she blamed her father for her dislike of certain housekeeping tasks. Her dad made her clean. This had been the source of much pain as a child, she always said, and she did not need any more of that. Ken remembered the debut of that excuse when he came home with a catch of fish.

"My dad made me clean fish one time," she announced. "I will *never* clean fish again."

Ken never doubted her childhood had been painful. He had heard many horrible stories through the years. But he was tired of the excuse involving her father being used as a catchall for anything she shunned. One day he extended his hand over a kitchen counter jammed with crusty dinnerware and milky glasses.

"Well look at this," he said to Jamie. "Grandpa must have made your mom do dishes one time, so she will never do dishes again."

He tried sarcasm. He tried humor. They tried dividing up the work, but he always found himself pleading for her to do her share. If he yelled, he only succeeded in disappointing himself. He hated to lose his composure.

Sometimes Ken wondered if Cathy's quirks expressed more about how she felt about him, and less about homemaking. They separated for six months in 1984. Then, she put up pictures, displayed knickknacks and bought a bookcase for her hardcover books. She kept the place immaculate. She reverted the day they reconciled.

In recent months, her favorite act of contempt involved one plate and one glass. Every day she ate in front of the TV, reclining in the big easy chair she claimed as her passive command post. She always left a glass and plate parked next to the chair.

"Cath, you're getting up to go to the bathroom, walking right through the kitchen," he pleaded, "wouldn't it be easy just to pick up the plate and drop it in the sink as you passed? Why do I have to always pick it up? Why do I have to trip over it?"

But almost trip he did, every night when he got home from work, whether she had talked sexy on the phone or not, whether he found her sitting or fast asleep.

Finally, he had stopped complaining about the house. He surrendered the night he planned to cook her a spaghetti dinner, but came home to find her asleep surrounded by squalor.

He woke her and tossed her a jumbo candy bar.

"To hell with it," he said. "Cath, I just don't care anymore."

Lately Jamie was picking up.

No, Ken had to face facts. Ken was twenty-seven. Cathy was twenty-four. If he was hoping for the traditional wife and mother, nearly seven years of marriage had not developed those traits in Catherine May Wood. He could no longer attribute it to her age.

He was glad she finally was accepting responsibility in other areas. She was taking business classes at Davenport College, and in August, would mark a year in at Alpine Manor. She made only $3.55 an hour, but he believed the nursing home had produced some real benefits. She worked nights. He worked afternoons. Someone was always home for Jamie. Cathy always had been a creature of the night. Now, he reasoned, she spent those hours with real people instead of book plots and mindless TV. As for the daytime, Ken had been asked to coach the Alpine's softball team for women. Cathy wanted to be an assistant coach, or maybe even a player.

Ken had to give Cathy credit. She had broken out of the cocoon she'd spun for herself in the years after Jamie was born. Earlier in the year she had bought herself her own vehicle. She picked it out herself on the lot of a dealer named Kool Chevrolet.

"Oh Ken, it's so cuuuuuute," she said, drawing out that last word. "I just love the color black."

Her model was called a Luv Truck. For her birthday, he bought her a custom-made horn that sounded tunes, including the bugle call for a cavalry charge.

Cathy liked trucks. She said she liked the way they drove. Most of all, she said, she liked being up so high.

"Oooooo Ken, I like the way I can look down at everybody else when I'm behind the wheel."

Chapter 3

Gwen glanced out the window nervously. Two hours airborne and she couldn't stop worrying about a couple of small metal plates riveted on the wing of the passenger jet. It was standard aircraft construction, but it looked like patchwork to her. She hoped everything didn't fall apart above the clouds, or when the wheels touched the ground.

Gwen had checked a ton of baggage. She had her own as well as everything her old roommate Fran Shadden had left behind in Tyler. She put all the stuff in boxes, wrapped them with tape and loaded everything into her mom's car for the drive east to Dallas-Fort Worth Airport. Tyler was friendly and peaceful, she explained to her mom during the two-hour drive, but it was downright boring to some. Fran just had her fill of Texas. That's why she left. That's why she moved back to Michigan.

"I just have to go, too," Gwen said. "Yep. I just have to go, I do."

Gwen had only eleven dollars in her pocket when she boarded the flight. Her mom had paid the fare.

Gwendolyn Gail Graham was only twenty-two, but already she had logged a lot of miles. She was born in Santa Monica. Then her family lived in Connersville, Indiana and towns in northern California before settling in Tyler when she was nine. At fifteen, she traveled to the East Coast with a teen missionary group, then on to Africa. At seventeen, after her parents split, she headed back to California to live with her dad. Three months into her senior year, she dropped out of Modesto High School and hitched up the Coast. She saw Oregon, then lingered in Santa Rosa, north of the Golden Gate. She was back again in Tyler at twenty. That's when she hooked up with Fran.

Folks might say Gwen got the wanderlust from her dad. Mack Graham was a railroad worker in Louisiana, a pressroom worker in

Santa Maria, a sheriff's deputy in Los Angeles County and a welder in Indiana. When he settled down it was behind the wheel of an eighteen wheeler. He'd been an interstate trucker since 1972.

By the time she was twenty-one, Gwen had laid brick for Christian dorms in Monrovia, Liberia, shuttled pizza in California, delivered the *Dallas Morning News* in east Texas, ran a cash register in the Stop-n-Go in the longhorn town of Flint and managed the Dixie Kwik Stop on Highway 64 in Tyler.

She had always dreamed of being a vet. She cherished animals when her dad dabbled in farming, but he always told her veterinary school was way too long of a haul. After earning the equivalent of a high school diploma, she tried the registered nurse program at Tyler Junior College, but dropped it when her work load mixed with some bad fortune.

After Fran left, she busied herself in her off-hours with her motorcycle, a Honda 450, candy apple red. She liked to ride it on the long, straight stretches of dead Texas road outside Tyler. She liked to wash and wrench-work it on her days off.

Gwen was looking through a cycle magazine when she saw the advertisement: "Become a Paramedic!" Davenport College offered the program. The school was in Grand Rapids, Michigan.

She called Fran. Paramedic. Emergency work. That was like nursing, with excitement. Gwen had seen a chance at some real direction.

And, the compass needle was pointed north.

Grand Rapids was not known for disappointing newcomers who sought an honest start. One lifetime Grand Rapids resident described her city this way: "It's clean and cultural and there's minimal corruption here."

By the end of the decade, the city of nearly 200,000 would become the fifth most moved-to city in the United States. An office furnishings industry boomed, but few people called it the "furniture city" anymore. Grand Rapids' diversified economy outperformed the rest of Michigan. Unemployment was minimal. The city was nearly recession-proof, civic boosters said.

In ways of the spirit, Grand Rapids bore some resemblance to Tyler. The Texas town of 80,000 was known for roses (the Rose Capital of America) and its Southern Baptist slant. In western Michigan, Christianity rang, from the bell towers of nineteenth century Baptist missionaries to the latter-day clamor of Jim and Tammy Bakker, who hailed from nearby Muskegon. In Grand Rapids no Christian flock influenced life more than the Christian Reformed Church. Ever since the Most Reverend Albertus Van Raalte established outposts in the Holland and Zeeland areas in the late 1840s, the area had attracted settlement by Dutch Calvinists. They believed in predestination, the doctrine that an all-knowing and all-powerful God had already decided the chosen. Good works by a man could be considered evidence of that status. Shunned in the Netherlands, Dutch Calvinists resettled in areas that included South Africa and western Michigan. Later, Dutch Catholics came as well. At the end of the nineteenth century, a third of Grand Rapids was Holland-born.

Grand Rapids' conservative reputation came largely from this ethnic group. It was not uncommon to see an entire family bowing heads in prayer before a meal at a public restaurant. Grand Rapids folk themselves perpetuated their own stereotypes with stories based more in myth than fact.

A suburban cop talking to a visitor at a Halloween party:

"Did you know that for years in Zeeland they wouldn't even sell root beer in the local drugstore."

"Why's that?"

"Because it had the word 'beer' in it. This is true. That's the way it is here around Grand Rapids."

Local folk also proliferated stories of Dutch austerity. Visitors were told to watch for blond-haired businessmen having authentic "Dutch treat" lunches. A local columnist once wrote that Grand Rapids was the only place in America where people bought underwear at garage sales.

Safe to say, Grand Rapids people valued free enterprise and hard work. Many working-class families had small real estate ventures, renting out flats and efficiency apartments. Others realized bigger dreams. Two Grand Rapids businessmen founded Amway Corporation, a soap-and-success giant with a marketing strategy similar to religious proselytism. Top executives were major contributors to the Republican Party and financed big civic projects as well.

Wealth fueled Grand Rapids cultural pursuits at a level above other cities its size. The Grand Rapids Art Museum featured 7,500 paintings, prints and sculptures. There was a Civic Ballet company, complete with a junior division. The city's symphony featured the first woman musical director of a regional orchestra, a French-born conductor with national acclaim.

However, artistic pursuits didn't necessarily translate into social tolerance. Abortion, homosexuality, minority issues and general permissiveness were eloquently damned and debated in the public letter section of the *Grand Rapids Press:* A suburb considered stopping Halloween and Valentine parties in schools because they're not educational. Another School district banned a book of modern poems dealing with racism and poverty, another a poem by e. e. cummings. Parents wanted a gay teacher fired.

Grand Rapids did have a substantial gay population, one that was becoming more public in 1986 with controversial plans for gay rallies downtown. One local gay sociologist theorized the city actually had a larger gay population than most cities because of the area's "intense gender roles." Men were dominant and women were subservient and restricted by local Christian cultures, she argued. Homosexuality was a way to break out.

Major crime, however, was more often covered under datelines from Detroit. Murder was still front page news in Grand Rapids. In most suburbs, a homicide was as rare as a lunar eclipse. Prostitution and street crime were considered problems for black neighborhoods on the southeast side and Division Avenue, a strip which also happened to feature some of the city's gay bars.

Such urban containment, and other factors, inspired many Grand Rapids folks to echo a common phrase. Visitors heard it over and over again, everywhere they went. It might as well have been the city's motto:

"Grand Rapids is a great place to raise a family."

Among the chosen, few argued that wasn't correct.

Gwen was no Hollander, but her appearance wasn't likely to hold her back. She stood two inches over five feet and was a stocky 140. She took her ginger hair and summer freckles from the Irish. Her father's stoic good looks had blessed her with an upturned nose and a strong lower jaw. She could display the furrowed brow of a troubled tomboy or the endearing twinkle of a bashful cherub. She often fluctuated between those extremes.

Gwen knew or cared little about Grand Rapids' civic character. She cared about Fran, and the kind of life she said she had there. Fran had told her she was working for a big newspaper company out of Detroit. She had a cozy new apartment, she said.

They talked on the phone before she left.

"After three months if I don't like it, I'm moving back," Gwen said. "Yep. We can both move back."

She looked out the window again as the airliner dipped, then circled. The flight was approaching Kent County Airport. Beyond the tip of the patched-up wing was a spectacular vista of the city and the Grand River valley. The earth was green with the new foliage of late May. The river was wide and brown with the tannin.

Later, Gwen would wonder if it was deep.

Chapter 4

An old schizophrenic named John maintained the sign outside the big dining room in Alpine Manor. It read in large letters:

THIS IS GRAND RAPIDS, MICHIGAN.
TODAY IS: TUESDAY.
THE DATE IS: MAY 20, 1986.
THE NEXT HOLIDAY IS: MEMORIAL DAY.
THE NEXT MEAL IS: LUNCH.

Down the hall, in room 207, Marguerite Chambers no longer was restrained. Her family had complained about the feeding tube. Her doctor ordered it removed. Nurse's aides were hand-feeding Marguerite her meals again.

Today she was rocking on her tailbone as she hunched forward in her bed. She rocked and rocked and rocked as two aides tried to lift her. She jerked forward with a sudden burst of strength, crashing headfirst into the metal bed rail. She wore a prize fighter's trademark. The laceration was two-and-a-half inches long, located just above her left eyelid.

A nurse, scribbling on a clipboard, wrote: "She has continual spastic-like movements and is difficult to care for . . ." She scheduled Marguerite to be taken to Butterworth Hospital for stitches.

Outside, an erratic wind toyed with the American flag that flew out front. Alpine Manor was a flat, one-story building isolated by a parking lot of jagged blacktop. To the south, wild grass merged into a small woods of wolf trees. To the west, there was another field and then some sparse commercial development. To the east, a complex of attractive apartment buildings outlined the view. They were Tudor-style cream and brown. To the north, a green water tower labeled "Alpine" rose out of the trees on the other side of Four Mile Road. This marked the boundary between the suburb of Walker and Alpine Township.

Try as they might, these surroundings and the name "Alpine" on signs everywhere did not conjure up Old World beauty. The area was one hundred percent American suburbia, an urban planning hybrid thrown together in the rapid conquest of once wide-open farmland.

In fact, Alpine was called English Hills when it opened in 1973. New ownership changed the name in 1984, but not the nursing station designations inspired by the old appellation. The stations were called Abbey Lane, Buckingham, Camelot and Dover. Conveniently, they corresponded with the first four letters of the alphabet, but everybody used the full names.

"I'm on Camelot, tonight," a nurse's aide might say. Or, "They transferred Mrs. Chambers from Abbey Lane to Dover."

Otherwise, nothing else inside Alpine resembled a "manor." It was a one-story brick and block construction, architecturally akin to a 1950s schoolhouse. The layout on a blueprint looked like two square buildings, joined together by a common side. Each square was hollowed in the center by a courtyard. Alpine had been built in two sections, the first with 123 beds, the second section pushing the total to 207 three years later. Every leg of the square was hallway. An average sixteen rooms, two patients to a room, lined each leg.

The British designations of the stations also included the halls and rooms. Abbey Lane covered halls 100 and 200; Buckingham 300 and 400; Camelot 500 and part of 600; Dover part of 600 and 700 hall. A room was broken down into beds "1" and "2." Bed 1 was near the window; bed 2 was near the door. A drawn curtain divided the two beds.

The halls and stations were color-coded: pink for Abbey, yellow for Buckingham, powder blue for Dover, and green for Camelot.

"Serene green," Jackie Cromwell, Alpine's director of nursing, liked to say. "Sometimes patients can't remember their room number, but they can remember their color."

The coincidence of her last name and the British setting did not escape the director. Nor did it escape the home administrator. She too was a Cromwell, Nancy Cromwell, though they were not related. Jackie Cromwell had been with Alpine just over ten years. The administrator was the owner's sister.

Jackie Cromwell sometimes conducted tours for families of prospective patients. There were many applicants. Nationally, one in two women and one in three men who reach the age of sixty-five were likely to one day stay in a nursing home. At Alpine, the applicant conditions varied: Cancer, Alzheimer's, organic brain syndrome, the incontinent, tracheotomy, muscle disease, severe arthritis and other disorders of aging. One in five in Alpine were psychiatric cases, schizophrenics, largely, transferees from state mental facilities when Alpine was seeking to fill empty beds.

Alpine was not a retirement home. Every patient needed nursing care. That ranged from daily medication, a good diet and supervision to the "total care" cases like Marguerite Chambers, who depended on nursing staff for most everything but a breath and a heartbeat.

Cromwell sometimes wondered who was in worse shape, patients or loved ones. Patient maladies varied. Loved ones, however, often were afflicted with two predictable conditions, defeat and guilt. On tours, she could apply some balm.

"Our patients do get up and get dressed every day," she said, touring one party through Alpine later. "We want it more like a home setting than a hospital. If they're in their nightie or robe all the time they tend to feel—well, ill."

She showed the beauty shop, the physical therapy room, the dining room, the three day rooms for activities and the two courtyards. She explained staffing. The number of supervisors, registered nurses, licensed practical nurses and nurse's aides amounted to more than seventy people across three shifts. This included a support staff that included a social worker and an activity director and her assistant.

As for costs, the rate in 1986 was sixty dollars a day for private-pay patients, give or take five dollars depending on the level of care. Those covered by government entitlement programs like Medicaid and Social Security paid about twenty dollars less. Private patients were kept on Camelot and Dover, though Alpine Manor, she always said, gave the same "quality care" throughout.

For the uninitiated, however, a trip through Alpine Manor or any nursing home could be a disturbing experience.

"And these," Cromwell said, opening the door to the day room near Dover station, "are the Dover Rovers."

Inside, a dozen patients were slumped around several circular tables. The surfaces were spotless, but also bare. There were no books, no magazines, not even the obligatory checkerboard. Most of the old folk just sat and stared, looking at the tables, gazing up at various spots on the wall. Men wore mismatched clothing. The white hair on many women hung straight.

However, in the middle of the room, at one table, four women sat upright in their chairs. Their silver hair was permed, their clothing finished. They looked as though they had banded together in a last stand against the human deterioration around them.

"The Dover Rovers are a group that meets every Monday and Wednesday, and then you decide what to do, right," Cromwell said.

"We have a lot of fun with it, us old people," said one.

"Oh c'mon," said Cromwell. "You're good for another one hundred years."

"With one foot in the grave," said another.

Indeed, a silent watch for the inevitable sometimes seemed to pervade all of Alpine. The large dining room, where the ambulatory ate their dinners, was a large version of the Dover day room. At lunch, nearly one hundred waited, but not one read or spoke. A Wurlitzer organ sat at one end, a baby grand on the other. Periodically, a patient was admitted who could play it.

"We had one lady who could play all the standards," said one resident. She broke the silence around her, but only after a visitor asked her about the piano. "But she fell and broke her arm. We hope she'll be back. She knew all the songs we liked."

The day rooms were used to feed the nonambulatory, wheeled there by aides. They waited in a variety of poses and positions. An old woman chewed on her hand as though she were teething. Another held her face in her open palms and moaned. There were women in pigtails and long gray ponytails, utilitarian styles seemingly unfitting for faces with so much character drawn by time. Men had well-defined, angular cheekbones and wild cowlicks. One chewed on his cheek and winced repeatedly. His head turned back and forth like a hyper rooster, ever vigilant for the first sign of any trouble.

When they were fed, those who were able to chew munched on a selection of whole food ordered by a dietician. Aides fed others a pureed diet, meals the consistency of baby food.

At the bottom of the dietary hierarchy were the tube feeders. Candidates were patients who choked easily, could no longer swallow or just plain refused to eat. Sometimes individuals went on hunger strikes, refusing meals until they were taken back home or some other demand was met. After the family was consulted, a physician could write a "tube order." The NG tube was fed down the patient's nose, sometimes with great difficulty. It was not a pleasant way to dine, but one way or the other, it stopped most hunger strikes.

Staffers tried to soften the sometimes torturous conditions of age and disease with activities and ambience. Some residents had TVs and telephones, provided by their families. Community education made classes in social studies and current events available. There was ice cream every Thursday, bingo on Saturday and church on Sunday. On Fridays there was a movie, rented from the local library. Often the star was little Shirley Temple.

Many of the activities in Alpine Manor were childish. "Crafts" in fact was usually coloring, with crayons in coloring books. Sometimes there was finger painting, sometimes cutouts. Every month workers decorated the dining room with these figures of colored construction paper. They pasted up leaves in September and shamrocks in March and firecrackers in July. Inside the cutouts were patients' names.

There was also the big bulletin board labeled "Resident's Birthdays" in a hallway between Abbey and Buckingham. There was Lester, sixty-nine, Lena, seventy-six, Mary, eighty-three, and a half dozen more. Each featured their face cut from a recent photograph.

All were riding in the same kind of vehicle. Everyone had his own baby carriage.

Training sessions for nurse's aides urged new employees not to talk to patients like children. With all the grade school stimuli, however, some aides wondered why more didn't fall into the habit.

Between meals, many patients walked the hallways—"ambulated," as staffers called it. They ambulated with walkers, or by hanging onto rails on the walls, or solo. They ambulated to the safe sounds of WOOD-FM, Grand Rapids purveyor of elevator music, piped nearly around the clock over the public address system. The old folks zigged and zagged, leaned and shuffled and cut other meandering patterns as they walked clockwise and counterclockwise in the rectangular building layout. Among them, nurses and nurse's aides pushed carts of medication or hygienic supplies, darting in and out of rooms as they made rounds.

Every thirty seconds or so, however, the kind of bleating alarm one hears from vehicles backing up on construction sites would interrupt a trombone solo of "Feelings" or violins from the Midnight Moods Orchestra. It was the sound of a call button, which also lit a red light above the patient's door. A repetitive beeping meant a patient was in distress.

Jackie Cromwell told visitors that staff worked to keep that to a minimum. She told visitors Alpine Manor was more than the typical American nursing home. It was a far cry from the roach-ridden facilities in large cities like Detroit. It was a standout, in fact, among the inspection and complaint files kept by the state health department that regulated it. Alpine Manor was one of the most trouble-free nursing homes in Michigan.

It was trouble-free by state standards, at least.

Chapter 5

Of all the people you talk to, please be careful about
Ken. I think he's a bit off.

—Catherine Wood, October 24, 1990.

Ken might have predicted something like this, had Cathy not been
so faithful in her studies. Two classes away from an associate degree
in management and sales and marketing and she wanted to flush
two years of work.

"But I want to go to nursing school now," she said.

"But Cath, you're just a couple of credits away," he argued. "Get
the degree, then go to nursing school if you want. But finish, for
Chrissakes. Think how impressive it would be for a nurse to also
have business degrees."

She did not want to discuss it. It was the end of spring term. Now
she had the summer off from school.

Ken had come to expect surprise developments in everyday matters with Cathy, simply because she was so driven by her fickle
moods. He also knew this: Every once in a while, Cathy took a major,
extended trip to left field. He hoped she wasn't headed there once
again.

"Cath, I'm telling you that if you blow off Davenport, you're
crazy," he said.

She needs help, he told himself. She really needs some kind of
help.

Ken Wood had believed this for years, and he did not mean it
figuratively. Cathy had seen a psychologist a couple of times when
their marriage was falling apart in 1984. They both had. Then the
therapist called them in for a joint session. Cathy stormed out ten
minutes into the appointment. She never went back.

"You two guys were ganging up on me," she had snapped.

The girl Ken had first come to know as Catherine Carpenter had been anything but combative when they first met. It was on the telephone. Cathy called Ken's apartment, looking for his younger brother, Terry, whom she had befriended in Riverside Park on the Grand River. Terry wasn't home, but Ken and Cathy began to chat. They talked for five hours, mainly about themselves.

Ken ran a wire extruding machine at General Motors, the same company that cut a paycheck for his dad, his mom and most of his extended family as well. Cathy went to school. Her dad drove a lift truck in a food warehouse. Her mother was a bookkeeper. Ken lived in Kentwood, a suburb to the south. Cathy lived in Comstock Park, a suburb to the north.

"What kinda teeth do you have?" Cathy asked.

"What?"

"Do you have good teeth?"

He laughed at other inquiries about his appearance. She was silly. She was also witty and irreverent. She talked effortlessly on any subject, even sports, a subject on which he considered himself an expert. He was surprised to find out she was only a high school junior, two months from her seventeenth birthday. He was twenty. He asked her out anyway.

They doubled with Ken's brother. Cathy told Ken to pick her up at Comstock Park High School, only a half dozen doors from her house. She said her mother would never let her go if she knew about the date. As he drove up to the high school, Ken wondered where she was. All he could see was a large guy, facing away from the street.

"Go ask that guy over there if he knows who Cathy Carpenter is?" he told his brother.

His brother returned with the stranger.

"So you think I'm a guy, huh?" Cathy said, poking her head in the window.

She was wearing a big parka, and her hair was tucked in a big fur collar. Ken tried to make a joke, but wanted to slide under the seat. His embarrassment increased when he saw her attractive face. Her features were soft and her smile spontaneous.

They saw *Every Which Way But Loose*. Ken widened the gap between himself and the stoic Clint Eastwood character in the film by committing more dating blunders. He kept calling her "Mary." He spilled an orange drink in her lap. She pushed his Chevy Monza when they got stuck on some ice. When he tried to kiss her good-night he collided with her jaw.

"You can call me later," she said.

This surprised him. He thought she'd never want to see him again.

"I had a great time," she said when he did phone, later that same night.

Catherine Carpenter was an unexpected delight in that first week of the new year, 1979. In fact, Ken considered her "a blessing from God," as he later told a friend. Two days before Christmas he had lost his grandfather to a stroke, a death that hit him hard. They were very close. Ken figured his grandfather always did the things for him his own dad should have done.

As for Cathy, she literally stood head and shoulders above her peers. She was a quarter inch shy of six feet and weighed 180 pounds. She was stocky, but not obese, and his size. Ken was six-foot, 250 pounds.

They had a lot in common. Both had hardly dated and were the oldest in their families. Both felt they had had troubled childhoods. Both agreed that they had raised their younger siblings, Cathy her sister and brother, Ken his brother Terry. Ken told her about his grandmother. She had always been his spiritual guide. She taught him about Jesus and all-forgiving Christian love.

On the lighter side, they both loved to laugh. He was the class clown. She was his audience. They liked to dissect TV shows and make fun of commercials and the hairstyles of TV newscasters.

After several more secret dates, Ken met her father and mother. Cathy's mother Pat did all the talking. Standing in her living room, Ken weathered a terse dissertation on what was proper and what was not. Despite his assurances to the contrary, they spent a lot of time from then on in his apartment. He couldn't afford to take Cathy out every night. They spent evenings just talking, eventually sharing fears and secrets.

Cathy had lots of questions. In time, Ken was able to detect a recurring theme.

"You say you love me, but you really don't like me, do you?" she asked him once.

"Of course I like you."

"No, people don't like me, 'cause they really don't know me."

"But I do like you, and know you."

"No, that's not the way you act sometimes."

"You're right," he finally admitted. "Sometimes I don't like you."

Sometimes, he just didn't know where she was coming from. She asked questions, then veered off on to unrelated topics before he answered. She told little lies, fibs aimed at making her look good. She giggled one moment, pouted the next. Her moods seemed hinged to no external stimulation. She set him up to probe, to find out the reason she was disturbed. Usually it was something harmless he had said days ago, something she had interpreted as a threat or a slam. At times he found himself confused, feeling guilty even, as he wondered what indeed he had initially said and meant.

"That's what I mean when I say I don't like you," he said. "It's not that I don't like you. I don't like the things you sometimes do."

He found out she liked to play mind games. She seemed to be testing him, with fire, and he did not like that at all.

He had to credit her ingenuity, however. One particular scheme was cleverly conceived and orchestrated. For weeks, Ken had been fielding phone calls from strange women. Actually, they were Cathy's friends, purporting to be girls he once met.

"Well, I just don't remember you," Ken would say.

But they were always equipped with background, just enough details about him to make him question his own memory, doubt himself. Later, he found out Cathy was listening on an extension. She apparently wanted to see what he was like behind her back.

She has never been loved, Ken decided. In real love you don't do things like this.

She wanted "unconditional love," she eventually told him, crying. She complained her mother did not love her. Her father, a Vietnam veteran, not only did not love her, he drank a lot and battered her around, she said. She did things for her parents, took care of her younger brother and sister, but "it is never enough," she said. They were cold and uncaring, she said.

This had created a great need in her, Ken concluded. He wondered if anyone could fill it.

"Who do you put number one?" she asked him one night.

He answered as thoughtfully as he could.

"Well, I'm no churchgoer, but I've believed in God since I've been a kid. Sometimes I talk to him. I'd have to put God number one."

She appeared hurt, disappointed. Even in his spiritual order of things, he decided, she needed the top spot.

Cathy often jockeyed for this position, with his friends, his family and his pastimes. Like the rest of the state of Michigan, he became caught up in the 1979 showdown between Larry Bird and Magic Johnson in the NCAA basketball finals. Cathy pouted, insisting he forsake one of the games.

"I'm tired of being third," she said. "Magic comes in first. Bird second. And I'm third."

He apologized.

"Look Cath, this is a once-in-a-lifetime thing."

A couple of weeks later, she suddenly stopped calling him. When he called her she was cold, hesitant.

"Cath, what's wrong?"

"My parents told me I can't see you anymore."

"Why? What have I done?"

"You're into drugs."

This made no sense. It was he, in fact, who had warned her that if she ever showed up with drugs, that would be it for their relationship. Ken began a slow burn as she explained.

Cathy never trusted her dad, she said. She had always feared he would hurt her one day, or come on to her. (This, she explained, was because he called her his "little princess" or "baby doll.") The other day, she went on, her father had taken her for a ride alone in his truck. He finally was going to make his move, she figured. Instead, he had a different request. He wanted her to get him some pot. Could she get him some? Cathy said she obliged, scoring from a dealer at school. Then, her mother found the marijuana on a routine search of her purse.

"Ken, she started accusing you," Cathy said. "She figured I got the pot from you. Now she won't let me see you anymore."

Ken raved to himself. Man, her dad didn't have the balls to stand up and take the heat from the old lady. Those sonsabitches. God, he was beginning to really dislike the Carpenters. No wonder Cathy was so messed up.

Ken steadied himself and thought it over. He didn't want to lose her.

"Cath, we talked about maybe doing this one day," he said. "I didn't think it would be this soon. But if you want, you can come live with me."

"Really?"

A couple of days after she moved in, she told him she was pregnant.

They had had sex a half dozen times.

"How do you know the baby's mine?" he asked.

She never forgave him for asking.

They had also gotten off to a bad start the first time he tried to enter her. She panicked.

"Get out," she said. "You gotta get out."

Yet she never complained in subsequent encounters. She was his first woman. He was her first man. And, *that's* why they had a problem the first time, she explained.

The details formed another incredible story. He was beginning to expect incredible stories from her now. This one she told a month after they started dating. She called him on the telephone in hysterics. She woke him. She was weeping. She sounded completely out of control.

"He's back! Oh God, Ken, he's back!"

"Who's back?"

"I haven't seen him. I used to know him. But now he's back!"

Who the hell was she talking about, he thought, trying to blink the sleep out of his eyes. She sounded like someone had a gun to her head.

"Is he trying to hurt you? Is he threatening you?"

"No, he's trying to get a hold of me."

"Grab you?"

"No, he's been around here, looking for me."

Ken tried to calm her. He assured her if anyone was bothering her, he sure could take care of some punk. He hung up the phone and sped north to her house.

He found her there. She was calm.

"You shouldn't have come over."

"I was worried about you."

Her mother was sitting in the living room.

A couple of nights later he pried the story out of her. She was fourteen or fifteen, she said, when she met the teenager named David. He had short hair, a childish smile and liked baggy jeans and sweaters. She said she went out with him for a year and a half. He lived in the little town of Lowell, a half hour away.

One day Cathy's mother arrived at David's house to pick Cathy up. She had a chat with David's mother at the door. There was no "David" there, only a "Debbie" the woman said. She told Mrs. Carpenter that sometimes her daughter Debbie liked to impersonate a boy.

"She told me if I ever saw her again she was going to put me in a mental institution," Cathy said, sobbing. "Ever since, I've been afraid of those places."

Cathy went on to explain that she herself could not accept that the first person she had loved in her life was deceiving her. She said they met again secretly and walked to a farmhouse owned by an old hermit they had befriended. They used a dark bedroom there. David advised her not to touch him below the waist. When he penetrated her it hurt, Cathy said. Later, she found out it was a dildo. Later, "David" finally admitted she was indeed Debbie.

David/Debbie. That's why she panicked the first time they slept together, Ken thought. Sex meant pain, physical and emotional pain. No wonder she had tested him. Everything that should have brought love in Cathy Carpenter's life—her parents, her siblings, her first lover—had brought her pain.

"Now, you don't love me," she said after the confession. "Now that I've told you."

She was crying again.

"No, that's not true."

"That's why I didn't want to tell you. I knew you'd never love me."

He put his arms around her. She was larger than a lot of his friends. But as he listened to her weep, she felt as tiny and fragile as porcelain. He feared how vulnerable she was right then.

He told her a few stories of his own. Nobody has a "normal" sexual development, he said. Everybody does something strange, at one time or another. She shouldn't feel shamed by David/Debbie.

"Then you don't hate me?"

"Cath, I'm not going to judge you for something that happened in your past, something that wasn't even your fault. You're a victim, for Chrissakes."

Indeed, he thought, she has been used and abused. He had only known her two months, but already Ken believed that Catherine May Carpenter had been wronged by her tragic past.

She was someone he could truly love, he decided. He wanted to make everything right for her, for the first time in her life.

* * *

Their wedding reception in August was held in a UAW hall. The two of them did all the planning and preparation, though Cathy was also having a terrible time with morning sickness.

Ken got a loan from his grandmother to pay for the wedding. Cathy's parents bought the wedding cake. Cathy's dad gave Ken fifty dollars for booze, told him to keep the change, then later wanted the change and liquor left at the end of the night. They were real tightwads, he told himself.

Yes, Cathy was right about her parents, he decided. He was not going to count on the Carpenters for any nurturing, financial or otherwise. Ken also knew he was damned forever as an outsider. Considering the way he figured the Carpenters had fallen down on their job as parents, this didn't trouble him at all.

Soon, however, Cathy's inconsistent feelings about her parents left Ken confused. She had become increasingly moody after she left home. She snapped at him as she curled her hair before school and gave him the silent treatment when he greeted her after work. This went on for days. Finally, he coaxed it out of her.

"Ken, I miss my mom," she confessed.

They moved to Comstock Park, just a couple of doors down from her mother's house. Cathy's grandmother lived across the street. Cathy and her parents had come up with the arrangement. Cathy's parents owned the house and rented it to Ken.

Soon, he felt like he was suffocating, but was doing so quite alone. The Carpenters never crossed the threshold. When she wasn't at a special school for pregnant mothers, Cathy was either at her mother's house or with friends. Proximity to the Carpenters and his wife's big mouth, Ken decided, was destroying his privacy as well. One night he drank too much and passed out in the bathroom. They found out.

"Oh Ken, they think you're a *drinker*," she said, drawing out the last word with concern.

"Well, why don't you tell them I'm not. That can happen to anybody one night."

She became matter-of-fact.

"They'll always hate you anyway," she said.

When Cathy wasn't visiting she was eating. She gained one hundred pounds during the pregnancy. He asked her about it.

"Cath, hasn't the doctor said anything about this?"

"Oh no."

She appeared bemused by the question.

She was approaching three hundred pounds when she was hospitalized three weeks before delivery. Her blood pressure was too high. Jamie was born via a C-section after three days of painful labor. As Cathy recovered, Ken convinced her that something had to be done about their home situation. He moved them to an attractive two-bedroom apartment on Grand Rapids southeast side. It was fifteen miles south of Comstock Park and the Carpenters. The complex was called Sutton Club on a street named Hidden Valley.

When she came home, Cathy's appetite became insatiable, for books as well as food. She had always been a reader, a quick study. In school she was undisciplined, but her fast grasp of the printed word alone earned her above a B average in Comstock Park.

In Sutton Club, she devoured mysteries and crime novels in one sitting. She also loved the horror genre. She read everything by Stephen King. She bought hardcovers of her favorites, but didn't limit herself to thrillers. She had works by William Shakespeare, Washington Irving and Harriet Beacher Stowe. She read a series of attractively bound American works: *Gone With the Wind, Moby Dick, Catch 22, From Here to Eternity, Wuthering Heights, Little Women.* She had three books by F. Scott Fitzgerald, including *The Great Gatsby.*

She collected popular contemporary titles as well, books by Joseph Wambaugh, James A. Michener, V.C. Andrews and many others. She gravitated toward stories of lust and crime. She liked complex plots laced with betrayal and revenge. Her tastes ranged from *The Other Side of Midnight* by Sydney Sheldon to *The Cradle Will Fall,* a page-turner by Mary Higgins Clark about a physician who murders a slew of patients.

She read nonfiction as well, from true crime stories to the irreverence of Erma Bombeck to the hip *The Diaries of Andy Warhol.* Some historical figures fascinated her. She picked up *The Life and Times of Gregori Rasputin,* a somewhat academic study of the monk who manipulated the royalty of Russia with his irresistible psychopathic powers.

Cathy's own imagination was active as well. One night she confessed to him that she had always wondered what it would be like to "stab somebody." She seemed excessively troubled by the fact that she had the fantasy.

"Cath, we all have those kinds of passing thoughts," Ken said. "It's just a curiosity thing."

Her concern didn't slow her consumption of horror plots. Deep into the early morning she read at Sutton Club, a book in one hand, food in the other. She ate chips and pretzels and corn chips and popcorn. She munched on reheated pizza and cold chicken. She ate tacos and potato salad. Then she washed it down with diet pop.

Ken knew he was partly to blame for her diet. She refused to cook, or shop, so he often brought home the fast food. Within two years, her weight neared four hundred pounds. Ken increased to two hundred ninety himself.

"I said to myself, I will never leave Cathy because of her weight," he later told a friend. "And I felt like a hypocrite, because I was heavy myself."

Cathy's weight justified more seclusion. She was reluctant to go out in public. She waited until after midnight to visit the laundry room. Ken bought her clothes at Roger's Big Men Shop. No one else had anything that fitted. When she complained to her doctor that no scale could weigh her if she chose to diet, the physician suggested she go to the local supermarket.

"Just ask workers to use the bulk scale in the stockroom," she reported he had said.

With advice like that, no wonder she won't go out, Ken thought.

While she feared the dynamics of life outside Sutton Club, Cathy grew accomplished within the static parameters of card and board games. She liked to play chess. Her favorite maneuver was "the fool's checkmate," a gambit designed to trap strategically handicapped players in just two moves.

Cathy had a twisted competitive spirit, Ken decided. She played not for the best score, but to best a particular player. When someone missed a question, or made a strategic error, she looked at her opponent and laughed.

This made her a bad partner, Ken decided. When friends took part in these games, usually her mark for the night was him.

Over the years Ken had tried to overlook her moods, her lies and her pettiness. He thought, I'm no saint myself. I can be too demanding and have a lousy temper. However, he never wanted to return to those reclusive years at Sutton Club.

This was why Davenport College and Alpine Manor had been such a Godsend. Her improved self-image was showing in her weight. Once pushing four hundred fifty, she now was poised to break three hundred pounds. Ken was still drawn to Cathy, obese or not. One day, he hoped to make her happy and help her lose not only weight, but her troubled past.

After seven years of marriage, that mission and other things attracted him. He still valued her intelligence. She also had a physical charisma he couldn't quite describe. The weight didn't show in her face. Her chestnut hair was soft and shoulder-length. Her eyes were green, or blue. Ken had always been intrigued by the way they changed color, green when she was mad or hyper, light blue when she was happy or silly. She didn't move the way a lot of heavy people did. She carried herself as though she knew she was really very attractive. She was never labored or out of breath. In fact, she walked so gingerly she could easily sneak up behind his back.

Cathy seemed to recognize her limitations. She chose the midnight shift at Alpine Manor because it required less lifting.

"The job is real *hard,*" she told him, drawing out the word. "But I really like it, Ken."

In the beginning, she told him stories about patients and medical procedures. Lately, she seemed more taken with the shop talk. Most of the aides were women. Cathy had a running narrative going about the personal lives of her fellow workers. He heard about aides leaving their husbands. One tired of her spouse's demands to have dinner on the table. Another was complaining her husband made her have sex with him every night.

"I'll tell you," she told Ken one morning, glaring. "No man is going to make me do that."

He found himself on the defensive.

"Cath, why are you getting mad at me? I've never made you do that."

Ken decided she just wasn't used to shop talk. At GM guys complained constantly about their wives and what burdens they shouldered as men. When he saw these macho types with their spouses, however, they were as skittish as squirrels.

He tried to share this perspective with Cathy. He also said sex often made up shop talk.

"Well, one girl now charges her husband for sex," she told him one day. "Ken, you could have sex with me if you paid me."

"Cath, I'm not paying you."

They both laughed.

Work discussions about sex, however, had slowly transformed into a commentary about sexual preference. Over time she had introduced him to a cast of characters from Alpine. Now she provided surprise character developments. Sometimes she couldn't wait to tell him, announcing the news as she came through the front door.

"Oh Ken, Paul is bisexual . . . and Ladonna is married, but she's really a homosexual."

One by one he learned about people he didn't care ever to know. So-and-so was sleeping with so-and-so. So-and-so had two lovers, and so on. Her preoccupation, he thought, was simply more evidence of how sheltered she had been all those years in Sutton Place.

He also couldn't help wonder about Alpine Manor.

"Gee, Cath," he asked once. "Is it in the fine print?"

"Whatya mean?"

"Does it state in the contract you gotta be gay to work there?"

In June, Ken met some of the Alpine workers face-to-face. He was holding regular practices for the Alpine women's softball team. Many of the aides, he decided, were very nice. Some he thought were just plain slobs.

Always serious about sports, Ken soon found the management of the team trying, to say the least. Players showed up late for practice. When they did arrive, they seemed incapable of listening. Some saw the diamond as an outdoor beer joint. Players took the field with a beer in one hand, a mit in the other. Some of these women, Ken decided, are messed-up in the head.

Cathy was involved, maybe too involved. On the one hand he was glad she had such an interest. It proved that his fears of her withdrawing again after dropping out of college were unfounded. On the other, she seemed obsessed with softball management.

The phone calls began coming at 4:00 A.M. and 5:00 A.M., jolting him always from the deepest part of his sleep.

"Ken, this is Cathy," she always said. "Did I wake you up?"

He knew she knew she did. She knew he worked second shift.

"We've got to do something about shortstop."

"Cath, it's five in the freaking morning."

"I know, but we have to."

He was so tired he never remembered the names. So-and-so wants to play short, she would say, but so-and-so thinks she's got the position.

Cathy's strategy, however, he could remember. She always was calling with inside information, to warn him that a player was planning to have a chat with him about something. She wanted him to be prepared, she said. In fact, Cathy usually was cutting the unsuspecting player off at the pass. Usually she had other plans for the player in her scheme of things. God only knows what that scheme is, he often thought.

"Now, Ken, we need to do this in a way where she doesn't know we have talked," she would say.

One night, awakened again, he was overcome with anger. He thought, why in holy hell this mattered so much, at this hour no less?

He interrupted her, as she chatted away.

"Cathy, for Chrissakes!" he snapped. "What in the hell is going on in there?"

Chapter 6

Soon after Gwen arrived from Tyler she took in a street fair with Fran. They walked through downtown Grand Rapids, browsing at craft booths and munching goodies from the food tents. Gwen liked the coolness she felt in the Michigan summer breeze.

Later, they visited the Grand River. Whirlpools and other evidence of the speeding current came into focus as she approached the shore. Beyond that, everything was dark and very blurry. Unless Gwen squinted her eyes, the Grand looked like a long, deep chasm cut through the city's heart.

Gwen was nearsighted. She refused to wear glasses, despite the urging of family and friends. Her vision had begun failing right after a motorcycle accident when she was seventeen. Some pea gravel swept her Honda out from under her on a turn. She landed on her rear, then slammed the back of her head against the pavement. It bounced up like a ball. She didn't see a doctor until her weight went up from one hundred eighteen to two hundred twenty pounds. The physician told her the accident had disturbed her thyroid gland. He wrote her a prescription, but she threw the pills away after they nauseated her. She walked the weight off, hiking three miles a day.

The bike accident wasn't her only injury. Once she was hit broadside by a hairdresser returning from a toga party. She lay unconscious for two days. Doctors put the bones in her left arm back together with plates and screws. Three months later she hit a parked car while driving her aunt on an errand late one night. She crawled from the wreck, kicked out a window and pulled her aunt to safety just as the car was engulfed in flames. A dentist replaced her front teeth right before she left Tyler.

"And you drove here?" the optometrist said, when she had her eyes checked.

She despised glasses, the way they looked and felt. Gwen also didn't mind having the perceptual limits of her own world reduced. Life, she sometimes complained, was too complicated as it was. Her bad vision, however, fed one of several persistent phobias. Large bodies of water terrified her, bodies like the Grand River.

"It's got dead bodies in it," she said. "There could be a lot of dead bodies floating down it."

She said it out loud, or maybe to herself, as she looked out for the first time at the dark outline of the Grand.

Within days, Gwen decided Fran had misled her about her state of affairs in Grand Rapids. She was not impressed with Fran's job, for one. She was delivering newspapers. The apartment was tiny and cramped, located above a sales office of a used car lot on Michigan Avenue. A guy named Billy lived downstairs, a full-blown boozer. He showed up the first night Gwen arrived, bringing with him a couple of beers, and every day thereafter.

This became old quickly. Gwen was broke, but so was Fran. She was eight years her senior, and had always brought some direction, and some money, to their partnership. Now, Fran's self-confidence appeared shattered. She could barely drag herself to work.

Fran had changed, Gwen decided.

Yes, she had, Fran finally confessed. She had been raped. She had been abducted outside a Grand Rapids bar and raped. Beyond that, she refused to elaborate. She was going to therapy, she said, twice a week to a psychiatric hospital called Kent Oaks.

"You're going there?" Gwen asked. "With the fruitcakes, Fran, for real?"

Soon, Gwen had jobs lining up. She could be a security guard. The local phone company had an opening for a worker in its food service. A third possibility came from Fran. A place called Alpine Manor did a lot of hiring. There was a lot of turnover, she said.

Gwen filled out an application. The phone call scheduling an interview came a few days later. On June 11, Gwen put on a pair of slacks, complementing it with a nicely pressed blouse. She picked one with short sleeves.

Over the years she had learned. It was best to get all the questions about her arms over with right up front.

Chapter 7

"What happened to your arms?" an assistant nursing administrator named Margaret Widmaier asked.

She could see circular scars, arranged in orderly rows on both forearms of the applicant. The girl named Gwen looked as though she had been vaccinated, over and over, in an effort to stop some persistent virus. The job interview for nurse's aide had to rule out serious disease.

"My father had a strange way with discipline," Gwen said.

Her head hung low, her eyes fixed on the floor.

Widmaier let it go at that.

The girl was quiet. Sincere.

"She seems so appreciative of the opportunity to work," Widmaier later told someone.

She also liked Gwen Graham's written responses to the questions on Alpine's application:

Why do you want to work this facility?
I am working (or plan to) my way through college and this
job can provide good experience since I plan to pursue a
medical career as a paramedic.
What can you give this facility?
I listen, learn, & work very hard.
What do you expect from this facility?
I expect nothing so that I don't get disappointed.

The applicant had a work history, references and ambitions for a future in the medical field.

As for the scars, Margaret Widmaier did not note them on her paperwork. If she would have counted them, she would have found thirty-one in all, nineteen on her left arm, twelve on her right. There were also more than a dozen less apparent marks, tiny lines of scar tissue at odd angles, all razor thin.

She wrote down a starting date: 6-23-86. Her pay: $3.35 an hour. She also addressed the health issue.

"Health problems: No known health problems," she wrote.

Chapter 8

Dawn Male cranked the wheel left, then right, never forsaking the immediate goal of butting her Camel Filter in the car ashtray. The notion of bringing everything back to center got overlooked somewhere around forty-five miles an hour.

When the car slammed to a stop, she was so drunk she thought she was mired in a ditch somewhere near Comstock Park. She floored the old station wagon but it wouldn't budge. The suburb was Rockford, and there was no ditch. Sometime after she crawled out of her door, the cops pointed out the tree imbedded in her front grill.

She blew a .017. She spent the night in the lockup, Sunday, June 22.

Well hello, Grand Rapids!

Dawn could have claimed she was celebrating a new job in a new town. Then, however, she would have had to find reasons for getting just as drunk last week or the week before. Suffice to say she was no longer living at home, but with her grandmother. She would have lived with anyone to get out of Lakeview, the little town sixty miles north, and light-years behind.

The Neanderthal strain in Lakeview had always harassed her, she complained, since early high school, when she displayed a fondness for leather and a stylish black beret. She liked the B-52s and the Dead Kennedys and Adam and the Ants. She more than liked Marilyn Monroe. She had every book she could buy on the star. She liked to read, period, preferably with a bottle of her favorite wine, Wild Irish Rose, both red and white.

Dawn had been kicked out of high school more times than she could remember, from pot to straight-up, balls-to-the-wall insubordination. Day school. Night school. Correspondence courses. She still hadn't been able to catch up.

All this would have been enough to give her circus freak status in the small farm town. But Dawn Male was also gay, a lesbian—the dreaded "L word,"she called it—or a dike, a *bull dike* as they might spit in Lakeview. Her last name helped keep the Neanderthal element well supplied with material.

She often thought: And people wonder why I don't like fucking men? Most were crude and ignorant and lacked any fucking feelings for anybody. She could include her father. He left when she was one. She'd seen him four times since.

Fuck it! Fuck him, and fuck them, too, she decided when she left Lakeview. And, she wasn't going back.

In Grand Rapids, it *was* different. For all practical purposes, she had been hired right off the street. Incredibly, the nursing home called Alpine Manor, for once in her life, didn't seem to give a shit the way she looked.

Dawn was only eighteen, but considered herself way ahead of her time. In high school, each ear was pierced five times. When she left town, she pierced her nose. Her hair was bleached white, or streaked with black, depending on her mood. She was known to shave a section or two also, if the inspiration struck.

Dawn Renee Male loved everything she was trying to become in the summer of 1986. But special effects aside, there was a major problem. It was not the jail cell she sat in. It was not her sexual preference. It was much deeper than that.

Dawn Male disliked herself immensely, right at the core, she would realize in a more sober time.

But suspecting as much now only gave her another reason to punch the accelerator, once she drew a couple more measures of inimitable uniqueness from the bottom of her favorite drink.

Dawn first saw Cathy in the break room, after midnight, on third shift. The room featured coffee, candy and pop machines—and other aides when shifts broke for lunch and snacks. She was sitting with a group. Dawn was off alone at a table when Cathy began to chit chat.

"You can come over and sit with us, Dawn," Cathy finally urged her.

"No, I'm okay right here."

"Oh c'mon," she said, drawing out the second syllable of the word, sounding very sad.

Later, Cathy and Dawn sat together at an empty table in the Camelot day room.

"So do you have a boyfriend?" Cathy asked.

"No one in particular."

"Do you date a lot?"

"Depends."

"Well, what do you do for excitement?"

"Depends."

Dawn thought, why is she making such a game out of this? She wants to know if I'm gay. Why doesn't she just ask? Dawn sensed it was not because the subject made her uncomfortable. She seemed to be skirting the issue just for sport.

Dawn's first two impressions of the girl named Cathy were in conflict. She seemed both spaced and razor sharp.

When Dawn did start joining Cathy in the break room on a regular basis, she became intrigued all the more. Cathy seemed exceedingly intelligent. She commented freely on every subject Dawn would pitch. Sports. Movie stars. Politics. Headlines in that day's paper. Her vocabulary was polished. Her observations about Alpine itself were acute and insightful.

"They always say a patient 'expired' here," she said. "They have so many euphemisms around here."

Euphemism. Cathy Wood used a lot of words like that.

But intelligence, Dawn thought, on planet earth. In Grand Rapids, Michigan, no less. This is why I moved. This is why I left Lakeview.

Dawn began to tell people: "Cathy is the most intelligent person I've ever met."

She also seemed quite sweet, Dawn decided, in a very vulnerable way. Cathy always asked permission to ask a question. She addressed elders with "Mr." or "Mrs." Everything was wrapped in pleasantries and gracious phrases: "Please." "Thank you." "Do you mind?" "Would it be convenient?"

"Oh, Dawn, I'm so sorry, I didn't say the wrong thing did I?" she quickly interjected at any hint of discomfort.

Or, she could be right down to earth if Dawn described something pleasing, or something sexy.

"Ooooooooooooo," she'd coo. "I like that."

In time, it became clear to Dawn that Cathy had developed quite a following in the little break room. People wanted to be with her, sit with her. No one could match wits with her, and few tried. She also knew everybody's business at Alpine Manor. She always was first with the latest gossip. And if somebody else had some new scuttlebutt, she often amended it, or amplified it with what sounded like the real inside story.

"When you were around her it was like she was the most popular kid in school, and you were the unpopular, maybe even deformed kid, who didn't have any friends," Dawn later told a friend. "You wanted very much for her to like you. You wanted to be able to do things with her. You wanted very much to be her friend. And if you were, you were very much proud of that."

In fact, the first night Dawn sat with Cathy and her companions in the break room she uttered her ultimate stamp of approval.

"Oh Dawn," Cathy said, smiling. "You're so *cuuuuute.*"

She drew out the last word so much it sounded as if she sang it. Dawn soon recognized the declaration as one of Cathy's pet phrases. It had little to do with appearance really, and everything to do with meeting her standards. She always said that to someone when they said or did something she liked.

"Oh, Dawn, you checked on Marguerite? You're so cuuuuute."

Cathy began opening up to Dawn on a very personal basis. She told her about problems she was having at home. Her husband was a tyrant, she said. He had ruined her life. She had a daughter, but wished she were a better mother. Her childhood was full of horrors, she explained. Her father was a drunk. Her mother made her feel insecure, fat, unwanted. She was just a fat little kid. She spent high school sequestered in her room.

Her problem, Cathy concluded, was that despite the rejection, she trusted people. She still trusted them, she said, and still they took advantage of her disposition.

Despite this, she remained exceptionally strong, Dawn decided.

"I don't want people feeling sorry for me," Cathy always said. "That would be horrible. I can stand on my own."

Dawn also observed how graceful Cathy was. When she sat or walked the halls of Alpine she moved more fluidly than many people half her size. It was as though there was another person—a willowy, confident dancer—trapped by fate inside that large body.

Yes, Cathy reminded Dawn of Norma Jean, the girl trapped inside her icon. And like Marilyn Monroe, no one had measured up to the task of making Cathy Wood happy. All the girl needed was love.

In no time, Dawn felt special because she was *trusted.* She was a chosen exception in a world Cathy considered unworthy of trust. She did not want to betray that.

One night, in the break room at Alpine, she found herself studying Cathy's face. Her features were fine, her cheekbones were slightly upturned like an all-knowing Buddha. She had penetrating eyes. Their color seemed a brilliant hue.

Cathy Wood was beautiful, Dawn Male decided. In fact, Cathy just might be the most beautiful woman she had ever met.

Chapter 9

Linda Engman felt as if she needed a good cry as she followed the ambulance with the logo LIFE written across it big and bold.

This is sad, she thought, just damn sad. There's no worse candidate on earth for a broken hip than my mother, seventy-eight or not. Walking was her passion, maybe even her obsession of late. Age hadn't curtailed that. Neither had Alzheimer's Disease or Alpine Manor. Until she fell ten days ago, she was walking miles in those pastel halls.

Now, hip repairs complete, the ambulance was transporting her back on a Monday in late June. Linda insisted on following the unit from Metropolitan Hospital. Ever since she found her mother tied up and doped senseless in the first nursing home she put her in a year ago, she trusted few in the health care field. She left little or nothing to chance.

"Pissed," Linda said to herself.

She gripped the wheel of her Cadillac tighter.

She thought, that's how mom would feel about this. Mae Mason, otherwise known as Maisy, would be plain *pissed off* about the broken hip. She knew in the old days it would have slowed her only long enough to heal.

Then she thought of her father, and Linda became depressed all over again. A broken hip and Parkinson's disease had forced Maisy to put him in a nursing home. He died there in 1965, less than twenty-four months later. Her mother went on punishing herself for the decision for many, many years.

Linda had vowed this kind of thing would never happen again. God, she thought, how many times did I tell my mother that, face-to-face. Those proclamations now only served to haunt her.

Both had given so much, she thought. Her dad's income managing two department stores in Tulsa, Oklahoma put her through

Michigan State, and her brother through law school. But Maisy's persona contributed more than tuition ever could.

"We're talking about one active woman here," Linda later told a friend. "At any age."

She always remembered the handmade dresses, in her school days.

"You need a new dress," her mother would say.

She made those kinds of announcements just before everyone else went to bed. Linda would detect the chatter of the sewing machine in the house's framing as she fell asleep. The next morning she would find a dress hanging, neatly pressed for school. Her mother never used a pattern.

Not by any stretch, however, was Maisy a homebody. She ignored cooking and housecleaning for other priorities. The theater. The opera. The arts. She took Linda everywhere with her, sometimes reminiscing about the acting contract she had been offered by a Hollywood agent when she was young.

Linda's father had left his widow very comfortable. For twenty years after his death, Maisy lived in a neighborhood among the upper crust on Grand Rapid's east side. She surrounded herself with living things there rather than possessions. Linda could barely get through the foyer, there were so many plants. She liked to put on rummage sale clothes and get her hands in the dark earth.

"Maisy," her neighbor once said to her, walking to the lot line, sporting a very proper blazer. "You're the only one in the whole neighborhood with the guts to get out and work on their own yard."

By sixty-five, however, she was bored. She lied about her age and took up interior decorating. She designed rooms for De Korne Ethan Allen Galleries and Dream House. She was a charismatic, consummate saleswoman.

"She could sell manure if she wanted," Linda recalled.

All this had translated into a very rounded upbringing and full adult life for Linda Engman. She had a spacious, glassy home overlooking the Thornapple River valley, a husband who was a successful attorney and two beautiful young girls, Stephanie and Sari. "Nanna," as the girls called her mother, had also worked her magic with the kids. As they grew, three weekends out of four were spent at her house.

"We're going to the library," Nanna used to tell them.

The first time they headed for the car.

"You can forget that," she said. "Girls, we're going to walk."

She left at a fast clip, the kids trailing. Their arms filled with books on the return leg of the three-mile hike.

When Linda picked up the girls on Sunday evenings they usually found everyone sitting on the floor, playing cards. There was Nanna, Sari, Steph, and later Gerry. He was her live-in boyfriend for years. She hooked up with him at age sixty-nine.

Every Friday night the two of them went dancing. *Every* Friday night. One time he showed up in a snowstorm. Linda watched as the two of them took off down the road. She was wearing an evening dress, but Linda thought she straddled that snowmobile like she owned one herself.

Gerry even picked her up at Alpine for the dancing, Linda remembered, up until just a month or so ago.

It was Gerry who first let her know how bad Maisy was getting when they lived together.

"Linda, I can't handle this anymore," he said, calling one night.

Maisy was pacing through the night, he said. When she did sleep it was with a blanket on the tile floor in the bathroom. She was talking nonsense about animals in her bed.

Two weeks later they moved her into their home on the Thornapple River. After the diagnosis, it was as though she were trying to walk away from the disease. They trained a German shepherd to go with her, leading her in one long circular hike on the country roads near Caledonia. Still, the police got to know her on a first-name basis. Once a squad car brought her back from Kentwood, eight miles away.

Linda never would have suspected that it would be her own resolve that would get sapped so insidiously. There would be no clear opportunity for heroism, no chance to pick up the two-ton fallen object off a loved one with a sudden burst of strength. Surrender would come in painful increments. It would not be glorified by one great failing moment. Linda faded with every police cruiser. She started losing hope the night Maisy was almost hit by a car. When her mother cooked the towels in the oven during a delirium, Linda began to know free-floating panic. When her husband John found Maisy standing dangerously close to the river, talking incoherently, all her best plans washed away.

She hoped she would never again have to live such a moment, when she realized that what was happening to her mother—what was happening to her—was bigger than she ever could have imagined. A lucid spell of her mother's the day they moved her into a retirement home made it a little easier.

"Maybe it's for the best that I no longer live with you," Maisy said.

Later came the incontinency, the nursing homes. Now, like her mom before her, she punished herself with her own shortfall: They took care of me in diapers, but I, however, am incapable of doing the same for her now. I have to protect my children, she told herself. It's no good for anybody if I go over the edge.

Linda Engman wheeled her Cadillac into the entrance of the nursing home.

She knew that there was only one way her mother would ever leave Alpine Manor. She tried not to think about what it would be like the day her mother would be dead.

Chapter 10

The day Mae Mason returned to Alpine Manor, Gwen Graham began a five-day class at the nursing home with nearly two dozen other aspiring nurse's aides.

Their instructor, a registered nurse, stressed the importance of the work. In Alpine, an aide was assigned a group of patients for an entire shift, caring for their needs as dictated by their charts. An aide could make the difference between comfort and misery. They were at the bottom of the Alpine pay scale, but they had more contact with patients than anyone.

The class learned the daily routines from the instructor and videotapes. They saw how to turn patients at two-hour intervals to avoid decubitus ulcers, or bedsores. They learned the stages of a deteriorating skin condition, when to apply a soothing balm called Sween Cream or spray open sores with an aerosol called Granulex.

They learned how to lift, feed and take vital signs. They learned how to apply restraints. There were different kinds, from the felt cuffs for legs and hands to the pelvic style that girded the lower body.

The instructor detailed patient hygiene. Aides gave sponge baths daily. Once a week patients received a complete washing in a "shower chair." It had an open seat, like a toilet, for lower body cleaning. The patient sat naked, restrained if necessary, while the aide employed a hand-held shower spray. Water temperature was critical. Still, some patients could be expected to fight the procedure in any case.

There were tricks of the trade. The aides learned special ways to lift and techniques to encourage a patient to swallow. A washcloth was a handy item. For a patient whose condition prompted him to clench his hands severely, washcloths could be rolled into tubes and placed in his palms. It stopped lacerations sometimes caused by fingernails.

During their second and final week of training, the aides moved from the classroom to Abbey Lane, Buckingham, Camelot and Dover. It was time for some hands-on work.

Gwen's solo on second shift in early July gave her more than the first day jitters. She was frightened. To her, some of the patients resembled the walking dead.

"I was scared, for real," she later recalled. "I'd never been around so many old people. The videos made it look like the patients were a day away from dying, but they sure weren't."

The woman named Marjorie demonstrated that quite clearly after Gwen wheeled her push cart to the door of her room. Her first job was to pass water.

"Would you like a drink?"

The patient didn't respond.

Gwen filled her cup anyway, handing it to the patient, who was sitting in a chair. Marjorie looked into the cup, then at Gwen.

"You need it more than I do."

Then she flicked her wrist.

The icy baptism covered Gwen's neck and shoulders. The water ran down her shirt and streamed between her breasts.

The first patient she fed dinner also brought excitement. Her assignment was waiting among all the other nonambulatory patients in the Camelot day room. The woman had upper dentures. Lunch was pureed and green. Gwen sat next to the patient, filled the spoon with the puree and lifted it to the old woman's mouth.

"There you go," Gwen said. "I hope it's good. I sure do."

The dialogue would remain one way.

The woman opened her mouth slowly. Gwen carefully guided the spoon inside, her patient closing on the helping. As she pulled the spoon out, the woman munched the liquid rapidly, as though it were solid. Finally, she swallowed and opened for another helping.

This routine continued for a few minutes, the cycle always completed by the woman opening her mouth again to reveal her useless upper plate. Gwen talked.

"I just don't know how you can eat this stuff."

Then, with no warning, puree exploded out of her mouth, spattering Gwen in the face. In seconds, the woman was jerking, moving like her chair had suddenly turned red hot. Her eyes bulged. Her mouth opened and closed like a goldfish as green puree dribbled out.

Gwen grabbed her by the shoulders, trying to still her. That's when she saw her bare upper gum. There were the colors of gum red and white swimming in the green puree deep in her gullet.

Gwen thrust her fingers inside, reaching. The woman pushed back at her with her hands. Gwen reached deeper, the patient's upper and lower gums pressuring the skin above her knuckles.

Then, she had it, between the print sides of her thumb and index finger. She pulled, pulling more supper out as well.

But she had it. She had the upper plate.

After Gwen cleaned both of them up, the old woman waved her off. She was done with supper. She wanted to go back to her room.

Gwen told Fran all about the emergency later. She was so excited, she forgot the patient's name. Sometimes, Gwen felt bad about letting the incident happen. She was jittery every time she fed someone for several days after that. Sometimes, she felt good she had kept her head in the crisis, like a good paramedic would.

She had almost killed a patient. But she had also saved that patient's life.

It was one. Or, it was the other.

Chapter 11

Ken Wood never would have suspected prayer could bring such fast results.

"God, make something happen in my marriage," he was praying. "Either make this work, or have Cathy leave me."

A born-again Christian at the GM plant had suggested the approach.

"Ken, your problem isn't about your wife, it's about you," he said. "You can't change her. You gotta be the one who changes. You gotta change from within."

He suggested to Ken he and his wife come to a series of seminars he was teaching every Sunday at a place called the New Wine Church. The subject was marriage. Cathy refused. Ken went anyway.

"You should treat your wife as Christ treats his Church," his message went. "You should be able to forgive, to understand."

After one of these sessions, Ken approached Cathy, deciding to make amends for years of shortcomings.

"Cath, I'm very sorry for the things that I've done, for putting so much pressure on you. And, I apologize for not being as good a husband as I should, and not always saying the right things, for saying mean things."

Her mouth dropped open.

"Wow," she said, half smiling.

That's when he started the daily prayer.

"Be careful what you pray for," the old expression went. "You just might get what you want."

By August 12, their seventh wedding anniversary, Ken Wood was worrying there was more truth to that saying than not.

Cathy was getting more far out. Her moods swung wider. She had more bad days with her mother. She had never really come to terms with how she felt about her, Ken decided long ago, even after his wife broke some apron strings at Sutton Club. Cathy often visited her mom, but not as frequently as the early years. When she did, Ken never knew what to expect. Their mother and daughter relationship was like having terminal cancer. There were good days and there were bad days. Sometimes Cathy returned from a visit pacified, serene. Ken suspected her mother gave her a lot of attention then. Other times, however, Cathy returned in a foul, hateful disposition. She complained her mother was irrational, petty.

"My mother has Alzheimer's," she would spit.

On other subjects, Ken noticed Cathy was rambling a lot, skirting something tucked deep away in her psyche. She kept saying she was "very bad."

"Ken, I'm bad. You don't know how very bad I am."

"Why, Cath?"

"I just am. You just don't know."

Or, out of the blue, she would say "I'm a terrible person," or "I'm a very dirty person."

He pressed for explanations. She only gave him vague illustrations that just didn't make sense.

Sometimes, she talked about her past. She confessed that she had made a neighborhood boy take his pants down when she was eight. She talked about a club she and David/Debbie had planned, one that would require girls to do mysterious taboo things before they could join.

"Cath, what in the hell are you talking about?" Ken asked. "What has brought this all on?"

"It's nothing," she said. "Just thinking."

Cathy, Ken had decided, already had a blurred perception of good and evil. In fact, he often wondered if she dismissed morality entirely. She never could face up to a minor flaw, let alone a major transgression. She deflected guilt, usually by turning the blame back on him, or someone else. She had a teflon conscience.

She could also be downright spooky. Once she told him about a "voice" she heard. The entity came to her, she said, after she broke up with David/Debbie. She was walking along the Grand River, alone near the rushing water at Riverside Park. She wasn't sure if it was from the ethers, or from somewhere deep within.

"There is no God," the voice supposedly said. "There is no devil. There is only *me.*"

When Cathy first told Ken this years ago he saw a countenance that came over her once in a very great while. Her head became motionless, her pupils fixed ahead. Her eyes were very dark and glassy, almost to tears, but she did not cry. Her expression was blank. She looked absolutely emotionless, void of any hint of feeling. It was as though she didn't know where she was or who she was. This look always disturbed him. It was as though someone had unplugged all her circuits.

"Cath, that's in your head, that voice."

She didn't respond. Then, she turned to him and glared.

"Ken, promise you'll never tell anyone about this."

So far, he had not. He also didn't plan to tell anyone about Cathy's twisted idea of a present for his birthday in October. He certainly didn't plan to tell his Christian friend at the plant.

Jamie had cued the subject, by asking out loud what he wanted when he turned twenty-eight. Cathy approached him silently, then spoke quietly up close.

"I know what you want."

He smiled.

"What?"

She squinted.

"You want to see two women do it, wouldn't you? You'd like to see two women. Or, would it be me that you would like to see doing it with another woman?"

He was floored. He had never known her to talk like that. Furthermore, for years their sex life had been minimal. They made love maybe twice a month at the most, always on her terms.

The gift of a threesome was no less shocking than a plan she proposed for a movie outing. She said she wanted to do something different.

"Like what?"

"The Velvet Touch."

She's kidding, he thought. The Velvet Touch was a pornographic adult store on Twenty-eighth Street. They had peep shows and sex toys and a clientele of men who always hustled into the place from their cars with their hands in their coats and their heads down.

He thought, it's a hole! No, he was not going to the Velvet Touch.

She responded in her quiet rage.

"Then I'm going. I'm gonna go there."

This, he thought, is the woman who wouldn't leave her own apartment just three years ago?

She continued, her voice full of contempt.

"I'll go with my friends. I'll go with my friends, or I'll go by myself."

A couple weeks later she confessed they went.

Her friends. He was wondering about them, too. She had become more and more involved in the social circle at Alpine Manor. The stories were getting increasingly bizarre. She talked about the girl named *Angie Brozak*. Ken had met Angie and her husband. They seemed like an okay pair.

However, Cathy said Angie had changed since undergoing a recent mastectomy. She wanted to jump the bones of anybody who would have her, Cathy said. She was chasing Alpine's leading "sleaze," as Cathy described the aide. She wrote him a letter, begging him to grab her by the hair and make her suck him. When she found out the aide was gay, she offered to have sex with the guy and his boyfriend.

Then there was Dawn Male, a new friend and aide at Alpine. He'd heard about her as well.

"Ken, I think Dawn is going to tell me she's gay," Cathy asked one night. "What should I do?"

He thought, how am I supposed to know? And, what kind of people are working there? Alpine Manor was supposed to be a nursing home, where old people went to die. She made the place sound like the set of a kinky soap opera.

Ken found himself seeing less of his wife. She insisted they take two cars to the softball games. She was leaving the ball field right afterwards. She flew out of the parking lot, sometimes with a friend, sounding the jingle on the horn of her Luv Truck. Ken and little Jamie walked the diamond alone, picking up game equipment they loaded in his car. Often they returned to the house on Effie to find it empty.

He wondered what took her.

Cathy usually said she was visiting with other team members.

"Why didn't you invite me?" Ken asked once.

"Oh, no, you wouldn't like it there. You wouldn't like these people at all."

Chapter 12

Belle Burkhard inhaled the cool, pure oxygen as the morning light penetrated her courtyard window on Abbey Lane. She was breathing easier now.

August had not been a good month. In the first week, her body contorted with seizures. By the third week, a respiratory infection labored her breathing and blanched her skin. Now her condition was improving. At seventy-four, Belle Burkhard was not ready to go gentle into that good night.

She hadn't come easily into Alpine Manor in 1979. Social Services had arranged her admission. She was living in a Grand Rapids apartment. Her brother, who lived nearby, reported she could not care for herself anymore. Her daughter lived three hours away. Belle limped through Alpine Manor's front door one cold day in December, leaning on a metal cane. Her teeth were decayed. Her nails were long and thick, her hair greasy.

Belle stood two inches over five feet and had eyes and hair as dark as burnt hickory. There was little gray and a bloodline that was three-quarter Chippewa. She grew up in Michigan's rugged Upper Peninsula, near the turbulent Mackinaw Straights. She lived for years in a house of fieldstone that overlooked a spectacular wilderness vista of another body of water called Silver Lake.

Moving downstate in 1935 brought different views. She moved to St. Joseph, married, raised one daughter. By the time she was fifty-six she had been widowed twice. She worked as a cook. She dreamed of moving back to the north. When she did, briefly, she complained about everything there. Like her late husbands, she was a drinker. Nothing fancy, but Belle had to have her beer.

Her admitting diagnosis at Alpine Manor was hardening of the arteries, arthritis and "organic brain syndrome," or "OBS." The term applied to any number of mental impairments. Relatives guessed Belle's drinking had finally taken its toll, though she had also abstained for years at a time. She was becoming confused and disoriented.

An Alpine doctor who called on many of the nursing home's indigent Alpine patients made the diagnosis of OBS after a brief physical in her room. At her age, Belle's symptoms could have been caused by any number of correctable conditions, ranging from thyroid problems to a hemorrhage between her brain and skull. Only a CAT scan and other tests could rule this out and confirm the nontreatable OBS, or "wet brain," as it was called by drunks. But Belle Burkhard neither had the money or sophistication to demand more scrutiny. By the time she got to Alpine, she'd lost the ability to write.

As for her limp, her right leg was shorter than her left. She made up the difference by stepping on her right toes. A car had hit her years back, fracturing her hip. A doctor told her she would not walk again. Belle had other plans.

Judging from her thick file accumulated in seven years at the nursing home, Belle was not in step with medicine as it was practiced at Alpine Manor either. Her first evaluation described her as "communicative," "cooperative," "friendly" and only "forgetful at times." Three days later she was found wandering in the parking lot without a coat. She was tied to her chair after supper. Over the next month she tried to escape repeatedly, hobbling out the front entrance and several exit doors. This only earned more time in the restraints.

Flight transformed into hostility. She swore like an ironworker, cursing aides when they woke her or strapped her into her bed at night. She sat apart from others during movies and Sunday Mass. She attacked staff with her cane. She struck other patients, knocking one to his knees with a whack across his spine. She snuck into other patients' rooms for chocolates and sweets. She took food from others in the dining room. She frequently shattered the silence there with a litany of expletives.

Meanwhile, an Alpine physical therapist was teaching her to walk correctly. She was fitted with a lift shoe and given a walker. It was too clumsy to swing. She used it to trip. She lurked in the hallways and tried to send passing staffers crashing to the floor.

When, three months into her stay, Belle scratched another patient, another kind of restraint was prescribed, this time a chemical one. The tranquilizer was Mellaril, a dose of 10 milligrams three times a day. She also was given Benadryl, a sedating antihistamine used to lessen side effects associated with Mellaril.

For weeks, the drug failed to have an effect. Further combativeness brought more bed and chair restraints. Belle frequently escaped them. Aides would find her walking in the hall, exercising her newfound ability to ambulate freely. One day, nurses tied her up in a chair next to the Abbey Lane station. She spent half the day cursing everyone who passed.

The medical file of Belle Burkhard's first year in Alpine Manor told the story of a patient besieged from several different directions. Therapists encouraged her to walk. Nurses applied restraints. The pharmacy would handle any inconsistency between the two.

By her fourth month, Belle was walking more than ever. She logged lap after lap on the facility's hallway circuit. She replaced the clumsy walker with an eating tray on wheels, pushing it in front of her. When a nurse complained that she was walking to the point of exhaustion, Belle was restrained again, not for inappropriate behavior, but simply to keep her off her feet.

During her tenth month in Alpine, her dose of Mellaril was tripled. Nurses soon noted in her charts "she's coming around to the program here." Another wrote she was "disoriented of time and place, but no longer fighting." By her first anniversary, her doctor noted in her file that "she does not walk as much as she used to."

By nearly her second year in Alpine Manor, despite her new elevated shoe, a nurse noted: "She's not as active. Needs to be encouraged to ambulate. No longer walking."

Through 1983 and 1984 her world continued to shrink. She stopped attending group activities. One day in 1985, she pushed aside her portable food tray and sat down in a wheelchair. There was a saying among veteran aides. Once a patient sat in a wheelchair, the patient never walked again. Belle Burkhard proved it true.

Belle was assigned to a new physician in late 1985, another doctor with many Alpine patients. He took her off the Mellaril and put her on Dilantin, an antiseizure drug, noting "she apparently has a convulsive disorder." Again, no CAT scan was ordered to determine the cause of this symptom, though it may have been evidence that Belle Burkhard was suffering from something quite different than OBS.

By 1986 Belle was confined all the time to her wheelchair or a bed, still restrained, but now the reason was to prevent her from falling out. Her brother visited sometimes, but no one had seen her daughter in years.

"Belle is a confused female," an activity staffer noted recently in her file. "She does not communicate her needs to staff. She cannot carry on a meaningful conversation. She enjoys watching TV in the day room."

Television, in fact, was her only diversion. On her activity chart, a daily log, the two letters "TV" filled a grid of little boxes, page after page, month after month.

Sometimes Belle did talk, though hardly anyone understood what she had to say. Her voice was slurred and her logic lacking. However, there was one aide, a new hire, who claimed she could understand her. Sometimes other aides would summon her to Abbey Lane just to get an interpretation of Belle's needs.

Some also noticed the new aide seemed to have a special rapport with the patient. She would look the old Indian in the eyes, make some kind of wisecrack and the giggling would start.

Both of them giggled. They were quite a pair, Belle and the new aide from Texas who went by the name of Gwen.

Chapter 13

Ken turned on the TV for his daughter and plopped down on the bed at the Cadet Motor Inn. He was wrung out, physically and emotionally. Now he knew the truth, but it provided little consolation.

"So this is it."

He'd been saying this for days, to himself or anyone else in the cosmos who might be listening.

"So this is the answer to my prayer."

His little family was history, his marriage finished. He was out of

Effie. So was Jamie. In good conscience, he couldn't condone his daughter living with her mother, not now. The two of them were miles from home, in the motel on Sixty-eighth Street. It was a warm Friday night in early September. School was starting any day.

But there was more, much more.

As past events played over again in his mind, Ken wondered what was fact, and what was his wife's sleight of hand. Honesty had always been in short supply with Cathy. Her lies were usually trite and harmless. This time, however, she had something of real significance to hide.

He wondered about the so-called "mandatory meetings" at Alpine Manor that Cathy claimed she had attended. She had come home one day and reported that a staffer had sexually abused a patient in the nursing home. The culprit was still unidentified, but the administration believed an accomplice was needed to pull off such an assault. They were having a big staff meeting to solve the mystery, she said.

At first Ken thought it was just one more fleeting installment in the never-ending Alpine Manor soap. But when the meetings numbered a half dozen, he complained to Cathy that Alpine was taking advantage by holding them in the early evenings on her time.

"They're trying to get to the bottom of it," she told him. "Ken, I *have* to go."

After one of the meetings, Ken got his first glimpse of the girl named Dawn Male. Cathy stopped by the house to tell him that she was giving her friend a ride home. She pointed to Dawn, who was standing outside by her Luv Truck. She was dressed in black and had leather wrist bracelets.

"She's kinda scary, isn't she?" Cathy said, excited.

"Kinda different," he said. "Kinda a punker."

After another meeting, Cathy failed to come home at all. He phoned into the early morning, looking for her. Her Alpine friend Angie Brozak said Cathy had last been seen with Dawn drinking at Cheers, a bar near the nursing home.

The next day, with Cathy still missing, Ken took Jamie to his stepmother's. He had to go to work. He returned to Effie to get ready and found Cathy asleep on the couch. They argued. He threatened to leave her, she begged him to stay.

"Cathy, I can put up with about anything," he said. "But when

you don't come home all night and we have a child to take care of,
and I gotta go to work, that's just too much."

When he returned home from work, she was repentant.

"Ken, I'm never going out with my friends again."

On Saturday, the next morning, Cathy announced that her
friend *Ladonna Sterns,* another Alpine aide, wanted her to go out
drinking with her one night next week. She only would go with his
blessing, she said.

On Saturday night, she said she wanted to make love. In the past
few weeks, in fact, there had been a regeneration of Cathy's libido.
She wanted him twice a week instead of twice a month. He couldn't
understand all the newfound interest.

On Sunday morning, she told him she would go out with
Ladonna whether she had his blessing or not.

On Monday, Labor Day, she had another announcement. It was
early afternoon. She was still in her nightgown. She stood with her
hands folded.

"Ken, I don't feel like I did anything wrong. I want to be able to
do what I want, when I want. So, you better leave."

She paused, then continued.

"Ken, I want a divorce."

That word had never been uttered before by either of them, in
all their previous disputes.

She can't accept the fact she was wrong in pulling that all-
nighter, he reasoned. Her teflon conscience had cooked up the
divorce threat simply to put him on the defensive. He slept in his car
in the big plant parking lot at work, figuring she would come to her
senses in a couple of days.

When he called the next day, however, she didn't budge. She
asked him if his grandmother could watch Jamie while she worked.
He picked up Jamie, took her to his grandmother's and booked the
room at the Cadet.

That night, he discovered the room's air conditioner didn't
work. As he tossed and turned in the muggy room, he thought of the
two big fans he had back at the house on Effie. He decided to get
one.

The first thing he noticed was all the lights. The whole place was
lit up, every bulb in the house, though Cathy's truck wasn't in the
driveway. He let himself in. He was almost out the front door when

he saw Cathy's truck pull up. He stepped back. She parked under a street light, illuminating her interior.

He saw Dawn Male. She was close to Cathy, right next to her. He watched Dawn put her head on his wife's shoulder.

Dear Jesus, he thought, what is this?

When Cathy came through the door he saw a hickey on her neck. A hickey, he thought, Cath would smack me silly if I gave her a hickey.

"Cath, where in the hell did you get that hickey? Did Dawn? For Chrissakes, did Dawn do that?"

He couldn't believe he was even asking. He felt his heart fall into some bottomless hole.

"No, Dawn didn't."

"Then why was she sitting next to you?"

"She spilled a beer on my lap."

He looked at Cathy's slacks. They were dry.

"Well, Dawn lost control of herself," she blurted.

"Then why didn't you control her? Why didn't you stop her?"

His thoughts careened from one memory to another. Her friend Angie. All the talk about gays at Alpine Manor. The conversation about Dawn. David/Debbie. The brimmed hat he'd found on their bed one day when he came home. He hadn't been able to shake the feeling that Cathy had someone over that day. Now he imagined them prancing naked around the bedroom with it.

He thought, what has been going on in my home?

He looked at Cathy. Her eyes were blank.

"Is this it?" he asked. "Is this what we gave up seven years of marriage for? So you could be with your little girlfriend?"

On his way out he said something to Dawn in the driveway. She looked miffed as he passed.

"Is she any good?" he said.

He sped up Effie, squealing his tires as he turned the corner. He raced through a series of side streets. When he reached the freeway he was crying.

He felt like the world's biggest idiot! For seven years he had endured her moods, her excuses, her lies, her irresponsibility—her weight. Everything he had tried to do was meaningless. Anything would have been meaningless.

The lights from oncoming cars made shadowgraphs on his face.

He thought, my wife has left me. She has left me for another *woman.*

He thought, she has no limits. Cathy has no limits. She will take attention wherever she can find it. She does not love me. She is incapable of loving me.

Ken doubted she could love anybody.

Unconditional love.

Bullshit!

The next day he came into work in a daze and left in a fury. The foreman he blew up at saved him by directing him to the medical office, where he was given a couple days health leave.

Later, however, Ken decided once and for all that he was not the one who was sick. He remembered his last heart-to-heart talk with Cathy, when he thought things were getting better, when he thought everything just might work. They had to be honest with each other, he had said.

"Ken, I'm not going to lie anymore," she said. "There will be no more lies."

She seemed so sincere, so determined.

Later, he would learn how deeply she had deceived him. There were no mandatory meetings at Alpine. There was no patient sexual abuse. There was no culprit, no accomplice. He would learn that many of her stories from Alpine were fabrications. There was no wild sex spree by Angie, no gay confession by Dawn.

The lies went back years, to the beginning. The very premise that brought them together as a couple was a half-truth, he eventually learned. Cathy duped him into inviting her to move in with him. Yes, she had bought pot for her father and had been caught by her mother. That much was true. But it had happened months before Ken and Cathy ever met.

More revelations would come in time. For now, Ken needed to think about the immediate future. He had to make some plans. He looked at Jamie. She had fallen asleep on the bed. He thought, how will she ever understand?

He wondered what Cathy was capable of next, now that he had taken the responsibility of motherhood off her hands.

Chapter 14

For five years they had been friends, roommates and lovers. Sometimes Fran thought she was as much Gwen's mother as anything, and that could be the most precarious role.

Now, Fran Shadden simply didn't have enough left of herself for that kind of turmoil. She had cautioned Gwen before she flew up to Grand Rapids. She had told her how turning thirty meant she had to find a direction for herself. She had told her about being raped, about her need to get back what the assault had taken away.

"I have to work on my life," she said. "And you need to work on yours. You need to work on it on your own."

She wasn't sure Gwen had ever come to understand that in the three months since she had arrived. Gwen had a way of perceiving rejection where none was meant. The result could go one of two ways: Unconditional love or outright anger. One or the other usually served as the foundation for all of Gwen's major stands. There was no emotional middle ground.

Over the years Fran had come to know two distinctly different personalities in Gwen Graham. She was saintly and possessed, innocent and jaded. She could be as vulnerable and trusting as a toddler, or as tough as a street hood. Fran had never known anyone so helpful to others who herself was in so much need of help.

This touched something in Fran at the start. Christian pursuits had inspired her to move to Texas in 1976 to join a fundamentalist missionary group. But after five years with the Tyler organization she was less involved with the all-encompassing forgiveness she had discovered in born-again Christianity and more involved with the worldly scramble of church politics and fund-raising. Disillusioned, she left, finding work in a convenience store called the Dixie Kwik Stop. She broke some fundamentalist taboos regarding beer and night life, including a couple of visits to a gay bar in Longview, forty miles from Tyler.

Despite all the Bible study, Fran couldn't recall any epic inner struggle when she discovered her preference for women to men. She did know she especially liked Gwen, the baby-faced girl who showed up daily at her store to give one of her employees a ride. Gwen had a bashful smile and practiced the Texas tradition of good-humored chiding called picking.

Gwen was her first. She lured Gwen to her apartment on the pretext of checking her oil. Fran had two bottles of wine waiting. Before noon they were both quite drunk and in bed. Fran was twenty-five. Gwen was only seventeen, but she was already experienced in the ways of love between two women. Gwen said she had been a lesbian as long as she could remember.

Soon they were spending all their time together. They cruised the long country roads of east Texas, making beer runs and dancing in juke joints across the county line. Fran never thought sex was the foundation of their partnership, no more than it would be for most heterosexual couples. Those kinds of misconceptions were some of the reasons why most gays stayed in the closet. Gay sex was the flash point for most straight people. Heterosexuals could not see beyond the physical act of homosexuality. It skewed all their perceptions and prevented them from seeing traits common to all people and relationships.

As for Gwen, the accumulation of contradictions that characterized her personality defied any stereotyping, gay or straight. Gwen fancied herself "dikey," butch or boyish, but wrote sentimental love poems. She sat tall in the saddle of her Honda 450, but illustrated her letters with fragile, childish images of hearts, birds and bows. She was a dominant sexual partner, but as a companion she was a follower. She was fearless in the face of real danger, but was terrified of harmless things like toilets and bathtub drains. She accumulated unpaid traffic tickets, but agonized over household bills. She told Fran she once robbed a store at knife point, but Fran found her scrupulously honest.

As she learned more, Fran found that there was even a kind of balance to the extremes. The subject was first brought up by Gwen herself, near the end of one night of drinking and frank talk.

"How come you've never asked me about my arms?"

No one could miss those rows of circular scars up and down her forearms. The damaged tissue seemed so incompatible with the sweet side of her disposition.

"I figured if you wanted to tell me, you would," Fran said.

"My dad raped me," Gwen said quietly. "I did these because of him."

Fran thought, did what? With what?

They were cigarette burns, Gwen explained. She burned herself with cigarettes. She said she did this because her dad raped her.

"I had to do something. I was frustrated. I sure was."

Fran guessed the scars were her way of never letting her dad forget the shame of his actions. Lord, she thought, the poor girl. She did nothing wrong, but hurt only herself. As best Fran could piece the story together, the incest had gone on over an extended period of time in her teens.

Fran also knew Gwen and her mother had been at odds for years. She suspected Linda had been demanding and critical of her oldest child. She heard stories of Gwen doing housework as a preschooler. She heard nothing about play or companionship, only dark memories of conflict and rejection. Fran believed for all practical purposes Gwen had been robbed of her childhood.

If they were her parents, Fran would have cut all ties. Gwen was still trying to make knots. Forgive and try to forget. Turn the other cheek. That was Gwen's way with most folks. She desperately wanted a relationship with her mother. She feared her father, but nearly enshrined the man. She told sentimental stories about their small farm near Tyler, how he raised fighting chickens and taught her about livestock. She fancied patterning herself after him. She often quoted his code of ethics on human relations: "Try to be reasonable. If that don't work, kick their butts."

"If you're not going to be reasonable, Fran," Gwen would say, "then I'm not either."

Fran and Gwen had their share of fights, specifically, drunken brawls. Whiskey, particularly Jack Daniel's whiskey, put rage into Gwen's fists. More than one morning the two of them woke up needing stitches. Gwen often blacked out when she drank whiskey, remembering little or nothing. Fran usually blamed herself for throwing the first punch.

Gwen's battles weren't limited to the two of them. Gwen scrapped with Fran's sister, knocking a chunk out of her front tooth. She took on a fellow student at Tyler Junior College in a fight over a parking space. She bragged of all the butt she had kicked on the West Coast.

Fran knew Gwen also liked to exaggerate. She suspected that the brawls and stories were Gwen's attempts to prove she was tougher than her past. In Texas, they agreed it was best to leave the Jack Daniel's in the liquor store.

"Gwen just seemed to be a mixed-up kid," Fran later told a friend.

In Tyler, she also became Fran Shadden's next calling. Rescuing her bordered on an obsession. There was so much worth salvaging, Fran thought. Gwen seemed so determined to make something of herself. She had never been without a plan, some way out of her station in life. She worked long hours and moonlighted. Hard luck and circumstances like her car crashes seemed to conspire against her best laid plans, but usually this only made Gwen more determined.

Fran knew her to be vigilant about others as well. She was the first to step forward to defend a friend or their honor. As a companion, she was warm and touching. She put Fran on a pedestal, making her feel mature and wise. Gwen made Fran feel she was playing a crucial role in life.

Fran also knew of no one with more charity. Gwen loved to care for children. She brought home homeless transients for a bed and a meal. She cancelled important plans to give relatives rides, not to mention pulling her aunt from a burning car on one such trip. She gave away money, usually to her mother and relatives. They argued about that sometimes. More than once Gwen gave away their household budget.

"Fran, everybody deserves a break," she would say. "Yep. They sure do."

The work at the nursing home was perfect for Gwen, Fran figured. She seemed to have exceptional concern for the patients. She came home devastated the first time a patient died on her station. She sometimes joked about the work as well, though Fran sometimes wondered about her sense of humor.

"I was bathing one of them today Fran, and I got all excited," Gwen said one day.

Gwen's desire to please had always made it easy for Fran to call the shots. This went beyond mundane matters like the choice of movies or where they bought their supper. Fran was now realizing that for years her attempts to make Gwen's life right had been a noble, but counterproductive diversion. By mothering Gwen, Fran had allowed herself to put off the more uncomfortable task of confronting her own demons.

Her rape and subsequent therapy was putting an end to all that. Fran had major repairs to make on herself, and she couldn't spare as much attention for Gwen. Maybe that's why Gwen was sulking a lot. Maybe that's why they weren't getting along.

Fran feared the consequences.

Once, several years back in Texas, Fran had told Gwen she was going to leave her. There was a big argument. Gwen had locked herself in the bathroom. She emerged with a new burn on her arm, and a series of tiny razor cuts as well. Gwen stood in the doorway, crying. Tiny streams of blood ran down her arms as they hung straight at her sides. Fran realized that moment how deeply the prospect of rejection could hurt her. She abandoned all thoughts of leaving.

This time, however, the outcome might be different.

If it did come to them splitting up, Fran just prayed Gwen wouldn't do something rash.

Chapter 15

From the first day she moved into the little house on Effie, Dawn Male heard about Ken from Cathy. The more she learned, the more she despised the man. He was everything Dawn hated about the male of the species.

Ken, Dawn figured, was like a lot of macho types. He would probably resort to anything to keep a woman down. He tempted her with junk food, Cathy said. He turned Jamie against her, too. He expected Cathy to be his handmaid. He barked orders and made unreasonable rules. He prohibited her from standing near a fan, she said, complaining she smelled. This Dawn found incredible. Already she could see Cathy was a meticulous housekeeper and was obsessively clean. She showered three and four times a day.

There were outright horror stories as well. Ken beat her regularly, Cathy said. He was a sexual tyrant, demanding her body frequently. Once, she sobbed, he snuck up behind her while she was doing dishes. He pulled down her pants and raped her from behind, right there at the sink, she said. Then he expected her to finish her housework.

By the time she met Ken face to face, Dawn was suited up psychologically for warfare.

On the advice of his attorney, Ken tried to move back in for thirty days to "protect my assets," as he put it. He didn't last twenty-four hours. His first night back, he took Jamie to the fireworks at a city festival called Celebration of the Grand. He returned just as Dawn and Cathy came back from drinking. Dawn watched as Cathy began toying with his mind. He was asking rather innocent questions about her new life, but Cathy kept asking, very sweetly:

"Well, now tell me Ken, what does that mean?"

He tried to explain. The two of them would giggle, then Cathy would say it again, drawing out words in that sighing manner of hers.

"Yes, Ken, but then what do you mean by *that?*"

Finally, he stood up and threw a cup of pop in his wife's face. Dawn was in his face.

"Ken, fuck you!"

He woke Jamie and left.

Another time, on an unannounced visit, he came crashing into the bedroom where Cathy had told Dawn to hide. For reasons unknown to Dawn, Cathy didn't want Ken to find her there. He did, in her pajamas. Ken backhanded her onto the bed.

"Fuck you Ken," Dawn spat. "Why don't you leave Cathy alone? You just come over here so you can start some shit."

Cathy, in the meantime, had scampered out of the house. She was still in her robe as she sped off in the Luv Truck.

Ken stomped out, muttering obscenities.

Cathy was right, Dawn thought. He is a creep, a pig.

In time, however, Dawn also realized Cathy had the uncanny ability to push Ken's buttons. One night she bragged she had controlled him for years.

"I can make him do what I want him to do," she said. "I can make him feel what I want him to feel."

Sometimes, Dawn suspected Cathy was making Ken feel like she still loved him, as though she might take him back any day. However, the way Cathy demeaned him privately, Dawn seriously doubted that she ever had those intentions. As for Jamie, Cathy was more concerned about her own conscience than her daughter. She said she didn't miss the girl.

"I feel bad because I don't care about Jamie," she said, repeatedly. "I just don't care about Jamie at all."

Dawn could see Cathy was undergoing a transformation. She set and styled her hair, eventually bleaching it the color of Marilyn Monroe's. She spent more time in front of the mirror with makeup. They drank, nightly. They hit the Radcliff and the Carousel, two gay bars near downtown. They had Alpine friends over for house parties. Cathy loved to see everybody get wasted, but always kept herself sober and in control, even when drinking the powerful mixed drink Long Island Ice Tea, her favorite.

Cathy loved to spin records. She had some strange tastes, Dawn decided. Mostly, she collected pop 45s. She had some semihip sides. She liked Loverboy and very early Beatles. But she also was horribly square, capable of torturing everyone by playing young Donny Osmond or even an album by the Partridge Family.

Cathy was addicted to crossword puzzles, particularly the one in the tabloid named the *Star*. She insisted Dawn do them as well, and that they race to the finish. Cathy always won, no contest. Yet the crossword races continued, not only with Dawn, but others. The whole point, Dawn eventually realized, was so Cathy could win. Winning excited her. Greatly.

So did Dawn's hamburgers. She cooked small hamburgers with Italian seasoning, and Cathy fussed over them as she gobbled them up.

"Oh Dawn, you're so *cuuuuute,*" she said.

When it came to lovemaking, Cathy could be ferocious. She was experienced, Dawn decided. She told her about David/Debbie. Sometimes matters got out of hand. One night Cathy got drunk (or faked being drunk, Dawn thought) and went into the bedroom with Dawn and another gay aide from Alpine named Ladonna. It was oral sex. They gave. Cathy received.

Another time in bed Cathy severely scratched Dawn's back. She dug her fingernails into her shoulder blades and raked downward to her waist. Later she wondered if Cathy did it in the rapture of orgasm, or just to leave her mark.

At work, their circle of friends was growing. Dawn discovered there were a number of gay women and men on the late shifts, many referred to the job through mutual friends.

Dawn hit it off especially well with the new aide from Texas named Gwen. They slept with each other once, but found they weren't all that compatible. They had too much in common. They both liked feminine women. They thought the same girls were cute.

They both had attitudes, and drank at every opportunity. They were sent home from Alpine once after power drinking at Cheers on their break and staggering back to work. Gwen bought an orange Volkswagen Beetle for four hundred dollars. Together they ran it through the paces of abuse. They laughed themselves delirious as they drank and picked off flashing barricade lights one after another on the freeway, sending them flying over the roof.

When Dawn told Gwen she was sleeping with Cathy, Gwen's eyes became real big. She pushed herself back from one of the tables in the break room.

"Dawn, for real? How could you? Lord, she's huge."

One night, in the courtyard between Dover and Buckingham, Dawn formerly introduced them to one another. They decided they would all have to get together. Cathy. Gwen. Dawn. Fran.

Dawn Male was all for it. Add Jack Daniel's, and it ought to be some kind of party.

Chapter 16

Even in light of Cathy's long record of mood swings, Ken couldn't believe how fickle her devotion to Dawn and her new life-style appeared to be.

She began calling him on the telephone. She needed to talk. She wanted to be friends.

"I don't know if I know what I'm doing," she said. "Ken, I'm confused."

He certainly agreed with that. He was astounded by the changes—her hair, the drinking, the night life. Cathy never liked to drink.

He suggested she go see the psychologist they had consulted about their marriage. She made an appointment and kept it. Later, he inquired with the therapist about Cathy.

"Well I can't tell you what she said," the psychologist said. "But I don't think she's having any kind of breakdown."

Ken shook his head. He never doubted for a moment what had happened. She wasn't honest, he thought. She had gone in there with that mask of sanity she pulled out on special occasions. No one was better than Cathy at sounding perfectly intelligent and rational. It had taken him years to discern her intentions. A psychologist wasn't going to see through her act in one hour.

For now, Ken accepted that it was over between them. Soon, he and Jamie would start their life together in a new apartment complex called the Foxcroft. But Ken Wood was not ready to let go, nor was he ready to give up.

Maybe God is testing me, he thought. Maybe Cathy and I have to go through this because I didn't do things right. We shouldn't have had sex before we were married. We should have taken our time.

Now, he wanted, he *needed,* to understand. He needed to know what Cathy saw in her new relationship. He needed to know what she found in this new atmosphere she'd concocted. Was she really gay, or was this just another way to get acceptance and attention? He needed to know what could be more important than her daughter and their marriage.

Ken wanted to know where he had failed.

For days she refused to even admit there was any kind of intimacy with Dawn.

"Oh *no,*" she said, drawing out the vowel. "We haven't even slept together."

He started to doubt his own conclusions. Cathy had always been good at that. She could make him doubt evidence before his very eyes. On one visit Ken found Dawn passed out on his bed. Clothed, half her body was on the mattress, half on the floor. The next time he found her clothes in the living room and Dawn naked in bed. The night he tried to move back, Cathy and Dawn announced they planned to sleep together in the basement.

At the same time, he had been receiving mixed signals for three weeks. Maybe she really doesn't want to be doing this, he thought.

One Sunday he asked if he could drop by to pick up their portable color TV so he could watch a football game. She was very reasonable. She wanted to talk things out. She was rational. There was no longer any need to fight. She wanted an uncontested divorce. They could divide everything in half.

He thought, this is the Cathy I can live with. She's sensible, intelligent.

She complained she was short on money, didn't have enough for food. He gave her cash. He began to do this regularly when she was in need.

"Well, come over to my place, I'll fix dinner and you can see Jamie," he also suggested.

She showed up several times, without Dawn. They necked passionately on the couch.

"Why are you letting me kiss you when you're with Dawn?" he finally asked.

"Oh *Ken.* Because you want to."

"Well, I want to make love, too."

"Oh *no.* That would be cheating on Dawn."

He was confused, but only became more so with time.

"I really don't respect Dawn," she confided one day. "She is so like most women. Women are such airheads."

She talked about hating women frequently. She liked men like Ted Kopell and Peter Jennings. She liked intelligent, sophisticated men, she said.

In an effort to be civil and rational, Ken invited both Dawn and Cathy to his apartment. He had just given Cathy another handout.

When they arrived, he handed Dawn a beer. He sat down in a chair and looked across the living room. God, he thought, looking at Dawn in her chair. Look at her hair. Look at her ears. He hated her pierced ears.

Jesus, he thought, she's got a pierced nose. There's a chain with a hook right through her nose.

Suddenly the thought hit him. I gave her a beer, and she's not even twenty-one years old. I hate her. Why am I giving her a beer?

"Look it, ya better go, okay?" he said, standing up.

They looked at him dazed. He was fast coming to a boil.

"Dawn," he said. "If you were a man I'd kick the shit out of you, right here, right now."

She squinted her eyes and came right back.

"Don't let that stop you, motherfucker."

As they sped off from the parking lot he punched her Luv Truck.

However, no matter who initiated them, his conflicts with Cathy dissipated as quickly as they came. They had more frank talks. She said she was arguing frequently with Dawn. They were not getting along. At the same time, Cathy bragged she was the queen of her new social circle. They were impressed with her, she said, because she had a house and was making it on her own.

She also said she was shocked by the morals of gay people. One night, she said, someone had suggested a threesome with her and Dawn.

"I told them we're not into that swinging stuff," Cathy said.

Likewise, to Dawn's face, Cathy was the picture of devotion.

"Dawn makes the cutest hamburgs, Ken," she told him once.

Dawn was sitting like a puppy on the floor at her feet.

"I don't care if I have to go on welfare, Ken," she also said. "I'm going to support Dawn for the rest of my life."

Soon, however, Cathy began to complain about Dawn's sexual escapades. She was sleeping with other women, Cathy sobbed one day on the phone. While Cathy was away at work Dawn was doing this, in her own house, she said.

That's absolutely crazy, he thought. This whole thing is absolutely crazy. My wife is with a bunch of sex-fiend lesbians! He couldn't believe this was happening to someone he knew.

Ken didn't realize how deeply Dawn's betrayal was affecting Cathy until he dropped by the house one afternoon about three weeks after the whole ugly affair began.

When he walked up the steps he found Cathy standing in her nightgown, just inside the front door. Her body blocked him from entering, but she started talking. Her eyes were fixed on some spot in the distance, behind him.

"There were dead people," she said.

He thought, what is she talking about?

"There were dead people, standing all around the foot of my bed."

"Cath, what do you mean? You're dreaming."

"No, when I wake up, Ken. They're standing there. Dead people, all around the foot of my bed."

Her eyes were vacant, like the time she told the story about the voice, down by the river.

Jesus, he thought. She's going over the edge. All these changes. These lesbians. She's finally losing it. He hoped it wasn't some kind of premonition.

Cathy believed in premonitions.

Chapter 17

The quarter rolled down Dawn Male's nose, ski jumped to the table and bounced into the cup. Everyone roared.

"Oh no," someone said. "Where did you learn that one?"

Dawn waited until the commotion died down, eyeing those

around the coffee table in Fran Shadden's apartment. Gwen was sitting in a big overstuffed chair. Cathy was right across from her on the couch. Fran was sitting across from Dawn.

"All right," Dawn said. "Gwen, it's you this time."

Gwen set her Marlboro in the ashtray, filled a shot glass with Jack Daniel's and slammed the whiskey down.

The game was called quarters. Everyone took turns trying to bounce a coin into the cup. Those who did could order someone else to drink. Cathy and Fran were playing with Budweiser. Dawn and Gwen had bought whiskey for the contest.

Another quarter bounced.

"Alriiiiiiiiiiiiiiight," said Cathy, almost singing with delight.

"Gwen," she said, pointing.

Gwen downed another shot.

"People are always picking me," Gwen complained later. "I must be pretty funny when I'm drunk."

It was a Thursday night in early September. The game had started early enough, but as midnight neared, the three aides from Alpine didn't want to break the party up.

Fran Shadden thought the contest was getting a little tiring. She was too old for drinking games, and from the moment they met she hadn't liked Cathy Wood. Fran thought her sweet, innocent demeanor was a facade.

"She's a phony," she later told Gwen. "That woman is nothing but trouble."

Gwen, however, was studying the face of the woman across from her at the table. Later she disagreed with Fran.

"I felt terrible about what I had said about Cathy, that she was so big," she said later. "I could see what Dawn saw in her. She was very sweet."

As eleven o'clock approached, Cathy and Dawn needed some kind of ruse. They were scheduled for the midnight shift at Alpine Manor, and neither wanted to go.

Cathy dialed up the night supervisor with a story. She said she was calling from near Howard City, thirty miles north. They were stuck at Croton Dam in the National Forest on the Muskegon River.

"The roads are washed out," she said.

Mother Nature already was providing more than its share of cooperation for Cathy's concocted script. For the past two days, a turbulent front out of the southwest had dropped the barometer to near hurricane lows.

As they drank and played, waves of thunderstorms hit Grand Rapids, lighting up the windows of the little apartment. Six inches of rain would fall. Water streamed down nearby Michigan Avenue and made the iron grids of the storm drains hiss.

North of the apartment, along the banks of the Grand, the bolts of lightning illuminated stretches of the river. Periodically, a fallen log would speed by, ripped away from a bank upstream.

Gwen Graham wouldn't remember the storm. She'd blacked out on Jack Daniel's as the storm waters swelled the Grand River to near-flood levels.

A current was building in the deeper regions, right where Gwen feared all the bodies of the dead.

Chapter 18

Angie Brozak listened to what she already knew to be true. She considered that a distinct advantage when it came to information from Cathy Wood.

"Guess what?" Cathy said. "Dawn's been fired."

In fact, a supervisor found her hanging onto one of the hall railings in Camelot. That's how plastered she was.

Yes, and that was really too bad, Angie thought. Dawn was basically a good kid, with a lot of problems, most of them measured by proof.

"Well, I'm not going to support some *drunken kid,*" Cathy sighed. "I'm in the process of kicking her out."

Angie wondered what the old Cathy Wood would have done. However, weeks had passed since anyone had seen the old Cathy Wood, the woman Angie once counted as a trusted friend.

She had never seen such a complete metamorphosis. There was

no hint of the quiet, bashful girl that came to work on third shift last summer. Cathy was so shy then she wouldn't sit with anyone in the break room. Now she ruled it. Angie, her husband Ken and Cathy dined and played cards together. Now Cathy told spiteful stories about how Ken had nixed her schooling and made her do housework in the nude.

Angie at one time had been able to count on Cathy. She was there for her when she came down with cancer of the breast. Cathy sat by her side as her doctor told her about the mastectomy. Unlike her own husband, Cathy was waiting for her when an orderly wheeled her back from OR.

Cathy nicknamed her Bon Bon. She really didn't like it, but Cathy thought it was sweet, like the candy. Cathy included her in big plans. She was going into business when she got her management degree, she said. She didn't know what kind, but they would make a fortune, Cathy said.

"And, Bon Bon, you can be my secretary," she added.

But everything started to change with the new aide named Wendell, though by no means was it his fault. He was a homely little man. He also was gay and affected and had a condescending wit. He and Cathy took a liking to one another.

One night Wendell took Cathy to the gay bar called the Carousel. She came back raving about how friendly the people were there.

"And gay people don't care what you look like," she said.

Wendell was the first homosexual Angie had ever met. At thirty-five, worldly seclusion had come in the form of raising four kids in a small town north of Grand Rapids, until her husband suggested she go to work. She was all for the idea. She had spent a good number of those years overweight and bored.

Soon, Angie was making excursions to the Carousel. Cathy recruited others as well. They offered up excuses for their husbands. Cathy always had a good supply of those.

The Carousel was a dumpy little place with a dance floor and a DJ. Its clientele furnished all the ambience. The crowd couldn't be defined by age or color. Some gay men and women came out as punks and cross dressers. There were flamboyant types in a lot of leather. There were sophisticated, handsome men.

Angie found the place refreshing and a long way from boring. Nobody asked how many children she had or what her husband did. She found herself at ease, not self-conscious as she was in most straight bars. Men did not hit on her, and neither did the women.

"You could wear anything you wanted," she told someone later. "You could be as wild as you wanted, or as conservative as you liked. You could be straight, and have a nice time."

Angie also liked Wendell. He was sensitive and refined. He knew about the arts. He knew all about classical music and opera. She loved to tune in opera on the public TV station. The music moved her, and only in opera could a heavy woman be an international star.

One day she got a letter from Wendell, inviting her to an upcoming opera scheduled in Grand Rapids. She wrote back she would love to go. Soon after, Cathy approached her at work, her eyes dark with rage.

"Isn't your husband enough for you? Do you have to go after what I have?"

"Cath, I didn't go after anything of yours."

"You didn't have Wendell, did you?"

"But Cathy, all I've done is talk to the man. We both like opera."

Angie thought, my God, the man is a homosexual at that, and Cathy, you're my friend.

Cathy left in a huff. It was only the first of the changes. At the Carousel, Cathy became a regular Hyde. Angie had never known her to drink much or speak crudely. At the bar she was rude, often vulgar. She sucked on other people's cigarettes and drank copious amounts of alcohol, with little or no effect. On more than one occasion Angie watched her down a half dozen glasses of Long Island Iced Tea, a concoction that would have put most folks in a coma.

One night, Angie begged Cathy to join her on the dance floor. She always refused to dance. Finally, Cathy rose from her chair and walked to the hardwood. The dance floor was slightly raised. She bumped her toe. She turned immediately and walked back to her seat. No one was the wiser, but she scolded Angie nevertheless.

"You embarrassed me in front of all these people," she spit. "Bon Bon, *you* made me get up there and do that."

She became petty and vindictive with aides at work. Once, another aide reached over and sounded the horn on her Luv Truck as Cathy was leaving the Alpine lot. The thing malfunctioned, sounding jingles all the way as Cathy sped home. She was so furious she never spoke a word to the aide again. She spread rumors about her among the staff.

One night at work, she confessed about her relationship with Dawn.

"You're going to hate me, Bon Bon."

"Why's that?"

"I'm going to have an affair, and you're going to hate me. When I tell you who, you're going to think I'm terrible."

"Well, who is it?"

Cathy made a ten-minute guessing game out of it, letting Angie name every guy she knew in Alpine. Finally she revealed Dawn's name.

"Oh, you're going to hate me, and never talk to me."

She pouted like Shirley Temple.

"Cathy, I wouldn't hate someone because they were gay."

Suddenly, she began pleading.

"Don't ever fall in love with me. Oh Bon Bon, don't ever fall in love with me."

"Don't worry."

"All I want is a friend who I won't have to worry about hitting on me. Don't ever fall in love with me."

Angie looked her in the eyes.

"Don't worry, Cathy. You're not my type."

And that, Angie decided, had nothing to do with sexual preference. That only became more clear as the drinking parties moved from the Carousel to Cathy's house after her husband Ken moved out.

One night, Angie slept on Cathy's couch. She was just too tired to drive home. Cathy worked third shift. The next day, after Angie drove home, Cathy called. She accused her of sleeping with Dawn while she was at work. Angie raced back to the house on Effie where she found Dawn passed out on the floor. She shook her out of her stupor.

"Dawn, wake up. Did I sleep with you?"

Dawn opened her eyes, looked at both of them and muttered.

"Fuck no."

Then she passed back out.

Apologetic, Cathy claimed somebody else at the party had told her this. The next day, however, Cathy was spreading the word all over Alpine: "Not only did she sleep at my house. She slept with my roommate."

Angie felt the cold shoulder from several aides.

"How could you do that to poor Cathy," one told her. "Angie, she's you're friend."

She protested, my God, I haven't done a damn thing.

Now, Angie just didn't know where Cathy was coming from most of the time. She decided to lie low rather than challenge her. She would be polite. It was best not to get Cathy worked up.

Cathy Wood, she decided, likes to hurt people.

By late September, Angie could see Cathy had new plans underway with the ditching of Dawn. She wanted a roommate, but a "platonic," relationship, she told Angie.

"Bon Bon, Gwen is just so miserable at Fran's."

Angie liked Gwen, as did most the staff. She was earnest, and had the cutest Texas accent. She was a perfect aide as well. Angie, working third shift, was often assigned the same patients Gwen had on second shift. She found the patients dry and turned and their rooms immaculate.

"It's such a pleasure following you," she told her once.

Angie couldn't say the same for Cathy's work. Increasingly, her personal schemes seem to take precedent over care. She could be short with patients. Sometimes she was indifferent to their needs.

One night, Angie took Gwen aside and shared some insights. Angie had seen how Cathy had led Dawn around. Perhaps it was no coincidence that Dawn had a chain dangling from her nose.

"Gwen, just don't get involved with her," she said. "She uses people."

She had one more piece of advice. It was based on a hunch.

"Gwen, if she decides she wants to keep you," she said. "I think she's the type who will never let you go."

Chapter 19

Ladonna Sterns had written the verse out:

> Without doubt your eyes hold poison.
> Since the first look you gave me
> I know I die of love.

She had shown it to Cathy, who claimed she didn't understand. But Ladonna knew, and she suspected Cathy did as well. All Cathy had to do was look at her, give her the nod, and Ladonna was hers, forever.

Now here she was, driving to Cathy's house like some kind of fool. She thought, I'm nearly ten years older, but I'm her little puppet. She pulls the strings and I come running.

She knew she wasn't alone. Others wanted to be closer, in her inner circle. They would all sit, a half dozen of them from Alpine. They would sit around in Cathy's living room, drinking, smoking joints, listening to the music. Sometimes, Cathy didn't even join them. She stayed in her bedroom, talking with Dawn or someone else. Sometimes her house felt like a waiting room.

"Ladonna, come in here with me and Dawn," Cathy would say, emerging. "I want to talk to you."

Ladonna didn't know why she jumped at the chance. She only knew that when she looked at Cathy, her sad eyes said: *I'm so big and I'm so ugly and my husband doesn't love me and he doesn't make love to me and he looks at other girls. And now Dawn doesn't love me and she doesn't understand me and she beats me up and she drinks and what am I going to do?*

Ladonna only knew that something deep inside her said: *All I want to do is hold you and touch you and tell you that you're so beautiful. You're everything your husband wants you to be, but he's too blind to see.*

And Dawn is blind, and not worthy. You are lonely, and you are miserable. I will hold you. I am worthy. I will end your misery.

So far, Cathy had only used the attraction as an instrument of emotional torture. Cathy wept the first time when Ladonna told her she had feelings for her.

"Why didn't you tell me?" Cathy said. "Why did you let me go with Dawn?"

Later, she lured Ladonna into an empty room at Alpine.

"Well, aren't you going to kiss me?" Cathy asked.

She invited Ladonna to the movies, to her little house. When Ladonna came running, she was never there.

Then Cathy told Dawn that Ladonna was chasing her, that she wouldn't leave her alone. One night Dawn called her, asking her to come over. Cathy was asleep in the bedroom and Dawn was livid.

"I'm going to beat the shit out of you unless you leave Cathy alone," Dawn said. "Stop calling her, damn it!"

Ladonna protested.

"I'm not the one who's calling."

Instead of fighting, they slept together.

Everybody was sleeping with everybody, and Cathy was helping initiate the frolic. She fancied herself some kind of matchmaker. Nights at the Carousel were a sex merry-go-round. Ladonna would meet Cathy in the bathroom where they would make out. Outside, Dawn would be hitting on someone else, while Cathy suggested partners for Ladonna in the crowd. They were all drinking heavily. Ladonna felt as if her double life was becoming even more fractured. She had five kids and a marriage of fourteen years, but had been having lesbian affairs for years.

Nothing, however, had been as crazy as this.

Sometimes, she suspected Cathy was concocting everything for her own amusement. She watched her manipulate her estranged husband, picking up the phone in front of her friends.

"What are you doing tonight for dinner, Ken?"

Hanging up, she would turn to the group.

"Well, *I'm* going to dinner and the movies with *my* husband."

Ladonna knew Cathy had a cruel streak. Once, she threatened to tell all of Alpine Ladonna was a lesbian.

"Why are you doing this to me?" Ladonna asked.

"Because you won't leave me alone."

Ladonna didn't understand. It was Cathy who kept making the

overtures. Finally, Ladonna took away her leverage. She paid another aide to make an announcement on the Alpine public address
during third shift.

"Ladonna Sterns is a lesbian. Ladonna Sterns is a lesbian."

Everyone told Ladonna: "She's only playing with you. She's only
using you to see what she can get out of you. She's only seeing what
she can make you do."

Without doubt your eyes hold poison . . .

When Ladonna arrived at Cathy's house, they sat in the living
room. The record player was spinning. Ladonna knew Dawn was
history. She heard Cathy had her eyes on Gwen. She saw one last
chance to make her feelings known. She would tell Cathy she really
cared about her. Ladonna thought, I, alone, can remove the misery
inside her that makes her play her vicious games.

Cathy was eyeing her cautiously.

Ladonna thought, she knows I'm going to say something stupid.
I'm going to say it anyway. Her mind overflowed with the language
of the Harlequin romance novels she read incessantly. She had to
say it, now or never.

"Cathy, I want you," she began. "I want to love you forever. I
want to love you forever and a day."

Ladonna Sterns was heartbroken as she drove away.

Chapter 20

They were looking out the bedroom window from the little apartment above the used car lot, watching Dawn and Fran walk to the
corner store for beer. That's when Cathy and Gwen kissed.

In the Alpine break room, Cathy had told Gwen how unhappy
Dawn made her. At first Gwen felt sorry for Dawn. She was so
devoted.

"Maybe Cathy was one of these women who decided she was

going to try it with a woman for a little while," Gwen later told a friend. "Maybe she realized she'd gone too far, kicking out her husband and her kid."

Gwen had been giving Cathy advice. She said she wanted help from a woman experienced in female relationships.

"I didn't know what was wrong with the girl," Gwen recalled later. "She was so unhappy with Dawn and didn't know how to deal with it. She was like a lost puppy."

They talked only of a financial partnership at first. Cathy told Gwen living on Effie was cheap. She bragged that she never paid her mother rent. They would split the few utility bills. Then Gwen would have enough for the paramedic program at Davenport College. Cathy could help in other ways, Gwen decided. She was intelligent and well-read.

They kissed on Sunday. On Monday, September 28, Gwen drove up to the little house on Effie. The back of her orange Beetle was packed with boxes.

In the beginning they didn't see a lot of each other. Cathy worked third shift, Gwen second.

When they were together, Cathy liked to play backgammon. Somebody proposed stakes. They bet household chores. The loser had to do dishes for a week. The loser had to do the laundry. Gwen didn't do well in these wagers.

"I hate doing laundry," she later complained. "But I lost the game so I really had no choice. Three months of laundry! I lost that one, for real."

Gwen didn't lose the wager about the lawn. Cathy was supposed to mow. When it was warm, however, Gwen felt sorry for Cathy, who was so big and so unequal to the task. Gwen took over the chore.

"You're so cuuuuuute," Cathy said.

Other times, when they were drinking, the stakes became silly. One night, after losing, Gwen had to pay off a bet outside. She had to do pirouettes while naked, under the street lamp.

Every week, Cathy brought home two *Star*s from the grocery store.

"Here. Let's race."

Later, Gwen complained the contest was unfair. Cathy went to her bookshelf.

"Here, you can even use a dictionary."

"She still whipped my butt every time," Gwen later said.

They preferred music to TV. Gwen did like cartoons, but only when she smoked a joint. Cathy loved her stereo. She back-ordered old 45s from the record store, storing them in vinyl carrying cases with plastic handles. Her favorite was "Hold Me. Thrill Me. Kiss Me," by Mel Carter.

"Make me tell you I'm in love with you," the song continued.

Cathy played the song daily, sometimes over and over again for hours.

The two of them had heart-to-heart talks. Gwen told Cathy about her dad. She told her about life on the farm in Texas and the burns on her arms. Cathy told her about her marriage with Ken.

"Lord, he treated you like some kind of stepchild," Gwen said.

Ken bought all her clothes, Cathy complained. Gwen could see only three pairs of polyester work slacks, three work blouses and a couple old sweatshirts in her closet.

"Let's go shopping," Gwen said.

Cathy cried.

"No there won't be anything. With my size, they don't make anything for me."

Gwen talked to an overweight aide at Alpine, asking her where she bought her clothes. She lured Cathy to a strip mall, walking her past a place called The Fashion Bug Plus.

"C'mon, let's go in here. Let's see if we can find you some clothes."

Cathy glared.

"I'm not going in there."

Then, several days later, she changed her mind as though there had never been a conflict. Cathy went into the dressing room. Gwen tossed clothes to her over the partition. She threw her stone-washed jeans. She picked out fashionable slacks and blouses in natural fiber. She found a shear, loose-fitting jacket in black. Two brightly colored parrots were on the back.

"Oh Gwen, I adore parrots," Cathy said.

Gwen preferred cuddly things to birds known for their mindless mimicking. She picked out a shirt printed with small teddy bears, and bought it for Cathy as well.

"Sometimes I regretted getting the shopping started," she later recalled. "Cathy just went all out after that. It was good, but it was expensive."

From the start, Gwen was enchanted with Cathy's quick mind. She had never been with a woman so smart. Cathy grasped matters that Gwen had always found elusive or complex. She used psychological terms when she discussed people. She read the finance section of the daily newspaper. She commented on the economy. Often, she cited latest stock quotes.

"I didn't go to business school for nothing," Cathy said.

"She was real smart, she was," Gwen recalled later.

But it was the little things that really delighted Gwen. She began finding little notes from Cathy on her cart when they pulled double together:

"Why don't you come over and see me?"

When Gwen thought she had Cathy's idiosyncracies figured out, Cathy would surprise her. Gwen did the washing at the coin laundry, always folding her towels in thirds and her washcloths in fourths. One day Gwen came home from work and found the laundry not only done, but folded her way.

"Cathy, why did you do it, and fold them like this?"

" 'Cause that's just the way you like it," Cathy said.

Gwen found Cathy's weight something of a mystery. She hardly ate. They rarely cooked. The refrigerator was stocked with beer and mix. When they weren't skipping meals Cathy was eating fast food, Taco Bell and Burger King. The closest they ever came to a well-rounded meal was a smorgasbord they visited every Thursday.

Gwen, however, carefully steered away from the issue of her weight. She remembered her own thyroid problem. She knew what it was like to be heavy.

Cathy, however, made an issue of her size. It started just after Gwen moved in. Cathy's shower was in the basement. Gwen was afraid of the cellar, specifically a drain in the floor. It was round, dark and just a few feet from the shower. She had never seen anything like it in Texas, where most everything was built on slabs.

"Cathy, take a shower with me," she begged.

She told her about her phobias. She didn't like toilets. She didn't like drains, even the ones in bathtubs.

"I feel like I'm going to break up into little pieces and be sucked into the drain, right through those holes around my toes."

Cathy said she had fears in the basement as well. She pointed out a small opening in the base of the chimney, a clean out for ashes.

"Ooooooo, that's what scares me," she said.

Cathy agreed to shower with her on one condition. Gwen would have to face the corner of the basement when she washed.

"I don't want you to see me naked," Cathy said.

For several days, Gwen stood, facing the wall, listening to the water running over her roommate's body. The frightful became the erotic. Finally, Gwen was overcome. She kissed her in the living room, touching the side of her breast with her palm.

Cathy reacted shyly.

"Oh no. I can't do anything unless I've been drinking."

Gwen sped down to the local grocery. She returned with a case of beer. Still, that night, they only held each other. Cathy still was too self-conscious.

The next night, Gwen tried again. Cathy was wearing her favorite nightgown, a flannel full-length with thin pinstripes in red, yellow, green and blue. Gwen wanted to go into the bedroom.

"Oh no, I just can't take my clothes off," Cathy protested. "You're not going to like me."

Then, several nights later, the subject came up again. They had both been drinking, but Cathy still was protesting.

"Ken never saw me take my clothes off and neither did Dawn."

"Cathy, don't you understand that I really don't care. Don't you understand that to me it doesn't mean a thing."

Gwen eyed the nightgown. It was so old the armpits were ripped. Below, Gwen was throbbing. Below, she was very wet. Gwen had run out of patience.

She reached out, grabbed the nightgown near the collar and in one swift motion ripped the garment off.

They climaxed together.

Nudity was never a problem after that. When Cathy wanted coverage, she wrapped herself in a white sheet. She looked like liberty's statue, Mother of Exiles.

Gwen loved fucking her. Gwen just plain loved to fuck. But Cathy was real vocal and loved dildos and cunnilingus. Gwen liked to administer orgasms.

"There are those who like to do, and those who like to be done," she later said. "I like to be the doer, though I don't mind being done."

It wasn't long before Gwen's back was covered with deep scratches. They left hickeys on each other's necks.

The marks were so numerous the other aides at Alpine began to notice them. They asked questions.

"Cathy did it," Gwen would say, giggling.

She began calling Cathy "my woman." Cathy came up with a nickname for Gwen. She called her "Bunny Foo Foo," named for the sound Gwen said her false front teeth made when she first got them.

The name also came from a nursery song:

Little Bunny Foo Foo
Hopping through the forest
Scooping up the field mice
And bopping them on the head.

When they were alone, Gwen called Cathy her "pretty girl."

Chapter 21

Cathy pushed Angie Brozak into an empty Alpine bedroom, slamming the door behind her.

"How could you?" Cathy seethed. "You slept with Gwen."

Cathy's eyes looked pure black.

Angie thought, she's going to beat the shit out of me. Right here. Right here on third shift!

"Cathy, you guys are just friends," she reminded her. "You told me you were just roommates."

Encounters with Gwen raced through her mind. Yes, she slept with her. In fact, Cathy matched them up. She put them together at the Carousel. Drunk, Angie was entertaining the idea of her first gay affair. Cathy kept whispering in her ear, right over her shoulder.

"Gwen likes you," Cathy urged. "Go on. Go Angie. She thinks you're pretty."

Angie slept with Gwen, at Cathy's house. It was before Gwen moved in with Cathy.

The next morning Cathy told her, "Oh I don't know what you did to her, but Gwen wants you to leave your husband. She's trying to figure out how she's going to support four kids when you come live with her."

Angie didn't remember Gwen saying anything like that. It was a crazy fling. Angie enjoyed it, but she didn't plan to take it much farther than that.

Weeks later, they slept together a second time, again at Cathy's house.

"Gwen and I are just friends," Cathy told everyone.

Now, Cathy would hear none of that.

"*You* took Wendell," she said. "*You* took Dawn. And now *you* are taking Gwen."

Angie's neck stiffened, preparing for the assault.

Air rushed out of Cathy's nostrils. Then she spun around, and scurried out of the room.

Angie stood there for a few moments, trembling.

She thought, did I disregard Cathy's feelings? No, damn it! I did nothing wrong.

Angie Brozak resolved to try to keep her distance from both of them. She suspected there was going to be more trouble, whether she was in the picture or not. At thirty-four, she considered herself a pretty good judge of people and their assorted appetites.

Gwen Graham, she had already decided, was the kind of gal who liked to sleep around.

Chapter 22

"I may have told many lies, and I may have played many games . . ."

—Cathy Wood, October 24, 1990.

A former Alpine aide named Tony Kubiak sipped on a soda in his Grand Rapids apartment and told a guest what it was like after he moved into the little house on Effie with Cathy Wood and Gwen Graham.

"I had some problems living with another roommate so I moved in for the first two weeks of October until my apartment was ready. It was just very hectic. I stayed out of Cathy's way as much as possible.

"I met them at Alpine Manor. My friend Paul Lopez got me the job there. Angie was a friend of mine. I was introduced to Ladonna. Cathy showed up in the picture. We all went down to the Carousel. More people were added into the group, and that's how Alpine got the nickname (Gay Manor). We would all go down to the bar in our uniforms. I would say the majority of third shift was gay.

"The scene at Cathy's was crazy. Girls were out in the middle of the street, making out. That's something I won't do. I may see a male friend and give him a hug, but I don't carry on. I don't care if it's dark out or not. You don't do what they were doing. Teenagers do that kind of thing. They were very pubescent. Hickeys, all that stuff. It was just a bizarre situation.

"There was also a lot of noise, people fighting late at night in the yard. A lot of yelling. It was usually over some relationship Cathy was involved in, whether it was Dawn cheating on her, or Cathy cheating on her, but usually it was somebody doing wrong to Cathy. Cathy was more dominant. Gwen was more of a passive person.

"One time Angie slept with Gwen, and Cathy found out about

it. I watched them have this real big fight. First Cathy said, 'How could you do that?' She looked like a puppy dog. It was her way of trying to butter Gwen up, make her feel sorry for her. But really, it was cold. Some people can see through that. Some people can't.

"Like I was saying, she had that puppy dog image. Then, all of a sudden, she was shooting off at the mouth. When Gwen tried to get away from Cathy, Cathy literally grabbed her by the hair on her head and pulled her back into the bedroom. They were in there fighting and screaming and slapping. Cathy had the upper hand. The next day I looked in the room and there's a nice big hole in the wall, twelve inches across.

"Cathy was very possessive. To tell you the truth I don't think she liked Gwen even talking to me. Gwen tried being nice to me. For Pete's sake, I had no interest in Gwen. She was a friend. She was a coworker.

"Another thing, I didn't whore around. I think that had a lot to do with the way Cathy felt about me. In a relationship, I'm monogamous. I didn't make turmoil in people's lives. I did not do what they did. That just doesn't work in a relationship, straight or gay. Cathy wanted a continual soap opera.

"Both Angie and Ladonna would get divorced while working at Alpine Manor, and Cathy had a lot to do with that. After Cathy divorced Ken what better way to get back at everyone than Cathy telling them their husbands were no good or they were not loving them enough. What's wrong with two women fooling around?

"Well, it's wrong if they're married. But Cathy meddled. She would call Angie's husband this or that, then turn around and tell him all kinds of bullshit about Angie. Cathy would go that extra step to make sure things were going the way she wanted them to go. She's crazy, but she's very brilliant. What is it they say, that there's a fine line between genius and insanity?

"Before I left, she accused me of ruining one of her 45s. It was left out on a table or something and she was just all pissed. She said I *owed* her for that. She made a bigger scene out of the whole thing than she should have. It could have been anybody. That house was turned around so many times with all the people coming over and partying. It was best that I got out of there. I left a day or two after that. Then, I met Jesse, who also worked at Alpine. Jesse is Ladonna's brother. And Cathy just got totally involved in this and that, trying to tear it up. She tried to tell me that Jesse didn't have the feelings for me. Then she'd go back to Jesse and say, 'Tony's not any good for you.'

"It was a constant jealousy thing. Cathy's life is not going good, so why should anybody else's . . . Cathy Wood just didn't want anyone to have a life of their own.

"But it was none of her business. She wasn't a friend of mine, or a friend of Jesse's. But Jesse is sometimes gullible and he'd sometimes fall for it. I think I was just too strong for her. I went up to her and told her to keep her head out of my business. I said, 'It's my business.' I said, 'It's Jesse's business. It's not your business.'

"Later I found there were people who she said she would get even with. In the break room she supposedly rattled off a list of people, and I was one of the people. Angie also was on the list. And here it was going through my head: What did I do for someone to hate me so much?

"At Alpine I found myself looking behind my back, wondering about everything I was doing. What puzzled me was how she was also able to turn everyone else against you. I just wonder what Cathy had on them. It was crazy that someone would let them control them the way she did.

"In December, we left Alpine and started working for Portamedic, a temporary agency. We started making money. They paid twice as much as Alpine. And there was also the friction Cathy was creating between me and Jesse. That's one reason why we left Alpine.

"If we wanted a life together, we couldn't be around that."

Chapter 23

Gwen saw her first patient die less than a month after her hire at Alpine Manor. Her name was Helen. The cause was pneumonia.

"I couldn't stand her," she recalled later. "I couldn't stand that woman. She whined all the time."

However, as Helen's life neared its end, one aide sat with her for nearly four hours. She talked to her and squeezed her hand as she came in and out of consciousness.

The aide was Gwen Graham.

When Helen expired, Gwen ran weeping to the bathroom. There, another staffer comforted her, holding her and patting her back. Back then they hadn't been introduced yet.

The aide was Cathy Wood.

No one knew Gwen Graham well enough back then to notice the contradiction. No one thought it odd that she was so shattered by the death of a patient she disliked so much.

By mid-October, Gwen was more familiar with the ways of death in Alpine Manor. From five to ten patients died at the nursing home each month, the higher numbers in the flu seasons of fall and winter.

Sometimes death simply came with no warning.

On October 14, a patient named June Lindenschmidt was up to her old tricks in the Alpine dining room. On a restricted diet, the sixty-nine-year-old patient often snatched food from the plates of other residents. She was a diabetic and an amputee. She was also quite mobile in her wheelchair.

Several aides witnessed what happened. At dinner the woman snatched a brownie from somebody's plate, slammed it into her mouth and quickly wheeled herself out of the dining room. She was discovered in her room minutes later. Word spread quickly. She had choked on the brownie. She had pieces down her throat.

"That's how she died, I'm sure, I'm positive," Gwen also recalled. "In her glass on her nightstand, the plastic straw, had brownie stuck all the way down it, like she had tried to take a drink."

Gwen and an aide named Paul Lopez, who discovered June Lindenschmidt dead, were assigned to prepare her body for the mortuary. The funeral home detail was disliked by many aides. They gave her a sponge bath, changed her bed linen and put on a clean gown and undergarments.

Death routines were entrenched. If a patient was expected to expire soon, a nurse notified the family so they could be bedside if they wished. The family also was given the opportunity to view the body before the patient's doctor was called. The physician released the body to the mortuary, later signing a death certificate.

June Lindenschmidt's death certificate with Kent County made no mention of choking. It was signed October 15 by a Coopersville physician, the day after her death. The cause was listed as "cardiorespiratory arrest," but the certificate described her demise as "natural."

Physicians seldom examined newly deceased patients at Alpine Manor. Doctors rarely examine the dead in nursing homes, as they do in hospitals. At Alpine a supervising nurse handled the duty. Doctors then based their findings on charts, often signing death certificates after the body was embalmed or cremated.

"I've never seen 'em examined by a doctor," Gwen later recalled. "No, they usually just send them on. What's the point? Old people are expected to die."

Autopsies were as rare as examinations. June Lindenschmidt's body would not be shipped to the county medical examiner, despite the nature of her death.

It was a practice known to many, including Gwen Graham and Cathy Wood.

Chapter 24

Cathy's liaison with Gwen came as a surprise to Dawn Male, but it didn't deter her from hanging out with them both. She saw them at the Carousel or stopped by the little house on Effie.

On Sundays Cathy came up with chores. She designated the Sabbath "Handy Dan Day." Dawn and Gwen were Dan. They found themselves fixing things around the house and cleaning the Luv Truck inside and out.

Sometimes the three of them went cruising in the truck around Grand Rapids, drinking and finding things to steal. They took a five-gallon bucket of truck-washing compound from the back of a pickup. They lifted lawn ornaments and yard materials.

One afternoon Dawn and Cathy cruised into a strange neighborhood, parked the truck and then walked up to a house, pretending to be new neighbors so Cathy could "borrow" a half dozen eggs. They returned that night with Gwen and stole a lawn mower they had spotted in the yard.

Alone with Cathy, Dawn thought Cathy flirted.

"After we split up we were just friends, but she would still make me feel like there was still a chance, that we could still be lovers," Dawn later recalled. "Then, she would tell Gwen that I was bothering her."

Dawn took a new job at a Stop-N-Go convenience store. She moved back in with her grandmother. Drunk again, she hit a parked car and got five more traffic tickets.

Liquor fueled Dawn and Gwen's rocky friendship. While Cathy worked, they made more boozy excursions in the VW Beetle, picking off more blinking caution barriers, and on another night, a bunch of shopping carts.

The unspoken competition for Cathy surfaced when the upper cortical regions of their brains belonged to Jack Daniel's. That's when they had their fistfights.

Often a tussle started in the living room, then moved outside. They punched it out in the backyard or stopped to brawl on the way home from the bar. All they needed was a patch of grass. Gwen went crazy if her hair was pulled. Dawn tired of eating dirt. Gwen was strong, and tough.

Once Dawn snuck a steak knife out of a kitchen drawer as they strutted together out the back door. She was on top of Gwen, holding down one of her arms with one knee and the other with her hand, when she pulled the weapon.

"At least you can be fair," Gwen pleaded.

"Fuck you."

"Cathy wouldn't really like this, would she?" Gwen said. "If you really love Cathy, you can at least be fair."

The struggle stopped momentarily. Dawn tossed the knife away into the darkness.

Then Gwen kicked her ass.

Ladonna Sterns decided somebody had to put a stop to this fight. These girls were really hurting each other. It was out of hand.

"You leave Cathy alone," Gwen had shouted.

"Whatya gonna do about it," Dawn had answered.

Now, they were beating each other to death under a street light in front of the Veteran's Facility, a government nursing center near the Grand River. Everyone had been at the Carousel.

Gwen threw Dawn against a large landscaping boulder. Ladonna heard the thud of her body against the granite. Then she heard laughing in the crisp fall air.

She turned and looked at Cathy Wood. She was in the shadows, giggling. She was delighted Dawn and Gwen were fighting over her.

"This has to stop," Ladonna said.

"No, let them go," Cathy pleaded.

Ladonna forced her way between the two women, wrestling them apart. Dawn was bleeding from the nose.

"Boy, you're so *strong,*" Cathy said, drawing out the word.

Ladonna took Dawn to her grandmother's, then went to Cathy's house. She had left her sweater there. As she looked for the garment, Gwen and Cathy were whispering to each other.

"We're gonna go fight outside, you and me," Gwen suddenly said. "We're gonna fight—in the nude."

"No, you're not," Cathy said, acting concerned.

That's when Ladonna became frightened. That's when Ladonna left.

Chapter 25

Gwen and Dawn arrived at the Halloween party in the same costume. They came as Alpine patients. They wore hospital gowns. Both had bound themselves up in restraints.

"You're so cute," Cathy said.

"Cathy came as Cathy," Gwen later said.

Dawn's chances of getting Cathy back were wishful thinking at best. By November, Gwen and Cathy's blossoming love affair had all the trappings of a couple of infatuated adolescents. They went to the zoo. They took long walks in Riverside Park. Cathy told Gwen she wanted to change her name to Graham. They skipped work to be together. They volunteered for double shifts to be together at work. Gwen also worked overtime anyway to help Cathy's finances. She was always short on money. They wrote poems and letters to each other from Abbey Lane and Buckingham, and Camelot and Dover.

One night, Cathy wrote:

> My sweet girl, I didn't want to leave you this morning . . . I used to love being alone. Now when I am, I just want to cry because you're not here. I understand you need to work. I'm so sorry I put you in a situation where you have to deal with my financial problems. I hope you don't hate me because of them . . .
>
> When Dawn was here I was always worrying about something or other, which I do anyway. But she made it so much worse . . . But now when I look into your eyes and they tell me you love me, I know anything will work out as long as I have you with me!

On another night, Cathy wrote a poem:

> I am always here
> to understand you.
> I am always here
> to laugh with you.
> I am always here
> to cry with you.
> I am always here
> to talk with you.
> I am always here
> to think with you.
> I am always here
> to plan with you,
> even though we
> might not always
> be together
> please know that
> I am always
> here to love you.

Gwen wanted to end the pain she perceived in Cathy's life. She had decided that Cathy was a victim of her parents, her husband and Dawn's drinking. One night she wrote:

I sure do miss you . . . One of these days I'm gonna grab you in the day room right in front of everybody. Sometimes it's all I can do to keep from it.

When I first came to stay with you I wasn't really sure about how things were going to turn out between us. When you and Dawn would come over I'd hurt for you 'cause I hated the way she treated you . . .

Then all of a sudden we're together. I like you. You're beautiful and I don't know what I'd do without you. I like everything about you. You make me smile. I've never beeno happy . . . I'm in love with you, and nothing can change that, so there. My love I hope you'll always be. I'd follow you anywhere . . .

Cathy began talking less of her past with Ken and Dawn and more about the future.

"You're going to leave me, I know it," she told Gwen.

Gwen wondered why she was so worried.

"You'll find some sweet thin girl and you'll be gone."

They talked about infidelity.

"Do all gay people sleep around so much?" Cathy asked.

"No, it's not that way."

Gwen confessed she had always had a problem remaining true. It had nothing to do with Cathy, she said.

"After a while I'm gonna be messin' around," she later explained. "I'm just that way."

They made an agreement. If one or the other wanted to sleep with someone else, they would have to tell each other first.

After Halloween the restraints Gwen had brought home for her costume entered into their bedroom play. They took turns tying each other up, strapping each other to the corners of the bed, embarking on long erotic teases.

Wagers entered into the practice. The winner at backgammon got to tie the other player up. The winner at crossword puzzles was the master of the bondage. Cathy used a dildo, but sometimes she employed other objects as well.

"She would stick ice cubes up me and leave them there until I begged for mercy," Gwen later told a confidant. "It hurt. It hurt after they had been there a while."

"Did you enjoy it?" she was asked.

"Yeah. I sure did."

Their lovemaking became more aggressive, with or without the restraints. They snorted a head shop item called Rush. The butyl nitrite dilated their blood vessels, delivered a surge of exhilaration and made their temples pound. Cathy pinched and bit Gwen. She pinched and bit right back.

"I didn't want to scratch her," Gwen said later. "She had real nice skin."

Cathy's scratching became more severe. She liked to tie Gwen down on her stomach. One hand would prompt multiple orgasms with the dildo, while the other raked her back.

One morning Gwen was sleeping off a night of Rush, drinking and lovemaking when she awoke to a discomfort quite different from a routine hangover. Pain was cutting a ragged path up her shoulder blades.

She opened her eyes to see Cathy, wide awake next to her, her head propped up by her hand. Cathy's eyes were fixed on her thumb and fingernail. She had the tip of one of Gwen's many long scabs. She was lifting, and slowly pulling.

"Good morning," Cathy said.

After Gwen spun away, blood trickled down her back.

Chapter 26

At first, Ken was relieved when Cathy told him Dawn Male had moved out. He had spies in his old neighborhood, and their reports had been disturbing. They told him of revelry, visits by squad cars and half-naked people wandering in the night.

"One hot evening, all the windows were open," one snoopy housewife told him. "We heard all these strange noises and I kinda wondered what it was. My husband said, 'Honey, that's just two women going to it.'"

Ken smoldered for days. He thought, can't she at least be discreet? Doesn't Cathy care about anything but her own pursuit of pleasure? Just about the time he would try to understand her new life-style, he would hear another outrageous report.

Cathy told him Gwen was just a roommate. In fact, Cathy said, Gwen was romantically involved with the temporary border named Tony Kubiak.

Ken met Gwen after one of many heated discussions with Cathy about visitations with Jamie. No matter what Cathy might be doing in the bedroom, Ken had decided, Jamie needed some kind of relationship with her mother. However, Cathy made this difficult. She dodged his phone calls with her answering machine. She came up with excuses when he proposed a visit. One day, he dropped by Effie to ask why she wasn't answering her phone, after spies had informed him her truck was in the driveway.

"I wasn't here, Ken," she said. "Gwen, tell him that I wasn't here."

He turned to see her new roommate coming through the doorway.

"No sir, she wasn't here," Gwen said, politely.

Her head was down. She glanced up only briefly.

She sure looks shy, Ken thought, even insecure. She was quite different from Dawn and all her bravado. He told himself, at least Cathy has someone decent, someone respectable living with her now.

Ken saw other signs of hope. Cathy continued calling him. She visited his apartment. She told him more than once that she wondered if she was really gay. She is only lost, he decided. She will find her way back.

One evening Ken drove to Howard City to see Angie Brozak, seeking guidance from her old friend. The story she told him broke his heart.

"Sometimes when she drinks she gets really emotional," Angie said. "She says nobody will ever really love her. She says stuff like that."

Ken thought, but *I* really love her. And when she sees how crazy everything she is doing is, I will be there to pick up the pieces. All she needs is some professional help. If only someone could nurture that rational side of her.

His plan only seemed more logical when she came over to his apartment one afternoon shortly after his twenty-eighth birthday in late October. She wanted to use the laundry. She complained her belt no longer fit, that she needed a new pair of jeans.

"Ken, I'm losing so much weight."

While her clothes dried she laid down for a nap. He sped to a department store and bought her a new belt and jeans. When he returned he found her in the darkened bedroom.

"Come in here and lay with me," she whispered.

They made love, the first time since the week before they broke up. Afterwards, she complained again she was surrounded by women who were mental midgets. The Trivial Pursuit game they used to play was now worthless, she said.

"Ken, no one can even play it."

Later, as she tried on the new clothes, he noticed bruises on her breasts and arms.

"Jesus, Cath, what the hell happened?"

"Somebody tried to rape me."

The attack came after she opened the door to a stranger, she said. She fought her assailant off with a knife. Her nightgown was ripped to shreds (Later, she showed it to him). Police came to the house. She made out a report.

She needs me more than she will ever know, he thought. He held her.

"Cath, let's do things. Movies, plays. Stuff like that. We'll start out as friends, and see where it goes."

"Really?"

"Yeah, I don't want a divorce. I'm not sure it's over."

Her mood changed instantly.

"Well," she said, flippantly. "You're the third person who's proposed to me this week. Girls are proposing to me at the Carousel. Ladonna wants to marry me. She wants me to go to California with her . . ."

"Christ, I'm not proposing, I'm already your husband."

A few minutes later he walked her to her Luv Truck.

"I don't want you to misinterpret what just happened," Cathy said coldly. "It was just sex."

"Oh, you mean you used me?"

He was trying to make a joke.

"And don't tell my friends," she added. "They would never understand."

A couple of days later, while he was visiting her at the little house on Effie, she had a confession to make.

"Ken, I've done something very bad."

He wanted to know.

"I won't tell you in person. Go home. I'll call you and tell you when you're home."

She was crying when she called. And damn it, he decided, she should be! She had written four hundred dollars in checks on his account for her auto insurance. She had kited them from a box of new checks he left behind when he moved out.

"Oh Ken, I don't know why I did it. Gwen said you would be mad. I'm so sorry."

He wasn't mad. He was furious.

"I'm coming to get the checks," he told her. "Don't be there Cath. Don't be there when I get there."

He found the two boxes of the checks on the front steps. Before he left, he took the ends of two wrought iron porch rails and bent them skyward, just to let her know he was there.

Cathy reported the damage to the Grand Rapids police. She accused Ken. Police declined to prosecute, saying she had no witnesses to the act.

By one weekend in early November Ken decided he had to go one step further to try and understand his wife. He needed to know what Cathy found so captivating about her new friends and new life. Once she'd suggested he visit the Carousel. Now, he decided to take her up on the offer.

There wasn't much left of Sunday night when he walked into the bar. He saw Cathy sitting at a table with other aides from Alpine Manor. Gwen was sitting at one end. Ken sat down at the other. Cathy looked at him in shock. Then she ignored him. Ken looked out at the dance floor. Two men were in each other's arms.

"Why are you here?" Gwen asked.

"I thought I'd come in and see what this place is all about."

"Do you like boys?"

"No, I don't like boys."

"Then why are you here?"

"Well, Cathy invited me."

Gwen looked confused by the answer. She sure seems right at home here, Ken decided. He thought, Cathy has been lying to me again.

He looked at Cathy. She was flirting with another aide, Paul Lopez. He was tall and thin, with classic Latin good looks. He was also gay, but that didn't stop him from sitting on her lap, then kissing her.

She's taunting me, Ken thought. She's rubbing my face in all this shit and taunting me. He thought of all her marriage proposals, the moans of women coming from his old house in the night.

"You're a slut," Ken said, standing up.

Everyone froze at the table in anticipation. He looked at all of them. He thought, they're so shit-faced they don't know their own asses from their elbows. Just get out, he told himself. Just get out of here before you end up doing something stupid.

When he slammed the door on his car he wanted to hit someone. Instead, he sat behind the wheel, surveying the parking lot. He steamed, I'd like to beat every fucking faggot that comes out that door. He sat and waited.

After the Carousel closed, he watched Cathy and Gwen meander to her Luv Truck, giggling. When they left, he followed. They headed through the main streets on the edge of downtown. He kept his headlights on her tailgate.

He thought to himself, why am I even wasting my time? Why am I following them?

He knew exactly when Cathy realized it was his Old's Sierra in her mirror. She scooted down a side street, then sped through residential neighborhoods. She headed back to main streets; then she ran a red light.

Ken pressed on the gas. He found himself enjoying it. Let her squirm for once, he told himself. Let her see what it feels like to be fucked with. God knows she can dish it out.

They raced into the city center, past tall office buildings and through the deserted streets of downtown. They roared up Monroe

Avenue, parallel to the Grand River. They went several blocks, then Cathy's Luv Truck screeched to a stop.

Cathy jumped out. So did Ken. She ran up to a lone motorist who had just parked his car.

"Help me, please. I've got somebody bothering me."

The stranger looked at Ken.

"Man, don't even think about it," Ken said.

Ken followed Cathy on foot. She was trotting, then running, down the sidewalk. He walked briskly behind her. Gwen never left the truck.

She turned and ran up steps. There were a series of them, separated by concrete plateaus. She scampered up the elevations toward the front of one of Grand Rapids' landmark buildings.

Cathy neared the front doors.

"Don't hurt me," she shouted.

"Damn it Cath, don't you realize how you hurt me!" he cried.

He looked up at the large letters across the building behind her. The Hall of Justice, it read. It was the courthouse, where criminals were tried and punished.

He thought, what is she going to do, go in there and tell them about her girlfriend?

Justice. There's no justice. Seven years of my life, he thought, and it's come to this.

He was disgusted with her. He was more disgusted with himself.

He turned and descended the steps. He muttered obscenities to himself and aimed his car toward the freeway that followed the Grand River.

As Ken sped away from the Hall of Justice, Cathy was halfway up the steps.

Chapter 27

Cathy scrawled the note to Gwen at work, the evening after Thanksgiving dinner at Cathy's mother's house in Comstock Park:

> Hi my sweet girl! It's terribly boring over here. I fell asleep in
> the day room. That's terrible! . . . Can we do a no show
> tomorrow? I'd like to spend three days with you. It seems all we
> do in two days is catch up on our sleep.

The day after Thanksgiving Cathy Wood called in sick. One of them was due. Since they had become partners, they were averaging one absence a week between them.

They feared no consequences for skipping work. Both Gwen and Cathy already averaged well over fourty hours a week. Cathy came in early and doubled on second shift with Gwen. Gwen stayed to double with Cathy on third.

"All of us were working tons of doubles," Tony Kubiak later recalled. "To tell you the truth, I think Cathy worked most of her doubles to keep her eye on Gwen."

Cathy and Gwen also showed no signs of quitting Alpine Manor. That alone scored points with management. Turnover was epidemic at the nursing home. In late October somebody filed a complaint with the state health department about staff shortages and turnover after a patient had been left in soiled diapers for forty-five minutes. It was one of only two complaints made that year to the state.

An inspector paid an unannounced visit and investigated. She reported the nursing home met state staff-to-patient ratios, but also noted a turnover rate of 66 percent. There had been one hundred twelve nurse's aides hired in the first nine months of 1986. By October, only forty-one of them remained. The investigator also reported that while Alpine trained its new aides, once they were on the floor they were on their own. Licensed nurses, she wrote, "had little time" to observe them or their work.

Some supervisors found third shift the most consistent crew, and the easiest to manage as well. Three licensed nurses were assigned to the stations. A night supervisor worked a twelve-hour shift which ran from 8:00 P.M. to 8:00 A.M. The supervisor walked the entire facility periodically, but she also shuffled a lot of paper in her office wedged between Buckingham and Camelot.

As for the aides, from nine to twelve they were spread across the four stations. Third shift offered a less demanding pace. Second shift already had changed and bedded everyone. Midnight aides passed fresh water and escorted residents to bathrooms. They cleaned wheelchairs and walkers. They watched an average of ten rooms each, making bed checks every two hours. Rounds took no more than forty-five minutes. Depending on the demands of the particular supervisor, third shift offered aides an opportunity to relax.

Sometimes Cathy and Gwen passed the slow hours on third shift reading. They read patient records. These included past histories as well as medical information. Also available were lists of relatives, their home phone numbers and such.

Sometimes, they found other things to do.

The pranks began on third shift and spread to the latter hours of second shift. Cathy masterminded many, with Gwen often carrying out her plans, other aides later said.

One practical joke was particularly effective on jittery new aides in a facility where death was a regular visitor. Gwen would ring a patient's call button, then quickly slide underneath the bed. When the aide arrived in the semidarkness to turn off the call light, Gwen would grab the new worker's ankle. There was ample time to escape as the victim ran screaming down the hall.

They pried screens out of patient's windows, creating escape hatches to the courtyard so they could set up more gags. They reversed patients' positions so their heads were at the footboards. Then, they began switching the beds themselves, mixing up patients from room to room. One night, Cathy restrained Gwen in a geriatric chair and left her in the Buckingham day room.

But the hazing wasn't limited to the lowest workers in the Alpine pecking order. Cathy dressed up a mannequin and parked it in a chair in the medication room. The startled nurse was none the wiser after she turned on the light. The room was off-limits to aides, who were not allowed to dispense medication.

"How Cathy ever got a key to the med room, I'll never know," Tony Kubiak later wondered. "None of the aides were ever allowed a med room key."

Cathy and Gwen made use of the Alpine intercom. They piped Christmas carols from a musical stuffed bear. They recruited a lisping patient to make moronic announcements. Sometimes, a nurse came running down the hall trying to catch them during these and other antics. They escaped out the windows or into the routine of their rounds.

Patients became entertainment. Once, Cathy and Gwen made a trail of Reese's Pieces candy for a confused patient fond of putting things in his mouth. It snaked through Abbey hall and in and out the doors of the Buckingham day room. A half dozen aides sat around a table and giggled as the patient shuffled by, hunting the candy piece by piece.

Reactions by night supervisors varied when they learned of some of the pranks on other aides. One complained to upper management. Another wrote them off as harmless initiations, a way of "welcoming" newcomers to the staff. There were no formal reprimands against Cathy or Gwen.

Complaints by patients were routinely discounted, especially if voiced by the mentally impaired. Some of Alpine's most disturbed residents were up and active after midnight. A woman on Dover always ambulated in the early morning hours. A former policeman made security checks, trying door locks and sometimes finding misplaced keys. Two World War II veterans chummed around the hallways, staying up until dawn. One added readings from hallway thermostats, and announcing the total as the temperature.

Sometimes, a supervisor tuned the radio to WOOD-FM, providing a backwash to the routine outbreak of moans and cries from patients in pain, or the delirious outbursts of others.

Because patients were often incoherent, Alpine staff guidelines demanded matters of patient abuse be reported by employees. By late fall, however, few aides wanted to brave the wrath of Cathy Wood.

Cathy usually was a step ahead of workers she disliked. She

complained to supervisors about the performance of other aides and set up those she didn't consider up to snuff. Gwen would pour water into the beds of patients, while Cathy would tell a supervisor that a particular aide hadn't changed patients on rounds. The unsuspecting aide was reprimanded and his or her credibility damaged.

"Cathy played mind games, inside the nursing home and out," Dawn Male later recalled. "The object of the games was not only to see if people would believe you, but to make it as entangled as possible. She liked to play with people for sport."

Many knew firsthand how believable she could be. Those in her inner circle watched her turn on tears for supervisors or cry for Ken when she needed a favor and had him on the phone. Once she unabashedly demonstrated her acting talent in the living room at Effie. As her friends watched, she picked up a stuffed lion, studied its eyes and soon began to weep.

A number of Cathy's friends were awed by her ability to disrupt the lives of others. Gwen once complained to Cathy that another Alpine aide named Lisa Lynch was being too chummy.

"Lisa is just bugging me to death," she told Cathy.

Cathy sat in her big easy chair and listened, then came up with a plan. First, she planted unfounded information around the nursing home that a pregnant girl in their social circle was carrying the child of Lisa Lynch's husband. Cathy settled a score with the pregnant girl as well. She suspected she had slept with Dawn Male when they were roommates. Soon, Lisa and her husband were headed for divorce and the pregnant girl was ostracized.

"She got two people in one game that time," Dawn later said.

Gwen later told someone how she was taken with her cunning.

"Everybody was scared of her. Cathy would fuck with ya. That was just her thing, and everybody knew it. It kind of made me feel good, because she was my girl. And, as long as she was my girl, nobody was going to fuck with me."

Chapter 28

The phone call woke Nancy Hahn one frosty morning in early December, just about 4:30 A.M. A young woman identified herself as being from Alpine Manor. She had information about Nancy's mother, Belle Burkhard.

"Belle isn't expected to make it through the day," the caller said.

Nancy lived in Buchanan, three hours to the southeast. She worked her shift as a waitress, then hit the road to Grand Rapids, her mind churning all the way.

Years had passed since she had visited Alpine Manor. Before, there had been many years of drinking, by both her parents. The drinking had brought the turmoil. The turmoil had brought a certain distancing, for survival's sake. There were some good memories: A prom dress her mother bought for her on layaway. Her help in raising four of Nancy's own children.

No doubt, she should have visited more. Her mother's admission into Alpine was only one crisis in Nancy's forty-seven years. Her husband had died unexpectedly at forty-one, leaving her with two children, a lot of bills and a streak of bad luck. It was partly that she simply couldn't spare the wear and tear on the car and the fifteen dollars the trip cost in gas. It was partly that her mother had already taken what she had to give long before her last six-month binge. Before her admission, Belle was found wandering the streets of Grand Rapids, unable to remember where she lived.

But Nancy was grateful for the call from Alpine. Her parents' drinking had forced her to grow up long before any child should have had to, but she felt she loved her parents nonetheless. Her heart softened when she told her dad that on his deathbed. He had dispelled many resentments with a squeeze of his hand.

When she arrived at Alpine Manor it was dinnertime. She walked into Abbey Lane, looking for her mother's room. She found only an empty bed.

Maybe I'm too late, she thought.

She walked quickly to the nurse's station, inquiring. Nobody seemed to know just where her mother was.

"Why don't you go back to the lunch room," one of the nurses said. "She's probably waiting to be fed."

"But I got a phone call. She's sick. Somebody said she's really sick."

Everyone looked bemused.

She walked quickly to the main dining room. Her eyes searched for the burnt hickory hair among the dozens of silver heads and tired bodies. Then she saw her mother, sitting in a chair. As she approached she could see her skin color was good. Her movements were sure and deliberate.

She's not sick, Nancy thought. In fact, she seemed eager to be fed. Her mother always loved to eat.

Nancy fed her mom herself, trying to make sense out of the mystery as she spooned supper into her mouth. She ate mechanically, her eyes blank, looking into the distance. She doesn't even recognize me, Nancy thought.

Afterwards, Nancy went back to the nurses' station. Again, no one knew about any phone call made from the third shift.

"But somebody said she was dying," she said.

A nurse looked at her chart. There were no problems, no threatening conditions.

"We have no reports of anything like that," a nurse said.

Nancy Hahn didn't know whether to feel relieved or angry. For the longest time, the whole thing just didn't make any sense.

Chapter 29

The young orderly named *Jim Shooter* had been flirting with Gwen for weeks. Gwen was flirting back. Every now and then, she liked to sleep with a man.

Hearing rumors about the orderly's advances, Cathy approached Gwen with a wager. She bet Gwen that she could not inspire Shooter to kiss her in the Abbey Lane tub room, where patients were given baths. They put up their weekly paychecks.

The plan unfolded one Thursday afternoon in mid-December, early in second shift. Cathy hid behind a partition, so she could be a witness. Meanwhile, Gwen had confided in Shooter himself about the bet. She wanted to win that paycheck.

Gwen and the orderly strolled through the door, only to find Cathy sitting on the edge of the bathtub.

Jim, undaunted, turned to Cathy.

"Cathy, I know about the bet, but that doesn't really matter. I love Gwen, anyway."

He reached over, pulled Gwen to his breast and gave her a passionate kiss. Cathy's mouth dropped open. Then she burst into tears and ran from the room.

When Gwen got to her station, she was told Cathy had gone home sick. Gwen told a nurse she had to have the rest of her shift off.

"Does this have anything to do with Cathy?" the nurse asked.

Gwen was putting on her coat as she headed for the door.

"No, I can't explain it to you. I *have* to go. I've got personal problems."

Earlier, they had come to work together in Cathy's truck. Gwen took off for Effie on foot. She went east in a brisk walk along Four Mile Road, the cold December wind at her back. She meandered through Comstock Park, Cathy's old neighborhood, then headed south on West River Drive.

She stopped at the North Park bridge. Gwen paused and looked at the walkway. She could see the brown waters rushing below. Her phobia had not lessened since leaving Texas. In Michigan, with all its lakes and rivers, it was only worse.

She made her hands into fists and walked quickly. For Cathy, she would cross the Grand.

Across the bridge, she turned south on Coit, skirting the edge of Veteran's Cemetery and its pitted monuments. Her face was numb when she reached the doorstep on Effie. It was nearly a four-mile hike.

The door was locked. Cathy opened it a crack.

"Gwen, you walked."

Cathy eyed her from head to foot.

"I'm *impressed,*" she continued, drawing out the word.

"It was just a bet," Gwen told her, after Cathy let her in.

"You hurt me, Gwen," Cathy said. "Everyone hurts me."

They talked into the night.

"Tell me that you love me, that you'll never leave me," Cathy said. "Love me forever."

"Cathy, I'm yours. I'm yours forever. I'll never leave you."

"If you do, I'll come find you. I'll find you, then find a way to keep you home."

December 23, five days later, Margaret Widmaier, the assistant director who hired Gwen Graham, wrote her up for leaving the job in midshift.

"A friend of mine was threatening suicide," Gwen responded formerly for the report. "It won't happen again."

Ultimately, the incident would be the only disciplinary notice in Gwen's work file. Just the day before, another kind of document was included as well. Gwen received a certificate indicating she had passed all the requirements for a state health department competency program for nurse's aides. She had scored 97 percent on a new written test. Answering one question, Gwen had put down the washcloth "handrolls" as a way to prevent skin breakdown in immobile patients. The Alpine staffer doing the grading drew an arrow to the answer and scrawled "good." She also penned a smile face and "great" on other pages of the test.

As for Jim Shooter, Gwen and the orderly put an end to their flirting. They met secretly in a vacant patient's room in Alpine Manor one evening. They closed the bathroom door behind them.

Any noise their lovemaking produced was obscured by the songs of WOOD-FM.

Chapter 30

Robin Fielder scampered back from the dance floor, giggling as she retrieved her black high heel. The handsome aide Paul Lopez had filled the shoe with champagne, drunk it up, then tossed the shoe to the gyrating crowd.

Everybody roared. Paul. Angie. Ladonna. Dawn. Lisa. Cathy. They all sat at one table. It was a Saturday night in December, and Alpine Manor was holding forth at the Carousel again.

Robin reached down to slip on her shoe, looking up at the dance floor as she did. She met the eyes of Gwen Graham.

Later, Gwen plopped down at the table, out of breath.

"Do you look at girls?"

"No, not really," said Robin.

Gwen tilted her head to one side and smiled bashfully.

"But you're lookin' at me. Yep, you sure are."

"I watch you cause you dance so different," Robin explained.

"Well, the dance is kinda like the Texas two-step."

Robin thought, just one more lesson in my continuing education. There's plenty to learn, especially with this group.

She took another sip of her vodka and grapefruit juice.

Two months past her twentieth birthday, Robin finally was feeling like she was prying apart the golden bars of her all-American cage. She was still "daddy's girl" and "momma's baby." But she was becoming increasingly uncomfortable staying in her parents' Walker ranch home, the one with the pool out back and the Notre Dame mailbox at the foot of the drive.

Other Alpine aides figured her family was loaded, especially after she threw a pool party for the people at work. They saw the basement her dad dubbed "the locker room," the elaborate recreation room filled with sports memorabilia. They saw wrestling and golf trophies and photos of her two brothers. They saw Robin's cheerleader pictures and awards. West Catholic High School named her its outstanding cheerleader.

"I've been a cheerleader all my life," she later told a friend. She said it as though it were a former occupation, years after the Friday night lights went out.

Robin had an exuberant, gap-toothed smile and hair the color of corn silk. A half a foot over five feet, her figure was full and voluptuous by Rubens' standards. For months she had been fighting the fifty pounds she gained after the cheering stopped at West Catholic. She countered the weight gain with snappy outfits and meticulous hair and makeup.

With Alpine Manor she had found career direction. She was studying physical therapy at Grand Rapids Junior College. She had been an aide at Alpine for twenty months, mainly on second shift. She loved helping old people, working little miracles with those who supposedly couldn't speak or walk. She inspired one woman to leave her wheelchair. She brought another newspapers and quelled her combativeness after she found out she was Polish.

"Just speak a little Polish to her," she would tell other aides. "Just talk to her nicely, and she'll be okay."

However, in matters of her own heart, Robin Fielder felt cheated. Recently, she had penned another of many poems she kept in a hardcover journal of verse:

Drifting on a quiet sea
I look upon the lonely me
Watching waves slowly ride
Adrift the shore side by side
Whispering breeze upon my face
A tear has fallen and left a trace
Far away my mind has been
Lost at sea my heart won't mend.

A ship will pass, I have faith
But for now I'll just sit and wait.

Despite her school popularity, Robin had never dated, until she
met Paul Lopez. They had been close companions for more than a
year. At first, she found him sensitive and gentle in a city that
seemed to have a shortage of such men.

"I just fell head over heels for him," she later told a friend.

They golfed and shopped. They took a vacation together to
Florida. Then he told her he was gay. This explained why they had
never gone to bed. For months she tried to change him but made
no progress.

Paul introduced her to the Carousel. When she saw Cathy and
several others there from Alpine she was shocked.

"My God, Paul," she said. "Look who's here."

Robin simply was curious at first. She wanted to know why they
were that way, and what they did. After a few visits and a few grapefruit and vodkas, she found herself comfortable, even enthralled.
She felt like she had tapped into the Grand Rapids underground. In
western Michigan, homosexuals seemed to be the only offbeat cul-
ture going.

The women were very nice to her. She began going to the little
house on Effie with the rest of the group to play quarters and listen
to Cathy spin her 45s. Cathy seemed to go out of her way to be
friendly. Gwen always looked at her with the cutest smile, always
tilting her head.

Many in the group were heavy, even overweight. By comparison
Robin was a beauty queen. Yet, no one seemed to resent that, at least
not yet.

"I didn't feel like I had to compete with anybody," she recalled
later. "And they always said, 'You're so nice. You're so good-looking, and you can have anybody you want.' It made me want to lose
weight. It made me want to take care of myself again. It made me
feel good."

Knowing everyone eased the work load at Alpine. In recent
months she had become discouraged. Some nights, Alpine Manor
seemed to be little more than a warehouse-sized waiting room for
the dead.

There was little time anymore for personal care. Supervisors
were always looking for aides to fill vacancies. Robin had been

working her share of doubles, averaging sixty hours a week. She had set some real work records for herself. During one two-week period she worked one hundred thirty-six hours. Once she worked eight weeks straight without a day off.

The pace put a strain on everyone. Some nights she put half a hall to bed, some fifteen patients. They had to be changed, turned, and put in night clothes. One night a supervisor had them put pajamas on patients under their clothes after dinner, to make everything go faster. Robin thought, if I wanted this I could work on a factory assembly line.

Friends made such frustrations easier to endure. Caffeine took care of the fatigue. Lately, Robin had been popping caffeine pills she found in a local carry out. They were called 357 Magnums, one equal to a cup of coffee. Vodka and grapefruit juice took the edge off a dozen of those at the end of a long shift.

Robin eyed the Carousel dance floor and took another sip. It was habit now. She certainly didn't need to get any drunker.

Robin felt her arm get hit.

"Robin," said her friend, Lisa Lynch. "Did you hear that?"

"Hear what?"

"They're talking about you."

"About what?"

"Robin, didn't you hear Gwen?"

Later, after she had sobered up, others helped her reconstruct what happened. After Cathy stepped away from the table, Gwen had been giggling and pointing at Robin.

"She's mine," Gwen had said. "None of you are gonna have her. She's mine, I said."

Dawn Male said later:

"Robin was just a very normal girl. She was real pretty, real popular. She was a nice girl—until she met us. We were just so messed-up back then. And anybody who came in contact with us, also got messed-up."

Chapter 31

Cathy was upset.

"Look, *this* is from my mother," she told Gwen. "No card. No phone call. No Merry Christmas. Nothing."

They found the large fruit basket sitting on the table. Her mother Pat apparently had let herself in while they were out and left the gift.

There were no plans for a holiday visit to Cathy's parents. They were divorced, her mother remarried. Her father lived somewhere in Grand Rapids.

"I wouldn't call him for anything unless it was the absolute last resort," Cathy said once.

Gwen, like others, had heard Cathy's frequent complaints about her mom. Gwen had met Pat and other family members on Thanksgiving and come away with a different impression.

"Her mom is a good-looking older lady," Gwen later recalled. "She looked very sure of herself. She sure was. She treated me nice. She treated me real nice."

However, Gwen's view of Pat changed the day after the holiday dinner. A group of aides were taking a break in the Alpine dining room when Cathy brought a fork and knife to their table.

"Show me how you cut your meat," Cathy said.

Gwen held her fork down, Southern style.

"That's wrong," Cathy said.

"Well, it gets cut, no matter how you do it," Gwen said, blushing.

"No that's wrong. That's what *my mother* noticed. She told me you cut your meat wrong."

"That's all she said?" Gwen said. "That whole visit, and that's what your mom told you?"

"That's my *mother,*" Cathy said, drawing out the word.

Gwen vowed never to visit Pat again.

Cathy, however, frequently did. Often, she returned upset.

After Gwen saw the fruit basket, she tried to console Cathy. When it came to the subject of mothers, Gwen could tell a few stories of her own.

Ken Wood had become increasingly frustrated trying to arrange a visit for Jamie with her mother for Christmas. He never could get Cathy to answer the phone. She had taken to putting music on her answering machine. She was crafting clever greetings around the dark organ rendition of the Bach fugue played by the Phantom of the Opera.

Finally, he called Cathy's sister Barb. She told Ken that Cathy had told her mother that he had refused to let anyone in the family see Jamie, let alone Cathy. The rule held for Christmas Eve.

"That's totally untrue," Ken told her.

He still was angry as he headed for a holiday gathering at his parents' house with Jamie. Our daughter will have a good Christmas, he decided. He only wished, for Jamie's sake, Cathy could have been decent.

She at least could have gotten her own daughter a gift.

Jan Hunderman pushed open the front door of Alpine Manor, her husband and four children close behind. They were bringing gifts for her mother on Christmas Day, whether Marguerite Chambers knew what day it was or not.

In late fall, she had been moved from Abbey Lane to Dover, one of the areas for private pay patients. Ed Chambers had sold the family homestead and was paying seventeen hundred dollars a month for her care from her forty-thousand-dollar-split of the proceeds. With his share, Ed bought a small mobile home and a new car to drive to his daily visits with his wife.

Both Jan and Ed were pleased that the nursing home had responded to the family's complaints about the feeding tube. After meeting with Dr. James Piskin, one of the physicians associated with Alpine, the nursing staff agreed to make another try at feeding her mother a blended diet. Now she had been without the tube for seven months. She was eating most of her helpings. She wasn't losing weight.

For the holiday, Jan wanted to eliminate any other remaining discomforts. Her mother's skin always felt cold. Often they found her in only a hospital gown and diapers. She was always shedding her covers with her incessant rocking. For gifts, Jan had bought her a pair of slippers and a pair of pink, flowered long underwear.

The kids brought something to cheer up her mother's room. They had picked out a dry floral arrangement. In the middle was a stick topped by a foil balloon in the shape of a heart.

The family turned into the room on Dover.

"Merry Christmas, Mom," Jan said.

They all crowded around her, as everyone began producing the gifts. She was awake and rocking.

"Look," Jan said to her husband Gary.

There was dried pureed supper around her mouth.

"They could do a better job of wiping her," Jan said. "I'm going to clean her up."

She walked to the bathroom and returned with a small damp towel. She wrapped it around her fingertips and lifted it to her mother's face.

When the tiny cotton fingers of the terry cloth touched her cheek her mother's body jumped. She twisted her head violently, trying to avoid the washcloth, the way children do.

"C'mon Mom."

Then Jan saw her eyes. They were exceptionally wide. Her head was quaking.

My God, Jan thought, she looks absolutely terrified.

She stopped wiping.

"It's okay. It's okay."

The reaction bothered her for a few moments, then she dismissed it. She thought, I must have scared her. Maybe I should have told her what I was going to do.

Had Jan looked at her mother's medical file she would have seen that through Christmas week her mother had been under the care of one aide more than any other. The day before Christmas Eve, Gwen Graham had the assignment for one third shift, but Marguerite was not one of Gwen's regular patients. On both sides of midnight, Marguerite Chambers was entrusted to Cathy Wood. She would be caring for her on Christmas evening as well.

Before the family left, Jan placed the planter of dried flowers on a nearby sill. Her mother was in room 614 now, at the bed near the window.

Jan arranged the balloon on a stick so the light hit it nicely. The foil gleamed, highlighting the big colorful letters across the middle of the heart. There was only one word.

MOTHER, it simply read.

PART TWO

1987

Chapter 32

She was crying on the telephone. It was late on a Thursday night, eight days into the new year, right when Cathy should have been reporting to third shift.

"Are you alone?"

"Yeah, I'm alone," said Ken Wood. "You know, I'm not like you."

He was bitter, but he listened. She didn't want to go to work, she said. She didn't want to stay home alone. She wanted to come over.

Gwen was cheating on her, she explained when she arrived at his apartment. Gwen was chasing another Alpine aide. She had found them together that very night.

"We were at a party," she said. "They were in the closet making out."

She dabbed her tears throughout the monologue. She didn't understand gays, she complained. She didn't understand all the running around. Gwen had told her it didn't have to be like that. Now Gwen had done this. Now Gwen was sleeping around.

She lay facedown, burying her face in the couch and sobbing more. Ken sat next to her, rubbing her back, stroking her hair. He felt sorry for her. It's only been a few months, he thought, and look at her. Two relationships already have come to ruin.

Then anger dried her tears. She stared into the distance.

"They're always sorry after I leave," she said. "*Then* they find out how much they love me!"

"Well, some day maybe you'll meet a nice girl," Ken said. "And you can live the life you want."

Ken tucked her into his bed. He slept on the couch.

The next morning, Gwen called, looking for Cathy. She had already instructed him to say she was not there. An hour later, Cathy called Gwen back. Cathy had a few words with Ken before she left.

"Well, Gwen and I are gonna talk," she said.

Ken would not forget that Thursday. It was some kind of milestone for Cathy and Gwen. From then on, there would be no more complaints about Gwen's cheating.

For some reason, Cathy never mentioned it again.

Chapter 33

A low pressure front had just pulled a white sheet of snow over Grand Rapids as Ed Chambers arrived at Alpine Manor for his Sunday night visit. Later, the mercury would hit the single digits, the kind of cold that struck when skies cleared in the dead of the Michigan winter.

Inside, he called Marguerite's name as he turned the corner into her room. He grasped her shaking hand once more. He spent about an hour with her, telling her things of little consequence, talking to her as though she were normal. He would never know if she understood. He stayed nearly an hour. It was between seven and eight o'clock when he rose to go.

On January 18, Marguerite Chambers was marking day 1,293 as a patient of Alpine Manor. She had been institutionalized nearly five years. Twelve years had passed since she had been diagnosed with Alzheimer's Disease.

Outside 614-1, aides were working from room to room. They were rounding up some patients, changing others and preparing all of Alpine Manor for the night. Most aides were occupied. Others were taking midshift breaks. At 8:00 P.M., licensed nurses would begin going from room to room, passing out evening medication.

As Ed stepped outside, he noticed there were few cars in the lot. Most of them belonged to employees. Three inches of snow had kept many visitors home for the night. There was little traffic on Four Mile Road. The snow creaked beneath his feet. A light wind made the snaps on the Alpine flagpole ring in hollow tones.

The clanging seemed to sound deeper in the cold.

How Marguerite had always loved the waltzes. She had danced them freely, dipping and sweeping across the floor—one, two, three . . . one, two, three . . . one.

Strauss had no equal. The Emperor Waltz . . . Vienna Blood . . . Tales from the Vienna Woods. She loved the Blue Danube Waltz. It rushed and wavered, moving the spirit along, as though it were being carried away by the great river.

The Blue Danube was playing regularly in 614-1, once a week as a matter of fact. A regular visitor brought the music. She was a new face for Marguerite. The chipper activities staffer brought a portable tape player. She plugged it in, and then the Strauss waltzes began.

One, two, three . . . one, two, three . . . one.

In her predictable universe, Marguerite Chambers had come to experience two changes beginning in the days before Christmas. One was the music, courtesy of a new in-room program. The other was an aberration, an intrusion. It did not soothe her like the waltzes. It quickened the fiercest of all involuntary impulses. It unleashed her raw will to live.

If she could have articulated the first incident in detail, she might have reported it as a quirk, a momentary loss of respiratory rhythm, like a chronic snorer stuck between breaths. Then, the cessation came suddenly and with much fury. There was unrelenting pressure across her nostrils and the underside of her jaw. There was terry cloth, its loop pile so compressed it dug into her skin like dull darts.

Without air, she lost consciousness.

When she awoke—when she survived—her mind may still have been capable of associating the experience with a familiar face or a pair of hands or the smell of Sween Cream. On Christmas Day, she may have associated the attack with the touch of terry cloth, the touch of a wash towel around the lips.

These remained Marguerite's secrets. Her nurse only knew that her pulse was running a little over a beat per second, that her blood pressure was in the normal limits for a woman of sixty years. She had been very restless the previous night, all through Alpine's third shift. Her limbs were exceptionally kinetic. She ran a fever of 101 the night before. All the movement could easily have been caused by that.

After Ed left, it began.

There may have been some notice of the intruder's presence. Or perhaps the attack came suddenly, and Marguerite was jolted from her sleep. The traverse rod hissed as a hand pulled the divider curtain. There may have been the sounds of a polyester uniform rubbing against itself. Two hands positioned her head, resting it squarely on the back of her skull. Maybe this was sudden. Or, maybe it was gentle, like an oral surgeon readying a patient for his handiwork.

Of one thing Marguerite Chambers was certain.

Air.

Quite suddenly, there was no air. There absolutely was none.

The terry cloth was rolled. One covered Marguerite's nostrils. The other was under her chin. One squeezed, the other thrust up, violently, pushing her toothless gums together.

Marguerite began to thrash. He groans were guttural, deep within her belly. As the need to breathe became more urgent, her cheeks began to puff and collapse. Her lungs were sucking for the pathetically few cubic inches of oxygen that were left there before her mouth was slammed shut.

Perhaps trauma stimulated memory, as can happen so near death. There was the old farmland in Walker. There was the nursery across the golden field. There were Ed, Jan, Gary and Ed Junior. The lake glistened at the family cottage. She loved waterskiing for the children, putting on a show. She loved scrabble and she loved dancing. The waltzes played. The Blue Danube. She was waltzing freely . . . one, two, three . . . one, two, three . . . one.

Perhaps not.

The muscles strengthened by her fetal rocking drew deep upon their incessant conditioning. In a great effort, she twisted her head.

But nothing could have prepared her for this.

Her last movements were spasmodic. In the end, in her final

moments of consciousness, her eyes couldn't help but look at the face above her. Michelangelo might have painted it on a Sistine Chapel cherub.

But it belonged to an angel of death.

Chapter 34

The sounds of WOOD-FM were interrupted by the Alpine public address: "House Supervisor to 614."

Veteran aides knew what the request usually meant. Someone had died in Alpine Manor. An aide or nurse had discovered the body, and now the house supervisor was being called to confirm that all vital signs had ceased.

A night house supervisor named Letitia Prescott had walked through the front door only minutes earlier. She was just beginning her twelve-hour shift. One of her office doors opened into Camelot Hall, where Cathy Wood was stationed. Cathy approached her, quietly.

"What's wrong, Tish?"

"I don't know, I just got here."

A few minutes later, Cathy asked her again about the call.

"Is it Marguerite?"

Before she could answer, Cathy quickly added, "Gwen told me she was sick."

Tish Prescott didn't have time to discuss details. The death had come right in the middle of reports, the busy meeting when supervisors exchanged information as shifts changed. A charge nurse was handling the postmortem routine. An aide doing routine rounds on Dover discovered Marguerite Chambers dead.

One by one the aides began to arrive to room 614. No one ever formally verbalized the tradition. It happened spontaneously with every body. Aides visited Marguerite's room, simply to satisfy their curiosity about the dead.

Gwen Graham didn't have far to walk. She was assigned to cover nine rooms in 700 hall, just around the northwest corner of the building past the Dover nurse's station. Neither did Cathy Wood. From her location on Camelot, Cathy could see the doorway to room 614.

An RN named Linda Dapore made the final entry on Marguerite Chambers' chart. She noted that when she arrived in the room at 8:30 P.M. she was not able to get blood pressure or a pulse. The patient had been dead for some time. Her color was "yellow-gray," she wrote, and her skin was "mottled." Her arms and hands were cold.

Nurse Dapore also noted that one call was made to the family of Marguerite Chambers, as was the Alpine routine. A call also was made to Dr. James Piskin, who released the body to the mortuary.

The body was cleaned up by two aides. One of them was Gwen Graham. When the hearse from Reyer's Funeral Home arrived at 10:00 P.M., four aides transferred the body to a stretcher. Gwen helped, as did Cathy, who lifted Marguerite's head. Both still had the midnight leg of a double ahead of them.

House Supervisor Tish Prescott later reviewed Marguerite's chart, making sure all the details were complete. Nothing on it warranted a call to the coroner. In fact, in her long career she'd never seen a nursing home summon a coroner. Dr. Piskin would sign the death certificate the next day. He would not be coming in to examine the body on a Sunday night.

Tish Prescott knew the doctors never did.

Something had drawn Jan Hunderman back to church that night. The thought was persistent: After all these years, this was the night she should go back to church.

"Mom was always after me," she later told a friend. "Being a Catholic, she was always going. I knew she would want me to go. Maybe I should do this for my mom. Maybe, it will make her happy after she passes on."

Jan and Gary Hunderman had just returned from services at Ideal Park Christian Reformed Church, where Gary worshipped. It was not the Catholic faith of her youth, but Jan felt good she had taken the step.

The phone rang not long after eight o'clock. Gary answered. The voice was of a young female.

"This is Alpine Manor calling," she said. "We're sorry to inform you that Mrs. Chambers passed away tonight."

"How?" he asked. "What happened?"

"We don't know, but we think she choked on her food."

Gary turned from the phone, telling Jan. The caller from Alpine continued. She was in a hurry.

"Where do you want the body to go?" she asked.

"I don't know," Gary said. "I have to talk with my wife. We have family to contact."

The caller was persistent.

"Look, the coroner is here," she said. "The coroner is here and he's ready to leave. Please call us in ten minutes and let us know."

As Gary repeated the details Jan was overcome first with disbelief, then confusion. She wondered out loud why she hadn't been called and told her mother was dying? She wanted to be there at her mother's side, as the family had been during her bouts with pneumonia.

"They said she choked," Gary said.

"No Gary, that must be wrong," she said. "Somebody always had to feed her. They wouldn't let her choke."

"They say the coroner is there," Gary said.

There was no way they could call back in ten minutes, she told him.

"They'll just have to wait," she said.

Curiosity was overcome by urgency. After a series of phone calls the Hundermans drove to Ed Chambers', about twenty minutes away. There, the phone rang again. Again, it was Alpine Manor.

"Dad, they say the coroner is ready to leave," said Gary's teenage daughter Dawn, who answered the phone.

Jan complained to her daughter about the call: They were having a family meeting. They were deciding. Why was the nursing home pushing like this?

There were three calls from Alpine in all, the final one at Ed Chambers', around 9:30 P.M. Gary Hunderman finally gave Alpine Manor what they wanted. The family's choice was Reyer's Funeral Home.

For the longest time, Gary had an image in his mind of a big black van picking up the body of his mother-in-law. The coroner's office must provide some kind of service, he thought. They must make rounds every night to nursing homes and hospitals, picking up all the bodies of the dead.

They gave her a Catholic funeral. There was an open casket on Monday, a Rosary on Tuesday and a Mass on Wednesday at Holy Trinity. She was buried at Rosedale Memorial Park. She wore a pink suit. They put a black rosary in her hands.

The bronze grave marker had Ed's name on it as well. "Together—Married Forever," it read.

After Jan Hunderman took care of the final business with the undertaker, he handed her an envelope. In it was the death certificate.

Later Jan read it. Signed by Dr. Piskin, it listed "myocardial infarction," or heart attack, as her cause of death. It was a consequence of "arteriosclerotic heart disease," or a thickening of the arteries in her heart, he wrote. He also noted she had "severe organic brain disease." In the appropriate box Dr. Piskin listed her death as "natural." It was signed January 19, 1987, the day after Marguerite Chambers died.

The caller must have been mixed up about the choking, Jan decided. This made more sense. She remembered several ambulance runs to her father's house when her mother would stop breathing in her sleep. One of her former doctors said she suffered from a "lazy heart."

"One day her heart will just give out," he said.

Later, she picked up her mother's belongings from Alpine Manor. There were clothes and other odds and ends accumulated through the many months, gifts like the dried floral arrangement. Jan had no reason to notice that the balloon was missing, the one with MOTHER across the heart.

However, for the longest time Jan Hunderman remained unsettled. She couldn't seem to find any closure. She thought, you would think I'd have been prepared for this. Mom was sick for so very long.

She couldn't shake the unsettling sensation of disorder around her death. Everything had happened so fast. There was so much confusion about the body, about the cause of death.

Jan felt cheated. It's not fair, she thought. I wanted to be there, next to her when she left us.

She found herself crying, almost nightly. The tears came when she talked about her mother with her own children. It happened when she tucked them into bed. Before she turned off the light she always asked them if they had any problems, if there was anything they wanted to talk about before sleep.

They usually were okay, but she wasn't. She started feeling sorry for herself.

"I wish I had a mom like you have," she told them several times.

Often she still was crying when she put herself to bed.

Both Cathy Wood and Gwen Graham were scheduled to be off on Monday, the day after Marguerite Chambers died. Tuesday, they were scheduled to work a double, beginning on second shift. Cathy called in an excuse for them both. Something was amiss in the basement.

"The water heater is broken," she told a supervisor. "We're waiting for a repairman."

Cathy and Gwen were home drinking. They were drinking alone.

The hot water heater was located in the center of the basement, not far from the sewer drain and the little chimney door. Cathy later said she was especially afraid to descend the basement stairs during those two days.

"I thought maybe Marguerite would be down there and she would get me," she said.

On Monday night, they played in the bedroom. One of them applied the wrist restraints, lashing the hands of the other to the bed. One of them took a pair of tube socks from the dresser, pulling them over her hands. One mounted the other, straddling the other's body with her knees. One squeezed the other's mouth and nose.

There would be no suffocation, only tears. The restraints rapidly were untied.

"I'm sorry," one of them kept saying. "I'm sorry."

Later, the 45 spun on the turntable. Mel Carter was singing once again.

"Hold Me. Thrill Me. Kiss Me. Make me tell you I'm in love with you."

"I'll love you forever," Gwen and Cathy said.

Chapter 35

On Thursday, her first day back at work, Cathy Wood was nearing the end of the first leg of a double when she reported an altercation with a patient, her second in the past four months.

At 11:00 P.M., she told a nurse she was changing the diapers of a patient in 608-1, the bed position near the window, when the woman reached up and clawed the left side of her face. She showed the nurse the scratches down her cheek.

In September, Cathy had been slugged in the jaw by a male patient she was putting to bed. Cathy went for X rays that showed no fracture. The patient was given more tranquilizer.

On Cathy's latest "incident report" a nurse noted that the Camelot patient who scratched her had refused her Benadryl earlier in the evening.

On Friday, Cathy was asked about the status of her injury for official records.

"Still hurts," she said.

Chapter 36

Ken Wood thought the crank calls at all hours of the early morning were childish. He would expect such harassment from a couple of adolescents, but not women in their mid-twenties.

Ken never doubted who the culprits were, though he heard no one on the line. The calls always came in the middle of Alpine Manor's third shift. He had switched to days at the plant, so he could better care for Jamie. The harassment was robbing him of precious sleep.

Cathy was still difficult to reach. When he phoned her house he heard more creative recordings from her answering machine. Some of the messages were strange. There was a poem about somebody named "Bunny Foo Foo." She was "out in the garden" looking for carrots with Cathy. A dog was minding the house. Ken had a couple of friends listen. He wanted witnesses, just in case he needed to prove his wife had gone over the edge.

A new recording, Ken suspected, was aimed right at him. It was the old Supremes hit, "You Keep Me Hangin' On." He was sure of this when he reached Gwen one day. She was downright rude, refusing to call Cathy to the phone.

Finally, they hooked up. Now he was driving to Cathy's after midnight, January 30. She had agreed to give him her W-2 forms so they could file a joint tax return, but she wanted him to drop by in the hours she was normally up.

Ken didn't know what kind of reception awaited him. He found it impossible to predict Cathy's behavior anymore. In the days after their encounter in front of the Hall of Justice they had come to another truce. A few days after the week of January 18, he invited Cathy and Gwen to his apartment for dinner. Cathy talked and joked with Jamie. Ken had a nice chat with Gwen that day. Cathy announced that her sister was getting married in Florida in March.

Ken offered to drive both of them south. He wanted to take Jamie to Disney World.

"Gwen could come with us to Disney World, while you were at the wedding," he said.

Cathy couldn't stop laughing.

"What's wrong," he said. "I like Gwen."

"But you and Gwen, at Disney World? I'll have to think about that."

Cathy was in such good spirits that night. He couldn't understand why now he was getting so much trouble on the phone.

When he arrived at her house, he tried to avoid all controversial subjects. He talked to Cathy in the living room. She was sitting in her big chair. Besides the W-2s, he wondered, could he also get his record albums still stored in the basement?

"Gwen," Cathy said. "Go get his records."

Gwen headed for the stairs.

"By the way, Cath, I don't appreciate those phone calls," he said. "You guys keep calling and hanging up. And, I don't like Gwen being so snotty on the phone."

The criticism set Cathy off instantly.

"Forget it! You're getting nothing now."

She shouted to Gwen.

"Don't give him the records."

Now, he was pissed.

"I'm not leaving without my records. You've hung on to them for months."

Ken headed down the basement stairs. Halfway back up the stairs with an armful of albums, Cathy turned off the light and closed the door. He was in total darkness. He set down the records, turned the light back on, but found someone leaning against the door. He pushed it open six inches. He got a glimpse of Cathy. She had a baseball bat in her hands.

Ken burst through the door, grabbing the bat from her hands. He tossed it into the living room. He held himself in check. Cathy was hysterical.

"Get out of my house!" she yelled. "This is my house!"

"Those are my records."

She screamed she had called the police.

"Fine," he said. "I'll wait for them. 'Cause I'm not leaving without my records."

He sat down at the kitchen table, leaning back in the kitchen chair. He propped one foot up against the wall.

"Get your feet off my wall!"

Cathy grabbed his ankles and flipped him over backwards to the floor. As he pulled himself up he could see her scrambling into the living room, heading for the bat. As Ken pursued, he was met by Gwen. She put herself between them.

"Leave her alone," Gwen said.

"Gwen, get out of the way or you're going to get hurt."

He pushed Gwen aside. He wanted to get that bat from Cathy. She was big. The bat was rock hard ash. She could do some real damage with that, he thought.

"Cath, whatya gonna do, hit me with that?"

He was walking toward her.

The noise he heard came from behind him. It was guttural, like some kind of primeval war scream. He turned to see Gwen. She was coming head first, airborne. She brought him down instantly with a perfect leg tackle at the knees.

He chuckled at first, just after he hit the floor. He thought, they're defending each other. God, this is ridiculous.

Suddenly, they were both on top of him. Cathy was coming at him, her mouth open. She was trying to bite him on the face.

He thought, they're really trying to hurt me!

He rolled over, barely freeing himself from Cathy's oppressive weight. He struggled to his hands and knees, but now Cathy was on his back. Gwen stood up. Gwen kicked him in the crotch. Gwen kicked him in the head. Then he saw Gwen scramble for the baseball bat. He clutched the Louisville Slugger just as she did, but he felt like he was in slow motion with Cathy on his back. He pulled. Gwen pulled. Then Gwen yelled.

"I love you Cathy," she said.

He felt Cathy's long nails penetrate his eye lids. He squinted, trying to protect his corneas as she dug deeper and scratched. He felt liquid around his eyes. Blinded, he heard Cathy bark an order to Gwen.

"Give me the lamp. Gwen, hand me the lamp!"

He knew there was a ceramic lamp nearby, a very large ceramic lamp. He pulled on the baseball bat. Gwen pulled back.

"Hand me the lamp!"

He thought, the lamp will crush my skull. They're trying to kill me!

Suddenly, he felt Cathy's weight lift. He was still in a tug of war with Gwen for the Louisville Slugger when he heard a man's voice.

"Drop the bat."

It was an order, from a Grand Rapids police officer.

Ken had neither the tax forms nor his record albums when the police asked him to leave the house.

Later, the same day at Alpine Manor, a retired sales representative named Maurice Spanogle was giving aides Gwen Graham and Jim Shooter a hard time as they walked him to the bathroom for a sponge bath. Slightly confused, the eighty-six-year-old patient often resisted daily care. They each held an arm as he strained against them, complaining all the way.

Once in the bathroom, Shooter removed his pants and set him on the commode. He was still struggling as Gwen removed his shirt. Suddenly his back stiffened and his head fell back. He gasped for air.

A Dover nurse, just outside the door, responded. They lay Maurice Spanogle on his back, where he gasped several more times. He was turning blue. Then his eyes rolled back.

Later, Gwen told Cathy all about the struggle. Maurice Spanogle died on the bathroom floor, at 8:00 P.M.

Everyone figured he'd had a heart attack.

Chapter 37

Robin Fielder broke into a wide smile when she saw her car. She could see the driver's license beneath her windshield wiper. It was their secret message in the Alpine Manor parking lot after second shift. It meant: "Meet me across the street, in front of Family Foods."

The picture on the license was Gwen Graham's. They had been seeing each other secretly since January 8. Robin would never forget that night. Cathy, Gwen and Robin had stopped by another aide's apartment for a round of quarters after a movie. When they started spinning records, things began to happen. Everyone wanted Cathy to dance.

"Dance, Cathy," Robin urged. "C'mon Cathy, dance."

"Not unless Gwen leaves," Cathy said. "Not unless Gwen doesn't watch."

Gwen locked herself in the bathroom. Cathy gyrated a couple of times to the stereo. Then Gwen came out.

"All right, how did she do it?" she said, giggling. "How did she dance?"

Robin tried to mimic Cathy, but probably looked pretty foolish. She was blitzed, as was Gwen. Cathy was stone sober. She had to report later to third shift.

Out of breath, Robin plopped down in a chair, kicking off her high heels. Suddenly, Gwen reached over and pulled off her knee-high nylon, running from the room.

"Give me that!" she shouted, laughing.

Robin chased her into the bedroom.

The item retrieved, Robin walked slowly back into the living room, Gwen close behind.

"Where's Cathy?" Gwen asked.

"She left—mad," somebody said.

Gwen sprinted through the door. Robin caught her on the stairs, just as Cathy's truck sped off.

"No, you don't need to follow her," Robin said.

Gwen was sulking.

"I'll walk."

"You're not going to walk. I won't let you walk home. You can stay here."

Gwen turned and looked at Robin. She smiled and tilted her head. Robin was a little astonished when she kissed her on the lips. They went back inside the apartment.

As drunk as they were, both accepted an invitation to spend the night. Robin and Gwen took off their blouses, then passed out together on the bed.

The next morning Robin woke to find Gwen laying next to her on her stomach. That's when she saw all the scratches and the scabs.

"Gwen, your back," she said. "What happened?"

"Cathy did it."

"But why?"

Gwen never answered.

After they dressed, Robin dropped Gwen off at Cathy's house. Later, she learned that Cathy had confronted Gwen about what had happened. Gwen had protested she was drunk, and couldn't remember much.

That morning, Robin didn't know what was more disturbing, the sight of Gwen's mutilated back or the sudden turn her life seemed to be taking. She had never slept with a man, let alone a woman. Her relationship with Paul Lopez had only taken a large chunk out of her heart.

One night, she and Paul had an argument on second shift. He had appeared to become increasingly jealous of her new female friends. After she told him she had made other plans when he asked her out for a drink, he handed her back the house key she had given him.

"If you want to be with your lesbian friends, then why don't you go right ahead," he said. "I don't care what you do."

He ignored her on the job after that. Robin had always been sensitive, overly emotional, perhaps. The snub hurt her deeply.

Robin considered Cathy Wood a friend, a person at work always eager to listen. But, she found herself attracted to Gwen. She had a childlike quality about her, an innocence. With her turned-up nose and big eyes, she reminded her of the teddy bears that lined her bed.

Robin desperately wanted someone to care about. The two of them met again two days after their first night together, ending up at the house on Effie while Cathy worked third shift. Robin tried to drink away a case of the jitters. They spent the longest time just holding one another. Gwen led her through the lovemaking, very slowly, very gently.

"Do you want me to stop?" Gwen asked.

"No," Robin said.

Afterwards she felt guilty, but not over the physical act. She thought, we're in Cathy's house, Cathy's bed. I must be insane. This can bring only trouble.

But she did not resist. Nor could she tonight as she aimed her Mustang toward Four Mile Road. They had been meeting secretly a couple of times a week, in the early morning hours while Cathy worked. It meant another night with no sleep. She would counter it by swallowing a couple more 357 Magnums.

Robin Fielder also was feeling a new kind of energy. She was falling in love again. Only, this time, someone was responding.

As she headed for the supermarket parking lot she saw the orange Volkswagen, idling. She kept telling herself not to worry about what already had happened, or what might lie ahead.

Chapter 38

The red light was flashing above the room of the patient named Clara Pierce. If was after midnight. Ladonna Sterns turned into the doorway, and the screaming began.

"They're going to kill me! They're going to kill me!"

Clara was restrained to her bed rails, her eyes wide with terror. Ladonna tried to calm her.

"No one's going to kill you, Clara. No one."

"No, they *are* going to kill me. They whisper to me. They whisper that they are going to kill me."

She escorted her to the bathroom, reassuring her again.

"Everything is fine. Everything is fine."

Ladonna considered it an unfortunate delusion of the eighty-seven-year-old patient admitted six years ago with a diagnosis of organic brain syndrome. She had always liked Clara, though she was marginally confused. The terror had only begun recently, in the winter, after she fell while walking. Her doctor had ordered bed restraints to keep her from getting up. She was prone to wander. She could injure herself again.

The ensuing nightly ritual had become nerve-wracking. Periodically throughout third shift, Clara rang the call light, demanding to be escorted to the bathroom, demanding a bedpan. Other times she found her in her bed, frantically trying to escape her restraints.

"You have to stay in bed," Ladonna tried to tell her. "You have to be tied down. If you want anything, just ring for it."

"But, *please,* you can't tie me up," she would beg. "Don't you understand? They're gonna kill me. They come in here. They whisper. They *are* going to kill me."

Yes, Ladonna thought, and down on Buckingham there's another patient who was screaming "rape!" She had seen Cathy Wood escorting an old lady to the bathroom during rounds and the woman was screaming, "She's trying to rape me!"

Patients said all kinds of crazy things. Patients did all kinds of crazy things. Patients ate bugs. Patients thought enemas were sex. One male patient liked to masturbate as he ambulated down the hall.

The murder delusion was a first, however. Ladonna had never heard one scream homicide before.

As Ladonna walked Clara Pierce back to her bed, she started up again. Her body was docile. All her strength was directed to her voice.

"They're gonna kill me!"

"C'mon Clara, it's okay. Please. It's okay."

Ladonna laid her on the bed.

"They're going to kill me!"

"Clara, shhhhhh . . ."

She wrapped the thick felt bracelet around her wrist.

"Please! They're coming to kill me!"

"Clara, please, shut up."

She looped the cotton strap through the bed rails, then fed it through the brass loops of the restraint, doubling it back and securing it.

"Please! Help me! They're going to kill me. They're going to kill me."

The noise filled Camelot. By February everybody was used to it.

Margaret Knipp aimed her mother's wheelchair toward her room.

"No, not there," Clara Pierce begged. "That's the room where they do the killing. They're trying to kill me in there."

She thought, this delusion is getting to be a real problem. She was complaining all the time. Margaret visited her mother frequently. She approached staff members about the problem. A nurse asked her about her mother's history.

"Did she have a scare when she was younger? Did something happen to her like that early in her life? Sometimes they revert back to things like that."

No, she knew of nothing like that.

Margaret Knipp's mother had forgotten the names of her grandchildren, but not her daughter's name. Sometimes she was confused. But usually she was coherent and quite feisty, at least vocally.

That made her more difficult to calm down, as the delusions continued for more than three months. Senility is a horrible, unpredictable thing, Margaret Knipp thought. There certainly wasn't any truth to what her mother was saying. Her room was always immaculate. She always found her clean and well fed, even on surprise visits during off-hours.

That's why she liked Alpine Manor. There, she figured, her mother received the very best of care.

Chapter 39

Ted Luce doubted he would ever see a daughter more devoted to a mother. His sister Hazel might as well have been paid by Alpine Manor, she spent so much time with their mother, Myrtle Luce.

For years sister Hazel visited seven days a week, sometimes twice a day. She fed, bathed and changed their mother. She did as many things as she could, usually staying an entire shift at a time. Hazel's visits had become legend around the nursing home. Hazel used to say she was only doing what her mother would have done for her. They had lived together most of the latter years of their lives.

Now, in recent months, Hazel's visits had dropped. She was seventy-seven herself.

Ted Luce believed his mother had started her slow slide when his father died. They were like two peas in a pod, everyone said. After sixty-five years of marriage, they ought to be, Ted figured.

His dad made him promise just before he passed on in 1971.

"Don't you put your mother in a nursing home. You have to promise me that."

He promised.

That was sixteen years ago. Such pledges were for the young. When Myrtle became incontinent, the care became too much, even for Hazel. Ted now was nearly sixty-five.

Still, Ted agonized over the decision. He finally decided, Dad must have been thinking about those old-age homes for the poor. In fact, Ted found a couple of yellowed news clippings about those old bug traps in his dad's wallet right after he died.

Alpine Manor was more like a hospital. Over the nearly five years his mother was a patient, the family had come to know the aides on the early shifts well. By no means was she in the company of strangers. Besides Hazel, Ted and his wife Maxine visited several times a week.

At ninety-five, Myrtle Luce needed plenty of care. God knows, Ted thought, she's spent her life giving it. She had worked as a sales clerk in her early years, but she had the heart of a missionary nurse. She took in a troubled teenage boy as family. She nursed her husband's two ailing sisters and a couple of very sick aunts. When she ran out of family, she worked as a volunteer.

The last twelve months had brought changes in her own condition. There was little resemblance to the good-natured woman with black hair and blue eyes who used to stand five-foot-four. She had stopped walking and talking years ago. Even so, she always recognized Ted. She used to pat his face and smile. Now, she spent most of her time in bed, usually in the fetal position. Now he leaned over and whispered words in her ear, but she rarely opened her eyes.

A series of small strokes had taken her mind. Her doctor called it organic brain syndrome. Ted figured it wasn't that much different than Alzheimer's Disease. His mother's old Abbey Lane roommate, Marguerite Chambers, had been diagnosed with that.

Ted Luce was an auto worker, not a doctor. But the way the situation appeared to him, his mother's heart was too strong for her own good. She had hypertension and arteriosclerosis, but her heart kept pumping, despite all the damage to her brain.

"She has a good heart," her doctor told him after a recent physical. "In some ways she's as healthy as a horse."

She could go on for five days or five months or five years, the doctor said. There simply was no way to tell.

Recently, however, feeding her had become difficult. Myrtle was losing weight. The way aides worked with his mother impressed Ted. They put her in a geriatric chair to feed her pureed dinner with a big squeeze syringe. They stroked her neck, urging her to swallow.

Recently he and his wife Maxine had purchased a sheepskin for Myrtle. It was supposed to prevent bedsores, though that had never been a problem. If aides didn't turn Myrtle, Hazel made sure somebody did.

Everyone was doing what they could for her. One day, they even played Strauss waltzes for her. The Blue Danube.

Ted thought, my dad would have approved of this.

* * *

On February 3, a registered nurse noticed a trickle of blood from Myrtle Luce's right nostril during second shift. She applied a cold washcloth, stopping the hemorrhage with little fanfare.

With all the NG tubes, tired capillaries and high blood pressure around, nurses didn't consider a nosebleed a curious event. Winter and heating registers sometimes made the atmosphere in Alpine Manor exceptionally arid. This dried mucous membranes and made patients more vulnerable.

Nosebleeds were not uncommon, especially when the air was so dry it crackled.

Chapter 40

"I have a tendency when I get around children to be a child abuser . . . I just want to slap them. I can't stand kids—even Jamie."

—Catherine Wood, November 23, 1988.

Cathy bought Jamie a parakeet for her seventh birthday on February 4. It was the first special attention she had shown her daughter in months.

Later, Gwen recalled the relationship she saw between the two:

"I knew she wasn't seeing Jamie. When I first moved in, that was obvious. Poor kid. She'd call over there all the time and Cathy would be either laying down or say, 'Tell her I'm not here, or I'm at work, or I'll call back later.' I'd sit there and I'd tell her that. All the time.

"Cathy said, 'Jamie makes me nervous.'

"Well, I thought it was unusual. It was her own daughter. How come she didn't spend more time with her? If I had a daughter I'd want to be with her, you know. I wanted her with us. And Cathy said she couldn't be around her. She couldn't handle being around her all the time. She made her nervous.

"Like when we'd go pick her up and stuff, she wouldn't want to be around her very long. Usually, Jamie would either be across the street playing with the kids, or I'd be playing with her and Cathy would be laying down. When she'd go to sleep . . . we'd talk, play games. Backgammon. She was a smart little kid.

"You know how kids are. They talk a lot and they want your constant attention and stuff like that. She didn't have the patience for her. You know how kids go through the stage where they're screaming at the top of their lungs, just to be doing it? Cathy told me how she cured it when Jamie was a little baby. She went into the bedroom with a glass of ice cold water and threw it in her face—in Jamie's face! She was standing there, holding the edge of the crib.

"And she said, 'That cured it.'

"Could you see that little face with ice water? That'd cure me, for real!

"Jamie does, you know, require a lot of attention. When we were over Ken's house for dinner, she was trying to talk to Cathy the whole time . . . She wanted all her mom's attention. Jamie loves her mother very much, and God she would try so hard.

"Cathy just didn't like kids."

By spring, the parakeet was dead, the victim of a cold draft from an open window.

Chapter 41

Night House Supervisor Tish Prescott parked the Amigo, the little electric scooter Alpine Manor supplied so she could roam the halls and ease the strain on her arthritic knee. Not that she didn't appreciate it. Sometimes, she needed to be on foot. Sometimes, she didn't want the girls to hear her coming.

She startled Cathy and Gwen. They were alone in a patient's room.

"Tish, you're walking," said Cathy. "Where's your scooter?"

She said it singsong, drawing out the last word.

"Well, you know, I just felt I needed the exercise."

She moved on, satisfied she had put them on guard. Tish guessed they were doing rounds together again. Another procedure ignored or altered, she thought. Around Alpine Manor there just was way too much of that.

At nearly sixty-four, Leticia Prescott was a double for Santa's wife with her round frame, granny glasses and hair in a silver bun. It was a misleading visage. With more than forty years of nursing behind her, she was all business.

Patients and discipline were paramount. That's the way she learned her profession as a post graduate student at Children's Memorial in Chicago. That's the way she had practiced it as a top pediatric nurse. Hospitals, private practices and nursing homes filled her long resume. She had been at Alpine since late 1982.

Now, in her third year as night supervisor, Tish felt she was struggling against forces unseen and beyond her control. She knew this: The system was breaking down. Patients were not getting the attention they should. It was a scramble to find bodies to fill out the two night shifts. Not only was staff turning over, regular aides frequently called in sick. Many were just plain exhausted from working so many double shifts.

This meant nurses spent more time doing hands-on care, Tish observed. This meant they spent less time overseeing the duties and whereabouts of aides. Even so, when Tish made surprise spot-checks of work habits, aides seemed to know she was coming. Word spread quickly. By the time she checked a room on Abbey Lane to see if a patient was turned, her whereabouts were reported on Buckingham, Camelot and Dover.

Tish found the scramble exhausting. She was working twelve hours a day, five days a week since the supervisor position had been made into two shifts from three. Alpine threw in the Amigo with the extra hours. She and other managers were urging upper administration to hire aides from temporary agencies and raise the base pay of current staff to hold them, but nothing ever came of that.

Something also was amiss among the existing staff, Tish finally decided. She could see symptoms of trouble, but had no clear diagnosis. Aides were sneaking around. Someone was up to no good. She could feel it.

At first she thought it was the pranksters. She knew about the aides hiding under beds. She knew screens had been removed from some windows. She had reports of aides banging on the glass to scare fellow workers. When she saw petrified patients, she became fed up. One night she called the police, who caught an off-duty aide from an earlier shift in the courtyard. The aide was fired, and that slowed the shenanigans down quite a bit.

Tish was troubled by some lesbian aides. She had reports from nurses of aides necking in linen closets, courtyards and the parking lot. She saw couples walking hand in hand on their way to breaks. Tish didn't consider the atmosphere appropriate for the elderly. Later, she began hearing the references to "Gay Manor" from nurses she met who worked elsewhere. She complained to upper management.

"Well, when they're on their lunch break, that's their free time, and there's nothing we can do about it," a superior told her. "Their private life is their private life."

Two aides who came to her attention more than others were Cathy Wood and Gwen Graham. Gwen seemed to be the more masculine of the pair, the strong, silent type. She was quiet and worked hard. But one night Gwen turned up so drunk on her shift she staggered. Tish sent her home and made out a report, expecting her to be fired by upper management. She was back to work the next night.

Gwen may have seemed masculine, Tish decided, but Cathy clearly was in charge. She had the upper hand with Gwen and much of the staff as well. Tish knew Cathy could be a regular Jekyll and Hyde. She was sharper than most nurses; she was working way below her potential. She could handle complex situations and directions. She could be meticulously thorough with her care. She could get patients to talk or follow instructions. When Tish assigned her to the critically ill, she remained graceful under the pressure. Cathy was known to volunteer to clean up the dead.

Cathy's problem was with the healthy, Tish had decided. She snapped at nurses and complained incessantly about fellow aides. She was outspoken about who gave "good" or "bad" care. There was bad blood between Cathy and several workers. One was named Pat Ritter. Cathy frequently hinted she didn't come up to her standards.

Cathy went beyond sniping. Other aides accused her privately of sabotaging their rounds, setting them up for a reprimand by tampering with their rounds. Once Cathy threw a tray across the hall in a tantrum. Another time she dressed down an RN with a litany of foul, hateful profanity. She was written up on both occasions. Word went around the nursing home that Cathy had vandalized an aide's car in the lot.

"Just don't ever get on Cathy's bad side."

Tish heard this more than once.

Cathy Wood did make Tish uneasy. She was too moody. Some nights she showed up beaming. Other nights she would sulk, not speaking to a soul until sunrise.

When Cathy and Gwen were together Tish felt their work suffered. She watched them dote in the halls, frequently stopping to whisper to each other. When they teamed up for rounds they sometimes worked quickly, but that left a cluster of patients unattended. Tish thought, that's not the way the system was set up.

Tish didn't want Cathy and Gwen on the same shift, let alone the same station. But when she put them on opposite ends of the building, they switched with other aides. The daily assignment records were not reflecting reality. When they couldn't switch, one or the other just left.

"Where's Cathy?" a nurse would ask, as a call light went unanswered.

As someone filled in, Tish would go off searching. She could count on finding Cathy where Gwen was assigned. Often she found them together with a patient. Tish received complaints from other aides that Cathy and Gwen were alone in rooms with the doors shut, another violation of nursing home practice. Everyone suspected they were making out.

"I'm just helping Gwen with her rounds," Cathy would say.

Tish guessed lately that they had been on the lookout for the telltale whir of her Amigo. If they heard her coming, one would scramble back to her assignment and avoid a scolding with some concocted excuse. Tish couldn't shake the uneasy feeling the two of them were up to something, something more than sex. Maybe they are secretly drinking, she thought, or worse, using or pilfering the prescription drugs.

Finally, she decided to take the matter to Margaret Widmaier and Jackie Cromwell, the assistant director and director of nursing.

She explained how she had been chasing Cathy and Gwen around the facility.

"These two are just no good for each other," she said. "They shouldn't work together. It's affecting care. Something has to be done."

They looked at her blankly. Most of Tish's complaints about staffing, discipline and employee conduct were already being ignored. She had written up several formal reports and heard nothing. Her complaints about Cathy and Gwen appeared headed for the same result. Tish Prescott was getting the message: All an aide had to do was be competent, show up regularly and pull a load of doubles.

Do that and you can get away with murder in Alpine Manor, she thought.

Chapter 42

During the longest nights of winter they began stalking the nursing home, looking to see who struggled greatly, and who did not.

They did this by constricting the noses of patients, Cathy later said. They clamped nostrils shut with their well-scrubbed fingertips, cutting off air briefly. They studied the result, hoping to predict how a potential victim would react.

One night they came upon an Abbey Lane patient named Donald Randall, age seventy-seven. He was a stroke victim with a combative recent history when it came to the application of the NG tube. He fought nurses who tried to put one in. He found ways to pull it out.

When his nose was pinched his eyes opened.

He heard: "You're going to die tonight."

His eyes became very big. His wrists were restrained to the bed rails.

". . . So we figured he would be easy," Cathy said later.

He was not easy. His jaw was too strong. It was impossible to hold his mouth shut long enough.

As January became February there was a rash of incidents in Alpine Manor. Six patients suffered falls in nine days, a high rate by Alpine's own average. Others were agitated, restless. One woman attacked staffers, hitting and scratching whoever came close. An asthma patient refused treatment, demanding to be sent to the hospital. One woman's bottom dentures disappeared. Another injured herself scrambling over the footboard of her bed in panic.

In and of themselves, none of the incidents were unique in the routine of geriatric care. None warranted undue suspicion.

On February 7, a house supervisor noted in the shift log that Donald Randall had a problem in the early-morning hours of third shift. He was in systemic distress, his blood pressure dropping to 96 over 42. Randall appeared to be suffering from "60-to-85-second periods of apnea," she wrote. His breathing was stopping, a condition that sometimes preceded death.

Randall, however, didn't expire. The condition wasn't reported again after that.

Cathy Wood and Gwen Graham had the next two days off.

Chapter 43

Cathy and Gwen were sitting together at the desk of the Abbey Lane nurse's station, making slash marks on paper. They were counting their past lovers.

"It took forever for Gwen to get done," Cathy later said.

They were only a couple of hours into third shift. They would do no wandering tonight. Both were assigned to Abbey Lane. On official records, Cathy had been assigned ten rooms in the 100 hall. Gwen had ten of the rooms in 200 hall: 210 through 220, the block farthest from the station near Buckingham. She was on the second leg of a double shift.

Neither was assigned Myrtle Luce. For virtually every night for the past three weeks, Myrtle had been assigned to the aide Pat Ritter, the third-shift aide disliked by Cathy Wood. Myrtle's room was just down the hall, just past the day room, not even twenty-five feet from the station where Cathy and Gwen sat. She was in 206-1. Her window location overlooked the courtyard.

"I'm going to do Myrtle," Gwen said, getting up from the Abbey desk.

It was nursing home slang for giving routine care.

At 2:20 A.M., an aide named Sally Johnson reported what she found to the Abbey Lane nurse, who made the page on the public address.

"House Supervisor to room 206."

An RN named Martha Slocum was the night shift supervisor on February 10. When she turned the corner into 206 she found Sally Johnson standing at the side of the bed near the window.

"I walked in and she was gone," Johnson said.

Myrtle Luce was on her back, lifeless on her sheepskin.

Slocum knew Myrtle had been deteriorating over the past year. She knew the patient's family, specifically Bud Dredge, the son of Hazel, Myrtle's devoted daughter. They had children in high school together.

The night supervisor wanted Myrtle Luce to look her absolute best, should the family decide to view the body before it was sent to the funeral home. She helped prepare the body herself.

Cathy Wood later claimed she helped clean up the body, Slocum would not recall her being there. Cathy said she combed Myrtle's hair. She later reported a rolled washcloth was left on Myrtle's bed, and something else as well.

"When I went to the room, I looked at Myrtle and her nose was . . . smooshed," Cathy recalled later. "She had a lot of mucus and things in her nose all of the time, and it was like it had been held there. No one noticed it but me."

Later, no one noticed something else. There was a discrepancy

on the "resident care plan" record, the sheet aides sign on a patient's chart as they made their rounds. The February 10 entry on
third shift for Myrtle Luce had a shaky, forced signature. It was close
facsimile of the authentic one, but featured handwriting inconsistencies in the "P" and the "R."

The last person to treat Myrtle Luce on third shift, according to
the signature, was Pat Ritter, the aide Cathy Wood complained
wasn't up to snuff. That was quite impossible. She was nowhere near
Alpine Manor that morning.

Earlier that night, Pat Ritter had called in sick.

Supervisor Slocum placed calls to both families shortly after 2:30
A.M.

"Bud, we weren't surprised," she told Hazel's son. "We were
expecting it at any time."

Dredge would break the news to his mother. She had a hard time
understanding. She recently had been diagnosed with Alzheimer's
Disease herself.

Ted's wife, Maxine, answered the phone at the Luce's house. She
explained the call from Alpine to her husband as he rubbed the
sleep from his eyes.

"They said she died in her sleep," she told Ted. "They said it
looked like a heart attack."

"What?"

They discussed what the doctor had said about her heart after his
exam. For some reason, Maxine couldn't shake the feeling she had
choked. She had seen Myrtle choke on her own saliva.

"Gee, I just can't imagine her dying of a heart attack," Maxine
said. "Her heart was so strong."

Maybe the nursing home had it wrong, she said, but did it really
matter?

"It's a blessing," Maxine said. "Now she doesn't have to go
through this anymore."

They decided to have her cremated and to hold a memorial
service. In her final months she had become drawn and rigid. My
mother wouldn't want anyone to see her looking like that, Ted
decided.

They had the ashes buried in Memorial Gardens. They sent a

card to the staff of Alpine Manor, thanking everyone for the fine care. Somebody posted it on a bulletin board.

The obituary had all the details. Myrtle's family tree had many branches. She was born on February 20, 1891. Her father-in-law had come halfway across the continental United States in a covered wagon. Two of her five children were dead, as well as her husband of sixty-five years, but there were ten grandchildren to carry on.

If she had lived ten more days, Myrtle Luce would have been 96.

Chapter 44

Linda Engman cut through all the bullshit and told her daughter Stephanie point-blank.

"Stephie, whether you like nursing homes or not is absolutely irrelevant. But, if you *don't* go see your grandmother, and God forbid, something happens, you're going to feel so damn guilty. I know what you're going to go through, but at least you'll be able to say you went."

Until the Alzheimer's, Stephanie and her grandmother had been inseparable. It started when Stephanie was in diapers, when her grandmother started giving Stephanie her keys for amusement. She kept a token on the key ring just for the kids.

Maisy was the key to her daughter's independent nature, Linda thought. She suspected that's what made the nursing home so difficult for her daughter. She has her grandmother's spirit, and seeing that siphoned away by disease was difficult to face at the age of seventeen. Confronting the continuing deterioration of her grandmother had kept her away from Alpine Manor for months. Stephanie complained she felt powerless over the disease.

"The worst part is there's not one thing I can do about this. I feel like I'm tied up in ropes. I feel like I can't move a muscle and there's no escape."

On February 2, both of them visited 207-1 at Alpine Manor. It was Mae Mason's seventy-ninth birthday. Recently she had been transferred from Camelot to Abbey Lane. They helped Maisy out of bed and walked her to the Abbey day room, each holding an arm. Since breaking her hip, the incessant walker had become afraid to walk alone.

Stephanie hugged her in the day room. She was crying when they drove away.

"Mom, I think Nanna recognized me. I think she did."

Linda knew how she felt. There were bad days and good days. On bad days her mother did not speak and did not appear to recognize anyone. On good days she did both.

In the beginning, she would say to a nurse, "This is my daughter Linda."

There was little of that now.

Sometimes, Linda would ask, "Do you know who I am?" Her mother would squeeze her hand. Sometimes when Linda asked, tears would stream down her cheeks.

Sometimes Maisy could be quite talkative, but her subject matter was disjointed.

"I love you, Mom," Linda would say.

"It's a beautiful day outside," her mother would respond.

Or, there would be a stream-of-consciousness monologue.

"The birds outside. Gee, that's a nice pad of paper. It's a pretty day. A Pepsi can, huh? I'd like to go for a walk. What are you doing with this pencil?"

There had been few good days in the last six months. The one constant was the music. Her mother still could hum and sing. "Spanish Eyes" was her favorite. The activities staff also played songs for her. She was listening to waltzes, and other songs.

Linda found her mother humming when she returned to visit a week after her birthday. She was sitting, bathed in light from the window near her bed. Linda sat with her and held her hand. She saw a tear run down her cheek.

She wondered, what does she think about? Where is she now? Where does she go with her thoughts?

Once, her mother had given them such a scare. It was during her last days with them at home. Linda's husband John found Maisy standing on the bank of the river that defined the edge of their yard. She was gazing into the rapid, brown current. She must have been hallucinating. She was talking about her dead mother. Everyone thought it was lucky she wasn't found dead downstream somewhere.

Here on Abbey Lane, Linda Engman thought, at least I don't have to worry about that.

Chapter 45

In the fall, salmon fought their way up the brown water, coming in from Lake Michigan to spawn as their bodies deformed and their skin spotted with age. When the Coho and Chinook ran, people came to Fish Ladder Park just north of downtown to watch. During warm months, they came to cool off on muggy nights. In the dark of February, the park was barren except for an orange Volkswagen that idled in the parking lot on many frigid nights.

Gwen Graham had discovered Fish Ladder Park with Cathy in a warmer month by the light of day. There was a fish-viewing ramp built into a modern sculpture that overlooked the ladder and dam below. They saw whirlpools and a foamy backwash below the barrier. There was a powerful turbulence underneath. A sign warned: Dangerous Undertow at Dam.

"If somebody went in there they would never come up," Cathy once said.

In the coldest months Gwen found herself drawn to the park alone. She sat in her Volkswagen, the doors locked. She brought a bottle of Jack Daniel's and two bottles of Diet 7-Up. She liked to drink alone in the dark.

"It was the only place I knew in Grand Rapids where I could just go to be alone to think," she later said.

The sounds of the water often conjured up images, images of the bodies. There were bodies of the dead floating down the Grand. They were deep in that water, in some kind of aquatic ravine. Gwen Graham couldn't shake that thought. She hadn't been able to shake the phobia for years. Her father Mack had put those bodies there, she sometimes told friends, along with other childhood images that still replayed in her head.

The big water, many years ago, was the ocean. They lived just a couple blocks from the Pacific in California.

"You! Don't go near the water at the beach!"

She knew who "you" was. He often called her that.

Mack later told her he wanted to make sure none of his own waded near the dangerous undertows of the big Pacific surf. He told them stories. They listened. Gwen listened. She was six.

"Just off the edge, beyond the surf, there's a big drop-off. There's a great ravine and it's dark and it's deep. You don't want to go in there. In the great ravine is where they keep the bodies of the dead."

Dead bodies, suspended under that water. She had never been able to swim comfortably since. When she tried, the brush of a blue gill could send her screaming from any water. She thought of the bodies clustered underneath her, touching her legs, her thighs, her privates. She had nightmares about someone forcing her to take a swim.

The phobia haunted her. But there were other childhood moments, snapshots that lingered too. There were memories of many animals, helpless animals, and they were always dying. They were always being killed.

"Hey you, you're going to learn about nature."

She remembered the snakes, the big boas. Her dad kept snakes in the house as pets in California. She was only five or six. He brought home white mice from the pet store and fed them to the snakes. They looked like they were choking as the white rodents struggled in their throats.

"Hey you. You're going to stay here and watch."

When it was over, the serpents curled up and slept, contented, the mice somewhere deep down their long throats.

"It was terrible," she told a friend many years later. "Us kids would stand there and cry. But, I think we got used to it. We got used to it, I guess."

In Texas, as she reached puberty, her father's lessons became more elaborate. "Country psychology," he used to say. He wanted children to learn responsibility and enterprise. He offered them profits from their own animal husbandry. She watched the slaughter of rabbits and chickens, the birds always running headless. She learned to castrate pigs and gut them and skin them.

Sometimes she begged for mercy.

"Has to be done. Has to be done."

She found the pigs the most traumatic. She raised some of them from little babies, nursing them with a bottle when the sow wouldn't give up her teat.

Two of them followed her around well after they had grown. One was named Bonita. She was bit by a water moccasin in the face. Half her jaw was rotting away when everyone agreed she had to be shot. Another, named Tex, died after her father swatted him with a two-by-four. He said he was just trying to move the pig along when he missed Tex's fanny and snapped his spine. Paralyzed the neck down, the pig just lay there and died.

She lost a lot of dogs as well over the years, about seven, as best as she could recall. Some were hit by cars, others died of disease. And then there was Misty and Hoagie.

She picked Misty out herself when she was fifteen, after spotting her in a pet shop. They became quite attached. If not for the mixed-breed toy, the house would have been empty after school. When she moved to Modesto after her parents split she received word from Texas that Misty was missing. She returned to Tyler just to look. Finally, her brother admitted he had killed the dog. Misty had nearly thrown a horseback rider with her barking, he told her. So he just shot her, he said.

Gwen found out where the dog was buried, and she dug up the bones. She hung the skull up in her bedroom until her mother ordered it down. Gwen removed all the dog's teeth and separated some of the small bones in its paws. She stored them in an alabaster jewelry case shaped like a heart, its lid carved with roses. When she came to Grand Rapids she taped the case shut and brought it along. She had always planned to make a necklace from that dog's teeth and bones.

Hoagie was a mercy killing when she was seventeen. The dog was old and limping. One day her dad handed her his double-barreled shotgun and pointed at the river that ran behind his California property. Her dad always said she volunteered for the task.

"Take 'em out back next to the river and shoot him. Then throw him in the water when you're done."

She would always remember calling the old mutt down there, luring him to his death.

"Here Hoagie. Here boy."

He sat there, next to the water, as the current swept by his face. She aimed, closed her eyes and pulled one of the two triggers on the shotgun. She heard only a click from a faulty firing pin.

She opened her eyes and aimed again. The dog was looking at her over the bead of the barrel, tilting his head. She squeezed the second trigger and turned his head into a mass of flesh and blood.

The carcass was warm and heavy as she dragged the dog by its paws toward the bank. She couldn't lift the dog to throw him. So she waded in, pulling the dog into the water. The current pulled at her legs as she sent the old mutt on his way. Then she sprinted back to the house.

She complained to her dad, how scared she was, about the dog and the river. Later that night, as she lay in bed, she was almost asleep when she heard it.

"Hoagieeeeee. Hoagieeeeee."

Fingernails scratched at the screen of her bedroom window like a dog wanting to be let in. They belonged to her father. It was his idea of a joke.

The Jack Daniel's stirred, then clouded, these memories, as she drank down by the fish ladder. She thought about things both past and present. She thought about Cathy and Alpine Manor. She thought about the girl named Robin. They were seeing more and more of each other, but her devotion to Cathy seemed timeless.

One night they had an argument. Cathy took off. Gwen drove to the fish ladder to sit and drink. Sucking on her Marlboro, she turned down the window in her car for more air. She could hear the current in the distance. She could see the silhouette of power lines sagging across the width of the Grand. The river sparkled at night from the city lights.

She wrote Cathy a letter, right there in the dark of the Volkswagen.

I don't want to be here alone. It's cold out there but it couldn't
be any worse than the feeling I have sitting here wondering
where you are and what you're thinking of me. I know you love
me. I'm far from perfect. My hair is a mess. I have scars all over.
I say and do infantile things endlessly, but I know you love me

anyway. It makes me sad, but I know sometimes you have to push me away or just be alone away from me.

I love you pretty girl.

I sit by the river because it's so deep, fast, exciting, scary. It reminds me of the way I feel for you. Frozen on top, underneath it flows so strong. Much warmer than the surface, you see. I could never tell you how much I love you. My eyes, my touch, my words could never express what my heart can barely hold for you. I'm a silly girl. Romeo could never have loved Juliet as much as I love you. But they'd never write a love story about us . . .

Please love me. You mean everything to me.

She ended it with an acronym: "OCINY"
"Oh Cathy I need you," it meant.

Chapter 46

Nurse's Aide Shawn Dougherty pushed with all her might, finally sliding her shoulder through the jam. Suddenly the patient's door swung open with no resistance.

Cathy Wood and Gwen Graham were standing inside in the darkness, lit by only the incidental light from the bathroom. They giggled, then scurried past her like a couple of spirits.

Cathy's eyes said: *Ha, ha. The joke's on you.*

Shawn Dougherty had been an Alpine aide not even a month, but she knew the two women had no business there with one of her patients. Also, doors were supposed to remain open on third shift. She later complained to a nurse. She never heard anything more about the complaint.

Cathy and Gwen were an odd pair, Shawn thought. Gwen was one of the most helpful aides, when she wasn't with Cathy Wood.

Most of all she was strong. When there was heavy lifting to do, or a difficult physical job, Shawn looked for Gwen. Gwen didn't worry about her nails or getting her hands dirty. She was always willing to help.

Cathy Wood, however, had become Shawn's tormentor. Cathy didn't like her from the moment they first met. Cathy was rude, domineering and condescending.

"Hello Miss America," Cathy always said.

Shawn always reported for work in a fresh uniform, her hair and makeup neatly done. She was twenty-one, tall and attractive.

"Oh, so how's Miss America today?"

Shawn hated that.

Once Cathy asked her where she lived. Shawn lied. Shawn found Cathy frightening. She was big, loud and demanding. She was short with workers, and with patients. She ordered both around. Once, watching her trying to roll a patient over in his bed, Shawn heard her complain to the patient:

"If you'd help me, this would go a lot faster."

Total care patients were a lot of work. Most simply didn't understand directions anymore. They looked at Cathy bemused. Cathy was snotty anyway. When Shawn heard an angry voice rising in the hallway, most often it was Cathy Wood's.

"She was Jekyll and Hyde," Shawn recalled later. "One day she was your long lost best friend, and the next day she'd jump down anybody's throat that got in her way."

Shawn Dougherty was making her 2:00 A.M. check of 207-1 on February 16 when she found Mae Mason awake and very active. She lay in her own bowel movement. Feces covered her hands and were imbedded in her nails. Shawn moistened a washcloth to clean her up. This only made Mae more active. She kept clutching at the towel, seemingly fighting the terry cloth.

It was Shawn's first such cleanup. Routine bed checks sometimes brought surprises. A woman on Buckingham later would take a swing at her with a deodorant can. She had concealed it like a weapon under her covers. The patient stopped when Shawn threw up her hands.

After changing Mae, Shawn repositioned her in the bed. She rolled her from her side to flat on her back. She tucked the covers around her, eventually leaving the room to continue with her rounds.

When Shawn Dougherty returned during 4:00 A.M. rounds she was struck by Mae's color, a grayish yellow. Mae was still lying on her back, but her hands were at her sides, her palms up. Her eyes were closed and her mouth was open. Her jaw was open and pushed down to one side.

Shawn shook her, trying to wake her. Then she tried to get a pulse. She grabbed a stethoscope from one of the other aides, but couldn't find a beat. Her own heart was racing. It was another surprise on rounds. She had never discovered anyone dead.

As the Abbey Lane nurse followed her back to Mae's room, Shawn couldn't understand why she was going so slow. She walked ten paces behind. Shawn thought they should try to save the patient. Maybe someone could try CPR. She had been so active just two hours ago.

The nurse examined her, looking at her blue fingernails. She responded flatly.

"Yes, we did lose Mae."

Then, in a few minutes, the public address system sounded.

"House Supervisor to room 207."

Shawn was shocked. She was so active, she thought. Did I do something wrong? Then, she began to cry. She said a Catholic prayer. She sat down beside Mae Mason and began to rub her arm.

"Shawn!" barked another nurse. "Don't ever rub the arm of a patient after they die. It could bruise and the family will wonder why she died."

Shawn remained with the body. She was so shaken her rounds were assigned to somebody else. She asked for the duty of gathering up Mae's belongings, items accumulated over the years. As was the ritual, most of the ten aides working that night stopped by to see the body. Shawn stayed with Mae until the funeral home picked her up.

One of the other aides working on Abbey Lane that early morning was Gwen Graham. Her partner Cathy was on Camelot. Cathy had been assigned Mae Mason more than any other aide on third shift in January and February. On February 16, both were working the last leg of yet another double. They had the next day off.

It didn't strike Shawn Dougherty until later, not until a couple of hours after the body left. Everyone had dropped by the room to see Mae Mason—everyone, except for Gwen Graham and Cathy Wood.

"So how's Miss America today?"

Cathy's subtle harassment became worse in the following weeks. Gwen remained pleasant and helpful. Shawn decided that was the problem. Cathy loathed anyone to whom Gwen showed attention.

Married, Shawn certainly wasn't some kind of lesbian threat. In fact, she and another nurse had become self-conscious about Alpine's growing reputation as "Gay Manor." They worried what people where they cashed their checks were thinking.

There were enough problems to deal with on the inside. After Mae Mason died, her roommate in 207 became paranoid. She insisted her bathroom light be left on before she would go to sleep. She had a request as well.

"Shawn, when you come in, will you wake me up and let me know you're here?"

She complied with both. She would touch her gently on rounds. The patient would jump, waking instantly poised and very alert.

"It's only Shawn, and I'm here," she would say.

Shawn would do this every night. It would take several minutes before the patient calmed down. Then, assured the light was on, she would go back to sleep.

They were often short of help. Cathy and Gwen wandered all over the building. Night Supervisor Tish Prescott was always speeding around the building on her Amigo, trying to keep everything in check, and Cathy and Gwen apart. Patient records were not being kept properly. If aides neglected their flow charts for individual patients, at payroll time nurses passed them out to have them signed well after the fact.

Despite these and other drawbacks, such as the $3.50 hourly wage, Shawn Dougherty still loved the patients and the work. If it hadn't been for Cathy Wood and some of her friends, she would have continued. She told that to Tish Prescott when she asked her how to resign.

"I do understand," Tish said.

Shawn hadn't worked in Alpine Manor ten weeks when she gave her two-week notice. The next day she didn't show up at all. She no longer wanted anything to do with the madness.

Shawn Dougherty just picked up her check and quit.

Chapter 47

When he was done, the Congregational minister turned to the gathering and asked, "Is there anyone who would like to add some words about Mae Mason?"

His voice reverberated across the tall marble walls of the Grace-land Memorial Mausoleum. Family and friends sat in chairs at the foot of the steps that led to the ecumenical altar. Everything in the mausoleum was stone. On February 20, the marble radiated a pene-trating chill. The minister continued.

"Well, if not, Linda would like to say some things."

Stephanie Engman watched as her mother walked to the front, her heels clicking on the marble floor and steps. She admired her mother's bravery.

"The reason I didn't tell all of you that I was going to do this is that I really didn't know if I could," her mother began. "But I just knew my mother would be so pleased if I made it through."

She watched her take a big breath. That's right, Stephanie thought. That's what Nanna would have said. Take a breath. Don't sweat it. You can do it. Be steady!

"My mother was my best friend. I have lost my best friend."

Everyone was listening.

"If I can remember any one word to describe my mom, it was, 'time.' Yes, she loved me. Yes, if we were short on money she was generous. But that's not what mattered. It was *time.* My mother spent time with me. Loving me was time, when she easily could have bought me a car and said, 'Go away kid.'"

There were several stories. Her mother had jotted them down the night before in the dark, Stephanie later learned, when everyone else was in bed.

Stephanie thought, yes, and I have lost my best friend, too. I lost her long ago to some shitty thing that turned her into a toddler.

Stephanie Engman wished she could remake the last half dozen years. She wished she could remake herself. She would have exterminated the twelve-year-old who had become so embarrassed by her grandmother when she was no longer herself. How, she thought, could I been that way to the most important person in my life?

She couldn't shake the memory of the way she treated her the day she walked into the house with a teenage friend. Nanna was cooking the laundry in the oven.

"God, Nanna, what the hell are you doing?"

The incident convinced everyone that Nanna had to be put in a home. Somehow, Stephanie felt it was all her fault.

What a stupid, selfish kid I was, she thought. Then, the stupid, selfish kid started getting drunk through junior high, sucking down liquor at the homes of a new circle of dubious friends. In high school, she found a more constructive escape in drama and debate, but the memories of her grandmother still nagged her nonetheless.

She thought, and now my best friend is gone for good, and I don't know how or where to say I'm sorry.

As she watched her mother finish the eulogy, she decided Nanna would have been so proud of her daughter. She wished she could have made Nanna proud.

But Stephanie Engman felt ashamed. She felt she had fallen so very short.

Mae Mason already had been cremated three days before the memorial service. She went to the crematorium on February 17, the afternoon after her death. Her ashes were buried next to her husband's grave in a plot in Graceland Memorial Park.

Linda Engman knew her mother's wishes. She had heard the continuing argument between her mother and father over the years. Mom wanted to be cremated. Dad most certainly did not.

"No sir," Maisy used to say. "The worms aren't going to get me."

While the crematorium was insuring they would not, her physician, Dr. W. Keith Conner, fixed his patient's official cause of death.

He listed it as a cardiac arrest. He described it as "immediate" and caused by a myocardial infarction, or death to a segment of heart muscle—the all-American heart attack.

Linda's husband John commented that the death certificate was pretty ironic. He had just seen the family doctor recently himself on a medical matter. Dr. Conner, he said, had mentioned that he gave Maisy a physical in Alpine Manor a week before her death.

"He said she was in great health," John told the family. "He said her heart was as strong as a racehorse's."

John chuckled at the irony.

"I guess that shows how much doctors really know," he said.

Chapter 48

Angie Brozak liked her new assignment to first shift. Not only was Alpine Manor brighter, she saw less of Cathy Wood.

Sometimes their doubles would overlap, the two of them working together. What started out as fun and games, now gave Angie the creeps. The patient's name was Ken. He used to ask the women for kisses. He asked them to take off their clothes.

"You give me five hundred dollars I'll take them off," Cathy used to tell him.

Now, recently, Ken had become a screamer. Angie didn't know if the shouting stemmed from fear, anger or delirium. But he frequently filled Camelot and Dover with noise. He was always yelling, unless Cathy Wood was around. She had developed a reputation for quieting him.

One night Angie and Cathy were working together on second shift when Ken began to get boisterous.

"Cathy, how do you get him to be quiet?" Angie asked.

"Watch," she said.

Ken was sitting in a chair. Cathy walked up to him and leaned over, whispering in his ear. He immediately shut up.

"What did you tell him?" Angie asked.

Cathy cracked a coy smile.

"I told him, 'Go ahead, scream one more time. But look at me. I'm bigger than you. I'm huge, in fact. You are helpless. I am not. You scream one more time, and I will kill you. And there will be nothing you can do to stop me.' "

Later, Angie wondered if she should have reported it to the supervisor. However, she had no desire to brave the inevitable revenge of Cathy Wood. Her ruthlessness had only grown. She persecuted not only enemies, but those she called her friends.

Cathy, Angie decided, smothered everyone near her with her insatiable compulsion to be the center of attention. A visit by her estranged husband Ken revealed she had been packing his head with lies. She had him totally buffaloed. She remembered what Cathy herself had said once.

"I can just snap my finger," she bragged to Angie once. "I can call him up and he'll come over, take me out to dinner, sleep with me—anything I want."

She liked to have that power with everyone, Angie decided, with Gwen, with Dawn, with Ladonna and a few assorted others around Alpine Manor. God help you if you didn't fall in line.

At Christmas Angie had unwittingly unleashed her fury. She lambasted Angie for buying Gwen a gift, an engraved Zippo lighter. She'd passed out the same present to other friends who smoked. She gave Cathy a ceramic goose for her kitchen. She also baked her homemade bread she'd once raved about.

Gift or no gift, Angie discovered just how deeply her old friend held a grudge. Cathy struck back at the Carousel one night. She secretly pulled aside a large, drunken black man. She told him that Angie not only liked sex with blacks, but liked to be forced, to be slapped around.

He staggered over to her table and asked Angie to dance. She declined politely. He pestered her. Finally, she paid a strategic visit to the bathroom. When she emerged, he grabbed her by the arm.

"I said no, I'm not interested," she said.

He reached over and manhandled her.

"Bitch, I know you like it," he slurred.

She was terrified. She thought, why doesn't this man leave me alone. She looked over at Cathy. She was laughing, watching the scenario unfold.

Finally, a group of people at their table, who knew about the setup, urged her to tell the man it was a joke.

"This has gone too far. Stop this Cathy," someone shouted.

The man backed off. Cathy pouted when her fun stopped.

Later, she listened to Cathy announce she was going to ruin the marriages and reputations of certain aides. She spread rumors among the supervisors that one aide was hanging out in seedy bars on South Division. Cathy seemed insanely jealous of anyone's happiness.

Cathy also had a mysterious effect on those who clamored after her attention, Angie decided. She saw it first with Dawn, then with Gwen. She had no doubt who was in physical and psychological control. Once, she watched Cathy explode into violence during a jealous rage. Cathy picked Gwen up and literally threw her over the couch. Gwen landed stunned against a door. Privately, Gwen complained to Angie that Cathy would no longer let her pick out her own clothes. Cathy wanted her to wear only men's clothing. In Cathy's presence Gwen was a parrot. She mimicked everything Cathy said. Once, after Angie had Ladonna Sterns over for dinner, Cathy sniped at her in the break room. Gwen was sitting at her side.

"I hear that you and Ladonna are having an affair," Cathy said.

"Yep," Gwen added, nodding.

"Ladonna told me you darn near raped her," Cathy continued.

"Yep," Gwen nodded again, her eyes on the table.

"Bullshit," Angie said, before walking out of the room.

Angie had discerned Cathy's technique of prying and lying. She was a master of half-truth, she decided. She habitually offered up probable speculations, looking for a reaction to see if she was on target. As for her lying, the main thrust of her information was poignantly dishonest, but it was always supported by an elaborate foundation of truth.

And, Angie thought, all of Cathy's concerns are so extraordinarily petty. She will do anything to remain the center of attention or to keep the upper hand. She'd have us all be like her restrained patients, depending on her for our care and every need.

During the latter days of winter, the behavior repeatedly angered Angie. She thought, why does she care what I do? Why must she meddle in my life?

Angie did have feelings for Ladonna. In January, she moved in with her and the kids when Angie and her husband separated.

Ladonna's years of a lesbian double life had ended when her husband found the two of them together in bed.

For months, Angie had been watching Cathy play Ladonna as though it were some kind of sport. She flirted with her, only to set her up so she could complain to Gwen that she was being pursued. She tried to make wagers in the break room on how long it would take her to seduce Ladonna into a kiss. Then, she complained privately that she didn't like her teeth.

None the wiser, Ladonna still went over the house on Effie now and then to party. As far as Angie was concerned, however, Cathy had become the Rasputin of Alpine Manor. She wanted to wash her hands of Cathy Wood and her court.

Recently, as Angie woke patients up for breakfast, Cathy had approached her before leaving Alpine Manor after third shift. Cathy held her hands in front of her, as though she were making a formal announcement.

"You know, you and I can never be friends again," she said.

"What are you talking about Cathy?"

"As long as you're living with Ladonna you and I will never, ever be friends again."

"Why is that?"

"Ladonna will lie about me, and you will believe Ladonna before you will believe me."

No kidding, Angie thought. Perhaps, she really was worried some of her own mind games would be revealed.

"Cath, you and I aren't much friends now anyway," Angie said, politely.

"But you and I *never* can be friends again," Cathy said.

She hoped it was one promise that Cathy Wood finally would keep. Still, through February all the turmoil was still too uncomfortably close. Cathy speculated Gwen was cheating on her and at first she thought Angie was to blame.

Angie knew Gwen was seeing her friend from second shift, Robin Fielder. Robin had confided the whole torrid affair to her. Angie could sense major trouble up ahead.

Angie thought, this is all so twisted. It's beyond childish. It's nuts!

By March, Angie was ready to get out, day shift or not. She wanted better pay in a better environment. She valued her own sanity and safety over two years seniority in Alpine Manor.

She felt that way the day she quit.

Chapter 49

Another quarter bounced off the table and into the cup.

"All right, who you gonna do?" somebody said. "Who you gonna do?"

Robin Fielder took another sip of her vodka and grapefruit juice, then went into her act. She chewed on her tongue, then held her hands and arms rigid to her sides. She acted strong, determined. She pretended she didn't want to be put to bed, a task that sometimes took two aides.

"That's Belle," somebody guessed. "That's Belle Burkhard."

Another night of quarters and drinking was underway in the little house on Effie. This time impersonations of Alpine Manor patients were part of the game.

By late February, Robin Fielder had become awfully good at another impersonation, one that she didn't find so humorous. I'm pretending to be Cathy's friend, she thought. If she only knew what was really going on.

She was reasonably sure Cathy did not know about her affair with Gwen. Robin sensed some coolness, but dismissed it. She found Cathy hard to read anyway. She was so saccharine. In fact, Robin was tiring of Cathy treating patients and friends like babies. She sometimes made Gwen wear her hair in childish pigtails. When she saw Robin was upset she would call her to her side like some caricature of a mother. Her lips would pucker, then smack open and shut rapid fire.

"Oh come here, Robin," she would say. "Let me give you kisses."

Robin herself was blocking out the affair mentally when she was in Cathy's company, and that was frequently. Cathy seemed to be making herself more available. She offered to discuss problems Robin was having with her folks. She even invited her to move in if she finally wanted to take the leap away from Mom and Dad.

Robin was suffering a double dose of guilt. She felt bad about betraying Cathy. Sometimes, she felt worse about what was going on between her and Gwen. She thought, I'm not gay. I'm not a lesbian. How do I know? I've never slept with a man.

The conflict held her back sexually. She never could give herself totally in her lovemaking with Gwen. She found her happiness in the fact that Gwen enjoyed her so much. Robin, however, felt no joy every Sunday when she stepped through the doors of her church. She was relieved she had always attended group confessions. She sure didn't want to confess all the details to a priest.

What appeared to be going on between Gwen and Cathy sickened her. Gwen's scratched back healed. Then she showed up again one night with it ravaged. She always was getting hickeys on her neck, as though Cathy were marking her with her personal brand. Sometimes, when they were alone and drinking at Cathy's, Gwen would ask if she could tie her up.

"No, you can't *tie me up!* And, your back is ridiculous. I just don't get into that stuff."

One day, Gwen promised she would ask Cathy to stop the scratching. Robin wondered, how can someone so sweet get caught up in something so kinky? Gwen deserved better. She was so warm, so touching, so loving.

Robin faced her own inconsistencies as well. Sometimes she wanted to run. Another part of her savored the affair. Gwen treated her like a queen. She complimented her constantly. Gwen loved her hair, her clothes. She loved her breasts. Gwen loved her "little Polish nose," the nose Robin always had hated.

"You're my pretty girl," she always said.

It made Robin want to lose more weight, and she did. Her body became more shapely. No longer a model for Rubens, she was now merely voluptuous by modern standards. She felt that she was being noticed, and she no longer wanted to hide. She began keeping a diary. She penned entries in a journal she sent away for from Virginia Slims, her brand ("You've come a long way, baby").

Robin was writing poetry again, about herself, about Gwen. She was fascinated with her lover. There was a childlike innocence and a certain sadness in Gwen's personality, something that drew Robin even closer.

She was confused. She was confounded. She was in love. One day she wrote in her poem book:

Boxed in
there's no way out.
Oh, how true
without a doubt.
Stuck in the dark,
tell me, where's the light?
All that I am doing
am I wrong or right?
Is there a way
that I can escape?
I feel so withdrawn, I'll just sit and wait
for a chance I have
when you are near.
I'll cry so loud that
you can hear.
Will you rescue me
from this mess,
Or is your love
just a test.

Chapter 50

By late February, Ken Wood was seeing a couple of familiar patterns. Cathy was ready for another truce, even after their big battle with the baseball bat. She also was dismissing her relationship with Gwen, the same way she had dismissed her relationship with Dawn.

Earlier, there had been more harsh words on the phone. Gwen refused once more to call Cathy to the telephone.

"Ken, what is your problem?" she told him. "Why can't you just leave Cathy alone?"

"Well, she doesn't act like she wants to be left alone."

"Get real!"

Ken hadn't been able to shake the impression left by Cathy the day she stood in her doorway, talking about dead people around her bed. He continued.

"Look it Gwen, I don't give a shit anymore who she sleeps with. But I'm afraid for her. She's doing crazy things. She's even seeing crazy things. Did she tell you about the bodies. For God's sake, she's seeing dead bodies."

Gwen came right back.

"Well, they're probably from hell, and they're introducing themselves."

Ken said he was serious.

"Gwen, I'm afraid my wife is going to hell."

"Well if she does," Gwen said, "I'll be right there at her side."

Then she slammed the phone.

Less than two weeks after their brawl in the living room Cathy called. She wanted to visit while Gwen was at work. Ken decided, I'm the only link to normalcy she has. That's why she won't let go of me. I'm the only thing keeping her from falling completely into the abyss.

Cathy was a study in rational behavior when she arrived at his apartment.

"We've got to try and control ourselves," she said.

He agreed.

They sat together at his dining room table, talking. She was matter-of-fact. She was insightful. He loved when she discussed things so intelligently. Cathy could be so smart. If only she could be that way always, Ken thought.

They talked about commitment and infidelity. Ken told her he couldn't understand why she thought he was such a bastard, when he had always been faithful. Yet she forgave Dawn and Gwen several times. They were a couple of cheats.

She was flippant.

"Oh Ken, I can leave Gwen anytime. Sometimes we're close, sometimes we're not. It's not that serious."

She paused dramatically, then leaned forward and looked into his eyes.

"Ken," she said. "You just wouldn't believe some of the things we've been doing."

"Whatya mean?"

"You just wouldn't believe what we've been doing."

Oh yes I would, he thought. My spies told me: The sex. The naked people running around in my old neighborhood. The fighting in the middle of the night. Then he realized, maybe she's not talking about that.

"Well, Cath," he asked. "What kind of things *have* you been doing?"

Her back quickly straightened.

"Oh, it's nothing really. It's nothing we can get in trouble for."

She waved the subject off with her hand, like a pitcher waving off a sign from his catcher.

He let it go at that.

Later, however, she piqued his curiosity again. They were lying together on the couch. She seemed preoccupied with something, but she gave no hints.

"You know, Cath," he said, "if you got a problem, you can open up to me. I'm still somebody you can talk to."

She looked at him coyly, but remained mute.

"No," he said. "You wouldn't tell me if there was something wrong, would you?"

She smirked.

After eight years, Ken knew Cathy well enough to know she was holding back a bunch of secrets. She was teasing him with them. Ken also knew she would probably tell him when she was ready.

She would tell him on her terms, not his.

Chapter 51

During the last week of February, the anticipation of death was widespread in Alpine Manor. More than anyone realized, the nursing home was under siege.

By midweek, many patients were heavily congested and running temperatures near 100 and above. Three had been sent to area hospitals for pneumonia. Another had died. Two patients were listed as critical. County health department would draw blood for cultures aimed at identifying the responsible bacteria or virus.

Night House Supervisor Tish Prescott was struggling on a couple of fronts. She still had not been able to convince her superiors to reassign Cathy Wood and Gwen Graham to separate shifts. Repeatedly, when Tish's shift ended at 8:00 A.M., she stayed at the nursing home to express her complaints to Nursing Director Jackie Cromwell and her assistant Margaret Widmaier.

"There was never any cooperation," Prescott later recalled. "I mean, I went in that office I can't tell you how many times and literally begged them not to let these people work together."

Cathy and Gwen not only were working together, they were spending more hours on duty than ever. They volunteered for overtime and jumped at the chance to fill holes in the schedule created by call-ins. In February, Cathy Wood worked six doubles and Gwen Graham, seven. The two of them were together for a total of nineteen shifts. Gwen's hours mounted. She worked twenty-eight shifts in a twenty-shift month. Cathy worked twenty-three.

A pattern had already developed by late February. Their work days were scheduled so that they doubled together—often two days of doubles, back-to-back, at a stretch. Then, at the end of the work binge, they both had a day off.

Another pattern was also taking shape, one that no one noticed. Their time off came after patient deaths. Unlike Gwen, Cathy often stretched her rest periods into two-day sabbaticals. She accomplished this by her scheduling, or by simply calling in sick.

After failing to get assistance from her superiors, Tish Prescott was willing to try anything to keep Cathy and Gwen from wandering from their stations. The problem was escalating. Other aides were not staying put either. Her solution was the nursing home's version of a cuss bank. Every time one was missing from their station she had to pay a nickel to a kitty. She hoped maybe a little good humor and food would persuade everyone. They bought pizza with the kitty.

It worked for a couple of weeks.

One of the patients on the critical list was a ninety-eight-year-old Grand Rapids widow named Ruth Van Dyke. Age had diminished Ruth long before her fever began taking its toll. She had logged eleven years in nursing homes, nine in Alpine Manor. She was senile and nearly deaf and blind. Still, she talked and took food in her wheelchair, until the microscopic intruder ravaging Alpine rendered her semiconscious in her bed.

The afternoon of Wednesday, February 25, nursing staff called family members, informing them Ruth wasn't expected to last much longer. Her son Al Van Dyke and his twin sister Lavina arrived with their spouses at 6:30 P.M. Two of her other children lived elsewhere. The fifth was dead. The two couples sat bedside, watching and waiting.

At sixty-five, Al Van Dyke was no stranger to the dead and dying. Retired five years, he had spent thirty-seven years as a Grand Rapids cop, seventeen as a detective, eight of those in homicide. He had also moonlighted for nine years as an ambulance attendant.

After several hours of the death watch, Al became anxious. He had been studying his mother's breathing. She was experiencing apnea. He decided to hold his breath when her respiration stopped. About a minute later, he blew out a lungful of hot carbon dioxide. Still, his mother hadn't breathed. Then, after he caught his breath, she started again.

"Well, I've seen this," he told everyone. "You know, you just cannot tell when they're going to go."

His mother was holding true to her lineage. She was a Beckwith. It was an old Grand Rapids name from England. Three of her farm-raised sisters had lived to ninety-seven, ninety-eight and ninety-nine. She had another sister in her early nineties. Ruth had been a short, strong woman of more than two hundred pounds, before age took her down to one hundred forty. Still, as she lay there silently, her eyes closed, she didn't look more than seventy years of age. There were few wrinkles on her face.

She's so *strong*, even now, Al decided. He always remembered that story his mom told. Mom, Dad and two babies were crossing the iron bridge over Black Creek with a wagon and a team when the wheel slipped off in the snow. She left those two children in the wagon, grabbed the rig and held it herself. She kept the wagon from slipping into the rushing waters as his dad ran to the nearest farm for help.

By 10:30 P.M., no one was moving in the halls. They had seen one staffer drop in during their watch. Lavina wasn't feeling well. Through the window next to her bed Al could see the snow falling.

The snow. The rushing water. The wagon, and his mother holding on.

"You know," Al said to his twin sister. "This ole gal could lay here a long time."

Everyone decided it was probably best they go.

At approximately 2:40 A.M., Al Van Dyke received another phone call from Alpine Manor. The death certificate would indicate she died of cardiac arrest.

Wednesday was Gwen Graham's scheduled day off. But for third shift during the early morning hours of Thursday, February 26, she had arrived at Alpine Manor for yet more overtime. She was working another shift with Cathy Wood. Gwen was assigned to the 600 and 700 halls on Dover, just a short walk from 100 hall, where Cathy was stationed on Abbey Lane.

One of the Abbey patients on the rebound that week was Belle Burkhard. Belle was in 112-1, the position near the window. Earlier, on the day side, the activity staff had paid a visit. Belle smiled when the music was played, the Blue Danube and all the waltzes by Strauss. Earlier in the week Belle had cold symptoms, but now her congestion was clearing and her fever was only slight.

The entry made on her chart eleven days earlier, on February 15, was more noteworthy. That morning an aide had found Belle with reddish bruises around her nose, right cheek and temples. The contusions, as a matter of routine, were reported to management and to her family. But, considering her history of seizures and Alpine's stainless-steel bed rails, the incident was dismissed with no further investigation.

For the first two weeks of February, Belle's primary aide on third shift was Cathy Wood. Unlike Gwen, she found the patient frustrating. When Cathy tried to turn her, Belle would grab the bed rails with an iron grip and refuse to budge. Often she did this and laughed.

"I really didn't like Belle," Cathy later admitted. "She was so hard to take care of."

However, she had not been Cathy's burden recently. For the last eleven consecutive days, Belle had been under the care of Pat Ritter, the new aide Cathy criticized so much, the one whose signature had apparently been forged on Myrtle Luce's chart on the shift during which she died.

During the 3:00 A.M. break, when many staffers took their lunch, the Abbey Lane station was left to the care of Cathy Wood. She sat quietly at the desk. She often chewed on her lip and gazed at her nails when she sat alone.

Soon Gwen Graham approached the Abbey station, from the Dover side, through 100 hall.

One of them sat at the station, watching the hall, while the other headed into room 112. The patient intercom linked the station to Belle Burkhard's room. Cathy later said groans and the rustle of sheets sounded over the intercom's speaker.

"I heard gurgling out loud, like dry-heave noises. I did hear that for a while."

Minutes later, the intruder walked out of room 112 and turned away into the hall. A washcloth hung out of her back pocket as she strolled down Abbey Lane.

Since starting at Alpine Manor in late January, Pat Ritter had kept her head down and her nose to her business. Withdrawn by nature, the forty-one-year-old aide found two fellow workers particularly troublesome. Cathy Wood and Gwen Graham both had hollered at her on several occasions about her work. Then, they reported to supervisors that she wasn't changing patients. She suspected they were the ones who were pouring water into her patients' beds.

Ritter was not far into her 4:00 A.M. rounds on February 26 when she stopped her cart outside the door of room 112. She planned to turn Belle Burkhard, as she had at midnight and 2:00 A.M.

She was yelling when she ran from the room. It was her first dead patient.

She darted through 100 hall, heading for the Abbey Lane station. She could see two staffers as she neared the counter, her field of vision bouncing up and down as she approached in a trot.

"Come check Belle out!" she cried. "Come check Belle. She's dead. She's dead!"

The station nurse walked briskly toward Belle's room. Standing next to the counter and watching Pat Ritter panic was the large, inanimate figure of Cathy Wood.

"House Supervisor to room 112."

Belle Burkhard had expired at 4:25 A.M., the nurse noted on her chart. The station nurse picked two aides to clean up her body. Pat Ritter later remembered that Cathy protested the assignment. She didn't want the duty. Cathy was nervous and upset as she nevertheless was saddled with the task.

Before third shift had ended, the scuttlebutt was already underway in the break room. Cathy and Gwen were telling others about one of their favorite marks. Somebody noticed how Belle Burkhard's arm was folded underneath her dead body, the story went, that it also appeared red and bruised.

"Pat Ritter probably didn't turn her right," one of Cathy's admirers said.

Cathy sniped away. Gwen nodded her head in agreement.

By sunrise, Alpine Manor was turning over its second body to an undertaker the morning of February 26. Through the clearing sky, a low sun cast long, jagged shadows with the bare trees all across the snow-spotted Grand River Valley. The black Luv Truck was headed back to the northwest side, putting time and distance between the two young women and their work.

When they crossed the Grand River's rapid waters on the rusty North Park bridge, there was some release. They were almost at the little house on Effie.

Both Gwen Graham and Cathy Wood had the next day off.

Chapter 52

The day she received it, Nancy Hahn put the little plastic box with her mother's ashes on top of a case in her bedroom. That night, she lay in the darkness, troubled and unable to sleep.

Belle had died on Nancy's forty-eighth birthday. Everything seemed so complete, so tidy now. But there were other ashes, other memories: A cigarette, Belle passed out in the chair. Her mother burning down their house. Nancy coming home to the flames from a date. Nancy screaming, wanting to go inside. Everyone finding her in the alley, wandering around drunk in her nightgown.

There were other funerals: Her father's, after her parents separated. Nancy begging her mother to attend, begging her to sign the estate papers. The nasty words.

Nancy was always there for the aftermath, as far back as the age of nine: Getting herself to school. Getting herself fed. Getting a beer for her mother. The hangovers. The lonely trips to her own bed.

Nancy thought, I have always been caretaker of the remnants.

The next morning, Nancy put the little box out in the family camper, a good fifty feet from the house. The ashes sat out there in the cold for six weeks, until the storms of winter cleared.

When they did, Nancy Hahn headed north. Her whole family came together for the trip, a caravan of three cars driving up the middle of the state. Nancy carried the little plastic box of ashes. In the trunk was a heavy granite stone that would mark her mother's grave.

Gross Cap Cemetery was five miles west of St. Ignace, not even a mile from Belle Burkhard's old homestead. The eighteenth-century graveyard was an ancient Indian burial spot, complete with its own historical marker. Graves marked and unmarked overlooked the tannin-rich waters of Moran Creek, right where they spilled into the big blue surf of the turbulent Mackinaw Straights.

Nancy and her family met aunts, uncles and others from St. Ignace there. Cold winds buffeted the gathering as Nancy placed the ashes in the ground. She put them next to her mother's parents. That's what Belle wanted. She wanted to be in the earth of her ancestors, in the peninsula where she was born.

They all said a prayer over her grave, then put the heavy stone in place. Nancy Hahn felt a great sense of relief. She thought, it is finished. Now, my mother's troubles are over. She goes to a far better place.

Now she rests in dignity, Nancy Hahn decided. In contrast to her days among the living, at least she died in peace.

Chapter 53

Fran Shadden watched her old lover Gwen Graham folding the clothes at the Grand Rapids coin laundry, or the "washeteria," as they used to call it when they lived together in Texas.

Gwen held up a giant pair of jeans. They were bigger than her entire body.

"Good Lord," Fran said.

Gwen peaked from behind the pants and giggled. They both laughed.

"Well, she's a wild one in bed," Gwen said. "She sure is."

Fran had discerned that on previous occasions when they met and chatted over the spinning clothes and towels. She had seen the marks all over Gwen's neck and the deep scabs on her back. No hard feelings lingered over their split-up six months ago. Forgive and forget. That was Gwen.

Fran harbored no resentments either. She was regaining her spiritual direction with a Grand Rapids church that ministered to gays. It was called Reconciliation. She was reconciling with God. She was getting right with herself.

Only the owner of the mammoth jeans had stirred trouble since they parted. Cathy, with Gwen in tow, had broken down the door of Fran's apartment to get the license plate that Gwen had used on her Volkswagen. Also, one night in the bathroom at the Carousel, she and Cathy nearly came to blows. Cathy was backed by a group of followers from Alpine Manor. Fran was saved by a friend, who pulled her quickly out of the bar.

Fran wondered now if Gwen finally was seeing the true nature of her roommate. Recently, in late winter, she was showing signs of discontent. Gwen complained Cathy was overly jealous. Cathy was acting petty, and she often wouldn't let her out of her sight, she said. Gwen almost whispered, as though Cathy would somehow find out.

"I sure wouldn't want Cathy to be hearing me saying this stuff," she said. "Nope, I sure wouldn't."

Fran thought, Gwen has found another mother to run her life and to put her on a schedule. She knew Gwen would never come right out and say that. But at least she's recognizing Cathy isn't the great love she once claimed. Gwen admitted as much before she picked up her clothes.

"Fran, I don't think I'm so deeply in love. No sir. I don't think it's love. For now it's just a place to be."

No, Fran thought, Cathy Wood sure wouldn't like to hear that.

Chapter 54

In the last throws of winter, the flu virus that hospitalized some Alpine patients with pneumonia and snuffed the breath out of others dissipated with the winds of March.

The winter death toll was comparable to that of the previous year. In January, Alpine lost five patients, one less than in 1986. In February, ten died, the same total as the year before. In March the list of dead dropped to eight, three less than twelve months earlier.

Few aides, however, were worried about the patient death count. More newsworthy were the sexual and emotional liaisons of people associated with Gwen Graham and Cathy Wood.

The overview presented quite an entanglement. Dawn Male had slept with Cathy, first alone, then in a threesome with Ladonna. Dawn did a one-nighter with Gwen, then one of Gwen's friends. Now she was eyeing Robin Fielder. Ladonna Sterns had been strung along by Cathy, had left her husband and now lived with Angie Brozak. Angie, after Cathy had tampered with her marriage, had been turned out by Cathy and Gwen and had now left her husband as well. She was sleeping with Ladonna. Robin Fielder, who had dated Paul Lopez, was now immersed in a secret affair with Gwen. Paul had been paired with Tony Kubiak. He left Alpine Manor with Jesse, Ladonna's brother, despite Cathy's attempt to break them up. On the fringe was Lisa Lynch, one of Robin's best friends at Alpine. Lisa maintained she was not gay and blamed Cathy for the destruction of her marriage.

If anyone was keeping score, Gwen Graham deserved the grand prize. Since coming to Alpine she'd bedded Dawn, Angie, Cathy, Robin and the young aide Jim Shooter, and had made several less noteworthy conquests along the way.

By late March, the latest gossip revolved around Cathy's newest psychological mark, an aide named Katherine Brinkman. The thirty-three-year-old mother of one had started working as an Alpine aide in December. Aides watched her seek out Cathy's friendship, clamoring for her company and attention. She wrote her letters and bought her jewelry. She bought her flowers, then vases to put them in.

"You're crazy," Angie Brozak had told her before she left Alpine Manor. "You're just nuts, 'cause she's just using you."

Dawn Male later recalled, "Cathy had Katherine in the palm of her hand. Meanwhile, behind her back Cathy called her disgusting, ugly, crazy. Yet, she bragged, 'Katherine will buy me anything I want.' "

The competition for attention and social dominance continued. Jealousy, often nurtured by Cathy's half-truths and her incessant stirring of the Alpine rumor mill, caused some in the group to angle for still more scores.

"We had all gone crazy," Ladonna Sterns later recalled. "We

didn't care for each other's feelings. We didn't care what hurt came out of it, or nothing. We didn't have any feelings. We simply didn't."

Since she had been dumped by Cathy, Dawn Male's life seemed to have unfolded like an old hand-cranked picture scope. Between the flicker of boozy blackouts there were snapshots of fights, car crashes and court dates.

She hadn't retained many memories, either, from her regular visits to the little house on Effie through the winter and spring of 1987. There were more quarters games and wild excursions with Gwen in the VW. There was an ongoing attempt by Cathy to match her with Robin Fielder. One night Dawn got blitzed, and, for reasons that later escaped her, knocked out Ladonna Sterns's front teeth. Reasoning, dates and days of the week were obscured in a chemically-induced haze conjured by reefer, beer and the formidable proof of Wild Irish Rose.

One day in particular, however, did stand out. Later she would not be able to pin down the date any more specifically than this: It was after she had left Alpine Manor in the fall of 1986 and before she would return to Lakeview in the summer of 1987.

The three of them were in the living room on Effie one day before Cathy and Gwen went to work. Out of the blue one of them brought the subject up. The two of them said they had smothered a patient at Alpine Manor.

"We did it," one of them said.

Dawn took a big sip of her can of beer and studied their faces. Gwen was sitting on the couch. Cathy was standing over her, smirking.

Another game, Dawn thought.

"Why the fuck are you guys trying to scare me?" she asked.

No, they were not trying to scare her or play a game, they took turns explaining. In fact, they said they had smothered more than one. Then Gwen named a patient, but Dawn gave so little credence to the story that she would later forget the name.

"I smothered her with a pillow," said Gwen. "Cathy stood outside the door and made sure no one was coming."

Dawn took another sip.

"Do you believe me?" Gwen asked.

"Fuck no."

"Why not?"

"I just don't believe you would kill somebody."

This is an ignorant joke, Dawn told herself.

"Well, I can prove it," Gwen said.

She followed both of them into the bedroom. There, from her shelf in the bedroom, Cathy picked up a sock.

"This is her sock," Cathy said, referring to the patient she mentioned.

There were more names and more souvenirs on the shelf. Later, Dawn's memory was hazy about details. There might have been an item of jewelry, a necklace with a cross perhaps. When it came to names she would draw a blank.

Cathy was known to snitch items from patients. Once she took a patient's rosary and hung it from her rearview mirror in her Luv Truck.

No, these were from the dead, the once-suffering, the two women said.

"Somebody had to put 'em out of their misery," Gwen said.

Dawn eyed the sock. It was an anklet. Cathy wore anklets. In fact, Cathy always wore anklets. You guys, Dawn thought, are so full of shit. A new mind game. A new, stupid fucking mind game.

It was time for another beer.

"That's no fucking proof," Dawn said. "This shit doesn't mean anything to me."

And, for many months it didn't.

Chapter 55

The planned excursion to Disney World and the wedding of Cathy's sister in early March never materialized. Cathy told Ken and Gwen she had been bumped from the wedding party. She didn't have the money anyway. Besides, probably not even a Las Vegas odds maker would have given them a chance at making it, the three of them all riding in one car.

Cathy's mother Pat did make the trip to Florida. She left her quaint New England-style farmhouse in Comstock Park in the care of Cathy and Gwen. They moved in for two weeks to house-sit. They spent more time in Alpine Manor than the home, though they did invite a couple of friends over as guests.

Like Ken, Gwen had witnessed firsthand Cathy's ambivalence toward her mother. She returned from visits to mother's preoccupied by how she had been treated, or just plain spitting mad. She complained her mother didn't love her, that she was impossible to please. However, when crisis hit, Pat was the first one Cathy called.

Pat always responded. Once, when Ken tried to retrieve some of his winter clothes from the basement on Effie, Cathy called both Pat and the Grand Rapids police. Her mother came screeching up the driveway first. She stepped out the car door, her shoulders back and her head high. She was a couple of inches short of six feet tall like Cathy, big-bodied but not obese. She was meticulously dressed in slacks and had smartly styled, short silver hair. Her brow was furrowed and her eyes piercing.

Pat brushed right past Ken as if he were overgrown landscaping, marched to the top of the steps and then turned and glared down at her estranged son-in-law.

"All right, mister," she announced. "Now, do you want to mess with me?"

She said "mister" real loud.

Ken looked up. Pat had her hands on her hips.

Then the police drove up.

Pat stood in the middle of everyone with her arms folded as they all worked out a deal. Ken was allowed into the basement for his clothes. He came out carrying a brown sack of largely useless items. Mainly, he had come for his thick down coat. When she saw the parka under his arm, Pat surprised him.

"I bought my daughter *that* coat," she said.

Her consonants snapped.

"Yes, that's right," Cathy quickly added. "That's my coat."

The police looked at Ken's size, then Cathy's.

"I'm sorry, sir," one cop told him. "You cannot have that coat."

Pat and Cathy smirked. Ken looked befuddled.

Anytime Ken was circling, she dialed her mother.

"Would you quit calling your mom?" Gwen finally said. "I can take care of Ken."

She didn't mean her fists. Their protection was leaning in a corner, an arm's length from their bed. After their brawl with the baseball bat, Gwen had called her father Mack, who now lived in Oklahoma. She told him of their troubles with Ken. Mack sent Gwen her old hunting rifle, an old gift from her late grandfather. It was a 6.5 caliber Mannlicher-Carcano, the Italian mail-order special, the same brand of rifle Lee Harvey Oswald used on JFK.

Gwen chambered a shell and showed Cathy how to use it. Well after midnight, Gwen fired a round into the Grand Rapids night from the back doorway. Cathy covered her ears. Gwen's ears rang for an hour. The shot drew complaints from neighbors.

"I don't know why they were so upset," Gwen later told someone. "What you do in your own yard is your own business."

Gwen put another shell in the chamber and left the safety on before she put it in the corner. She said they didn't need the Grand Rapids police, or Cathy's mother Pat anymore. Just take the safety off first, she said.

"Cathy, if Ken breaks in, don't even bother to aim. Just point it in his direction and shoot."

Gwen didn't know what to think about Cathy's mother. Face-to-face, Pat's treatment of Gwen exceeded politeness. Once, Gwen went to the hospital emergency room with severe stomach pain. Pat stayed with her there while Cathy went to work. She took her home from the hospital, then babied her.

"She treated me just like a little kid," Gwen later recalled. "She said, 'Now get undressed, and get in bed.' She cooked for me. She stayed until Cathy got home. It was just so cute."

On the other hand, Gwen resented the way Cathy seemed to be so hurt after her private encounters with Mom. Cathy harped about the fruit basket at Christmas. Other than that, Gwen could not offer any more specific examples of Pat's coldness. But if Cathy said Pat was cruel, to Gwen's way of thinking, her word was good enough.

"I just didn't like the way she treated Cathy," Gwen later recalled. "Just from what Cathy said. She was just real impersonal—real impersonal with her."

Not long after Pat returned from her Florida trip in late March, Cathy returned once more from a visit to her mother's. She was nearly hysterical.

"She's cleaning," Cathy said.

She was weeping when she first told Gwen.

"She's *cleaning*. She's cleaning *everything.*"

The floors. The carpets. The dishes. The furniture.

Both of them had gone out of their way to leave the home as neat as they found it. It was early April. Gwen speculated Pat was simply doing her spring cleaning.

"No," Cathy said. "It's contaminated. Don't you see. She's cleaning because we stayed there. She thinks it's contaminated."

A couple of days later, Cathy told Robin Fielder about the flurry of housework. Robin had paid a visit to the house. Cathy had conducted a little tour, proudly displaying pictures of her family. She had talked about everyone's love of dogs. She had showed off her mother's knickknacks.

Now she was sniping.

"It has to be disinfected," Cathy said, coldly. "Robin, it has to be disinfected. She's doing it because we were there."

Cathy sounded crazy as hell over the whole affair.

Chapter 56

The orange Volkswagen idled in the parking lot of Fish Ladder Park, its valves tapping with the sound of the rapids in the night.

The river . . . the dark water . . . the bodies.

More Jack Daniel's. Alone. Thinking. Cathy. Robin. Pledges. And lies.

And trust.

There always had been so little of that.

First memories: A grandmother's house. In Indiana. Living with grandma. Mack in a car wreck. Mack in the hospital. A mother living somewhere else. On a farm maybe? But with grandma now. Hugs. And kisses. On the porch. An ice cream parlor across the street. The ice cream. The music of Johnny Cash. Somewhere, there was the music of Johnnie Cash.

She didn't want to leave there. No sir. Then she wanted to go back. They never did. But she remembered the porch. And the ice cream. And the music.

No, she was stubborn. She wasn't like Corey. She wasn't like Robert. From the start, as a baby, she refused to be held, they always told her.

She grew stubborn and hateful. She was a stubborn, hateful brat.

Mom said, what's wrong with this child?

She's stubborn. She was one little goddamn monster. For real! She sure was! Gwendolyn Gail was that.

The mirror. Maybe four, or five years old. She was looking in the mirror. She was looking at herself in that.

"Give me that mirror!"

No. Stubborn, and hateful. She pulled away.

Smash it!

Mother smashed it. She smashed it on her head.

"I won't go. No. I won't."

The toilet: Oh Lord Jesus, the toilet. No, please. Don't put me in that. Urine. The smell of old urine. Chill. The water. The swirling water. Don't suck me down. Please! Don't let me be sucked into that!

"I'm going to run. I'm going to run away."

Five years old: Still stubborn, the girl who refused to be held.

"I'm going to run, and go away."

"So, go you goddamn brat!"

Out the door. Slam. Alone, and very small. Out front of the house. The big front door. Closed. The street. Cross the street. No, that's forbidden. Run! No, don't cross the street. Go inside. The door is locked.

Locked out.

Mother.

Alone. Very alone.

Then, there was laughter. Lots of laughter. Laughter and the dead. Laughing at mice, and snakes, choking. There was laughter in that, and in old Hoagie.

"Hoagieeeeeeeeeee. Hoagieeeeeeeeee."

And the baby calf. There was the calf she and Mack brought to the table. She was twelve, thirteen maybe, at the vet's.

"I want to be a vet."

"You. Hey you. You hold the head!"

The vet working, trying to save it. The head is heavy. It's heavier. It's slipping. Dropping it.

"I killed it! God, I killed the calf."

No, it swallowed a plastic bag, the vet said.

But they were laughing. They were all laughing and giggling, she remembered.

"I killed it."

"Hey you. It takes too long to become a vet."

Mack. Laughter. And trust.

"You can trust me," he said.

But she *was* going to love her mother, Mack said.

Fifteen, sixteen years old, maybe: "You hug her and you kiss her and you tell her once a day you love her or I'm gonna beat your ass."

One day. She lasted one day, the girl who refused to be held.

"I'd rather have my ass beat," she said.

And then the two of them, mother and daughter, alone in the field. Fighting. Rolling in the dirt, in the wallow. Hitting her. Hitting her. Hitting her.

Yes, I'm goddamn hateful and stubborn. And I *don't* want to be held.

But Mack, and laughter. She wanted to be like him. She wanted to be like old Mack.

"I'll be reasonable," she told the boy in the neighborhood.

"I'll be reasonable," she told Fran.

But if they weren't, she would kick all their asses.

When Mack left, she wanted to go. She wanted to hunt deer. She wanted to drink whiskey. She wanted to leave Tyler.

California. Mack, here I come!

And there was whiskey. They were drinking. Together. She and old Mack. The Marlboro man. He looked like the Marlboro man.

She passed out, and woke up. Her shirt was off. Mack had his face in her breasts.

"I trusted you! Trusted you, for real."

Running. Hitchhiking up the coast.

And alone, now so alone, every night. Trusting no one. Feeling nothing. Feeling absolutely nothing. A bunch of pieces, floating. In pieces, ready to be sucked down any drain.

And then just a game of chicken. That's all. Drunk one night with a friend. For real! Just a game.

"Bet you can't put a cigarette out on your hand."

Yes.

Afterwards. Better than bets. Feeling. It brought feeling.

Alone, now, another cigarette, again. Feeling. Grounded. Hang on to that point. Hang on to that burning point. My limbs, pierced like Jesus. Healed. In pain there's feeling . . . there's healing in burns, in cuts, in punches to the ribs.

Feelings, and warmth, for the child who refused to be held.

Now alone, again. Locked in the car. The river. The bodies.

Still locked out. Run away! Cross the street!

The little child: A stubborn, hateful brat.

A mother.

"Hold Me. Thrill Me. Kiss Me. Make me tell you I'm in love with you."

"Hold me, Cathy."

"I didn't trust my mom," Gwen said, out loud, later. "I just didn't trust anybody."

Trust—forever, and longer.

The little girl who refused to be held might have done anything for that.

Chapter 57

The smell not only filled Abbey Lane. Some aides claimed they could detect the odor the moment they stepped through Alpine Manor's door.

By April, everyone knew how bad the gangrene on Edith Cook's toes had become. They not only smelled it, they heard Edith. She was pleading throughout the nights with the soft sounds of WOOD-FM.

"Please. Oh please, God, help me!"

Nurses were quick to respond with painkillers. At the age of ninety-seven, Edith Cook was Alpine Manor's reigning grand dame. She was also one of the most popular residents in the nursing home.

> One. Two. Three.
> Grandma caught a flea.
> Flea died.
> Grandma cried.
> One. Two. Three.

Edith used to sing her nursery song to the young aides, instructing them as though they were her little children. But by April, her mind clouded with codeine, Edith now was reciting letters, like a young school girl practicing her spelling. The teacher had become the student. The adult had become the toddler. The parent had become the child. They were familiar transformations in Alpine Manor.

"Please. Oh please, God, help me!"

Since her admission in 1981, Edith Cook had delighted staff. Despite considerable personal tragedy and hardship, she treated her residency as though it were a special privilege. The "social history" in her medical file provided some of the details. The social worker who took it wrote:

> Birth date: November 28, 1889. Committee diagnosis: General arterial sclerosis. Information and social history was given to me by Edith herself.
>
> Background: Edith was born in upper Sandusky, Ohio. She was one of three children. She did have two brothers, Vince and Perry. She was the middle child. She lived in the city with her parents. Her father worked in a furniture store with his brother. He died at the age of 32. Her mother was born in Ohio, and of German descent. She remarried and had one son, Frank.
>
> Edith was married January 28, 1913 to George Cook. He was a salesman. He died in 1940. A year before his death they started a restaurant. She ran it for two years and sold it.
>
> They adopted one child, but the child died at the age of 14 months.
>
> She went through the sixth grade. She also stated she went to trade school for millinery for 12 months. Four years before she got married she worked at Foster Stevens in the silver department.

She belonged to the senior citizens' group and was a registered voter.

Her interest is Bingo.

Medical history: Edith is alert and oriented. She feeds herself and is ambulatory with a cane and some assistance.

Events preceding admission: Edith was living alone. Her brother Frank would stop in and check on her often. She stated she is 92 years old and has no children and when Frank goes to Florida she has no one to look after her, so they began looking and talking about nursing homes.

Edith wasn't worried about coming into the nursing home because, "it is a government institution." [sic] Her feelings are: "This home is grand. The food is wonderful. And everything is all very lovely."

In Alpine, her enthusiasm did not deteriorate with her health. She hiked around the nursing home, visiting staff and holding long conversations with other patients. She attended all the activities.

In 1985, she developed breast cancer, but refused surgery. The carcinoma did not spread. By 1987, she could still stand with assistance, though she mostly was shuttled to and from activities in a wheelchair. In February, she survived the killer flu. Then, one night, a third shift nurse found her lying with her legs through her bed rails. There were indentations on her feet and legs from the bars. Sores developed on her foot.

By mid-March her feet were turning black. By early April, bedsores had appeared on Edith Cook's shoulder and hip. Her appetite was gone. She was losing weight. She weighed only ninety pounds. Some staffers suspected she wasn't being turned by squeamish aides put off by the pungent odor of her dying feet. Gwen Graham received her as a second shift assignment in April's first week.

On April 5, Edith Cook still could sit in a wheelchair for a visit from her nephew's family. They were her only relatives left. Eating, however, had become a difficult proposition for a woman who had always fed herself. Still, she insisted on wearing her upper plate, even keeping her teeth in when she slept.

As the days of April became longer, adding a few more minutes of daylight from the window next to Edith Cook's bed, she relied on staff for meals. A veteran aide later would say she fed Edith her last meal.

"Please. Oh please, God, help me!"
Her name was Cathy Wood.

At the midnight hour, as the morning became April 7, an LPN named *Marianne Conner* dropped by to check the patient in room 219. Edith Cook was spelling words again. Reassuring her in a calm voice, the nurse applied an antibacterial cream called Betadine to her toes.

On third shift, Marianne Conner had three aides working under her on Abbey Lane. They included Gwen Graham and Cathy Wood. Gwen was working the second leg of a double. Cathy was in for her regular shift.

Marianne considered Cathy and Gwen efficient aides, but their positive contribution to the atmosphere in the nursing home ended there. As a team, they constituted one clever bully—Cathy provided the brains; Gwen provided the brawn.

The thirty-six-year-old nurse refused to be intimidated. She would not forget the frightful scars on Gwen's arms or her first and only confrontation with Cathy Wood. Cathy had falsely accused her of making up the name the "Gay Bobs" for Alpine's woman softball team. Marianne had calmly explained she had done no such thing.

"I don't think it's very funny," Cathy said, glaring. "And you're going to be sorry."

Marianne looked her right in the eyes.

"Cathy, you don't scare me. You're not going to control me. I don't want anything to do with you."

From then on, they passed on opposite sides of the hall and discussed only work. Control, Marianne had realized, was what Cathy Wood was all about. She had her big table of friends. "And the select few that didn't buy into her circle of control were outsiders," she later said.

A crafty personality like Cathy Wood, Marianne decided, could flourish in Alpine Manor. After a dozen years of hospital work with the elderly, Marianne had taken the job there in January while her husband started a business and she finished her RN schooling. She would rank her six months in the nursing home as the worst professional experience of her life.

The basic problem was the help.

"There was a lot of people in there that didn't respect themselves," she explained later. "So how are they going to respect anyone else, patients or employees?"

Marianne saw aides who refused to do basic duties. Families who were concerned about loved ones often were dismissed as "bitchers" by both aides and supervisors because they haggled staff about care.

Specific incidents stood out. She found an aide doing his rounds with a radio on his shoulder, blasting music in the early morning hours down the hall. She confronted him. He uttered a litany of expletives. She saw aides throw food at patients who were having trouble eating. She watched others get in pathetic boxing matches with residents over food. She repeatedly intervened and wrote these incidents up for superiors, but never saw results. Only once she did see an aide fired for inappropriate behavior with a patient. The aide was hired back four weeks later.

"I was trying to break my butt for these old people and Alpine just wouldn't stand behind anything," she later recalled.

Ironically, Marianne Conner found the position at Alpine while looking for a nursing home for her father, a stroke victim. After she began working there the family decided not to put him in a facility.

"I'm glad Dad's not there," she told her mother. "The people just don't get good care."

At 2:30 A.M., Cathy Wood approached Marianne Conner with some news about one of her assigned patients. The nurse had just come off her lunch break. Cathy had just come from room 219.

"I think Edith is dead."

Marianne walked briskly to the room. It was on the opposite end of the hallway from the Abbey nursing station. Cathy appeared apprehensive.

"I've never seen a dead person before," she said. "I'm scared to go in."

Edith Cook was flat on her back, her face to the ceiling. She was pale. Her arms were at her sides. Her limbs were still supple, suggesting that if she was dead she had just expired.

As the blood pressure cuff confirmed what Marianne Conner already suspected, she noticed the large figure of Cathy Wood standing in the doorway. She lingered there for a while.

"I've never seen a dead person before," Cathy said again.

Then, as though she had to get up the nerve, she tiptoed to Edith Cook's bedside. She seemed nervous.

"I've never seen a dead person before," she said once more.

In a few moments the Alpine Manor public address sounded with hollow tone of a turned-on microphone.

"House Supervisor to room 219."

One by one, the aides began dropping by the room. Some lingered longer, a tribute to Edith Cook's popularity. Among the visitors was Gwen Graham.

Meanwhile, the assignment of packing up Edith Cook's belongings was given to Cathy Wood. As her body was picked up by the undertaker, one very personal possession was already missing. Marianne Conner didn't notice it, but the mortician did.

Edith Cook was no longer wearing her false teeth.

Chapter 58

They scrawled more letters, words and poems on nurse's notes stationery as they passed time on Abbey Lane, Buckingham, Camelot and Dover.

Cathy had a preference for the secret acronyms. They riddled her letters to Gwen. She could pledge her love and, in the same line, complain about her nails being dirtied by the feces of incontinent patients. It went like this:

Gwen,
I love you! MM—right now, right now, right now. IWK. IWH, IWL, IWCN!! Especially IWCN.

Cathy.

Translation: I love you! Marry Me—right now, right now, right now. I Want Kisses. I Want Hugs, I Want Love, I Want Clean Nails!! Especially I Want Clean Nails.

There were others. OGINYK: Oh Gwen I need your kisses. RN: Right now. WWK: Warm wet kisses.

Gwen, meanwhile, toyed with a new nickname for Cathy—"Rat Woman," an animal image to go with "Bunny Foo Foo," the killer rabbit in the nursery song. Cathy had complained recently about someone snitching on her about nursing home pranks.

"Hand them a piece of cheese," Gwen had told her. "Let 'em know they're a rat."

One night, as the Alpine Manor death count began to drop with the advent of spring, Cathy wrote:

I can love you Gwen
I think your great
For this afternoon
I cannot wait.

That's when we'll wake up &
That's when I'll kiss you
That's when I'll hold you
Oh Gwen I miss you.

Bunny hop
Over here
And let me lick you
On the ear.

I want to get married
Right now right away
Don't make me wait
Till the day.

When you're mine
Oh please say
You'll be mine
Forever and five days.

Gwen's poetry lacked the order of Cathy's. Her verses streamed across the page without stanzas or other forms of poetic organization. But she picked up on the "forever" theme, amplified from its origins with Cathy when Ladonna Sterns quoted the words of a Harlequin romance back in the fall of 1986.

Gwen wrote:

"Just sitting and wishing you were near, so I could kiss your cheek and nibble on your ear. You make me crazy, you make me wet, you make me wanna smile—just think, I can take you home for WWK's in just a little while. When we lie down I want to be in my favorite place, so you can hold me close or even lick my snotty face. Forever and 5 days, yes, I'm happy that it's true, you my little Rat Woman, me, your Bunny Foo Foo."

And, it was true. For a little while longer, at least.

Chapter 59

Gwen saw Katherine Brinkman's car parked a block away from the little house on Effie. Gwen had left work fifteen minutes ahead of Cathy. She turned her orange Volkswagen around in the driveway and headed back up the street.

Gwen stepped from the Bug.

"Whatya think you're doin'?"

"I'm waiting for Cathy," Katherine Brinkman said.

Cathy had been complaining about the aide. Gwen approached her.

"No you're not—waiting. It's time for you to get lost."

Gwen slammed her into the car for emphasis.

A few minutes later, when Cathy came home from work, Gwen confronted her about Katherine Brinkman's waiting up the street. Cathy brought up their agreement about being honest if one of them chose to pursue someone else. Gwen later recalled:

"Cathy goes, 'Well, I've been wanting to talk to you about Katherine Brinkman. I want to go out with her.' I just lost it. I was crying. I was hurt. Not that I had been faithful myself to her, but the fact that she *wanted* to go with her had me really troubled. I begged her not to go."

Cathy agreed.

A few days later, as Gwen, Lisa, Robin and Dawn were drinking in the living room, listening to 45s, when Cathy brainstormed a plan.

"Oooooo I know, I'll get Katherine Brinkman to meet me on K-Mart Hill," she said.

"What is K-Mart Hill?" somebody asked.

Cathy knew the location in detail. She had obviously done some research and given the plan some thought. The hill was just south-west of the K-Mart parking lot on Alpine Avenue. A two-track led up to a bluff there, one that overlooked the I-96 freeway.

"I'll get Katherine to meet me there," she continued, "and Gwen can hide in the bushes."

When she and Katherine arrived at the top of the hill, Gwen could stroll out from the cover. She told Gwen what to say.

"You say, 'Cathy you get on home.' Then, Gwen, you can take care of her."

She didn't mean anything gentle. The scenario would lead Katherine Brinkman to believe she and Cathy had been caught unexpectedly by Gwen. The aide would have to face the consequences with Gwen alone, while also being led to believe that Cathy would be reprimanded later.

"Fuck it," Dawn Male said. "I wanna be there too."

They all would be there. Robin and Lisa would wait in a car in the parking lot. The plan was a trademark Cathy Wood mind game, Dawn later explained to a friend. To all appearances Cathy would appear blameless, when, in fact, she had masterminded the entire scheme.

The only cars left in the K-Mart parking lot belonged to the stock boys when Gwen and Dawn walked up the two-track. They giggled as they walked, blowing warm whiskey-breath into the April night.

On top, the two surveyed the area. There was a clearing. There was a stand of trees. There was some illegally dumped trash. The place was just like Cathy said. They stepped back into a stand of young, twisted wolf trees. A damp spring chill penetrated to the marrow and considerably lengthened their wait.

Finally, they could hear two cars, then voices. There was no mistaking the chatty, singsong delivery of one of the two women ascending K-Mart Hill.

Cathy stopped at the top, pointing out the All-American city that sprawled below her feet. Katherine Brinkman looked at the broad vista of the Grand River valley and the distant glow of downtown. It was a beautiful spot, save for the garbage and the dominating roar of another huge truck that powered by on I-96 just below.

Gwen cracked a twig under her foot as she stepped out of the darkness. Her arms were arced at her sides like a linebacker's.

"Cathy! What are you doin'? Who you with?"

Katherine Brinkman turned to look.

"Cathy! You get on to the house."

Cathy took quick, tiny steps down the hill, her breasts bouncing.

"What are you going to do, beat me up?"

Brinkman's voice had fear.

"That's right, Katherine. I tried to be reasonable. I told you to leave her alone. Apparently you have not. I tried to be reasonable. But if you're not going to be reasonable, then neither am I."

Dawn came out of the trees, talking shit.

"We're not only going to beat you up. We're going to throw what the fuck is left of you down to the freeway."

Gwen pushed Dawn away.

"She's mine!"

Then she let out a guttural scream.

She slammed her knuckles into Katherine Brinkman's rib cage, instantly doubling her over. Then she went to work on her body and her face with a smothering flurry.

In no time, Brinkman was on the ground. Dawn ran up to her body, giving her a couple of swift kicks.

Brinkman lay there sobbing, vomiting, her knees drawn into her breasts. Dawn staggered around in the darkness. Gwen clenched her fists again.

Suddenly, Gwen stopped. She looked at the body below her, then the night vista, then shuffled down the hill.

Dawn Male urged Katherine Brinkman to get on her feet.

"You better get out of here," Dawn said. "She'll kill you."

For several minutes Brinkman couldn't get up. When she did she was met by Gwen Graham halfway down the hill. Gwen was holding her arms out.

"Would you please forgive me?" she said.

Gwen said it again, over and over.

The two of them limped down the hill, Dawn staggering not far behind. Gwen helped the woman into her car. She sat her behind the wheel, pushing a mess of hair away from Katherine Brinkman's bright red cheeks.

"I don't know how to say I'm sorry," Gwen said.

Then she turned away and began walking.

The plan called for Cathy to pick Gwen up, but Gwen wasn't going to be waiting. She was angry, but no longer at Katherine Brinkman. She was angry at Cathy. She walked off into the night alone, heading toward the one-story building on Four Mile Road.

Maybe from Alpine Manor she could find her way home.

Katherine Brinkman told Margaret Widmaier she had snuck in Alpine Manor's back door so no one could see her. She was sitting in Widmaier's office. It was the next day. Her arm was in a sling, her eye was black.

"Gwen Graham did this," she told the assistant director of nursing. "She beat me up on K-Mart Hill."

Besides the lacerations and contusions, she said she had a cracked rib. She had already been treated at a local medical center. Now she needed some time off. Widmaier granted her request.

When the aide did return to work, she told everyone she was sitting in a tree when she was hit in the eye by the ball of a spring golfer. Reportedly, one of Brinkman's friends showed up at Alpine Manor during third shift a couple nights later, looking for Gwen Graham. He had a baseball bat with him, but Gwen had the night off.

Margaret Widmaier confronted Gwen and asked whether she had assaulted the aide.

"Margaret," Gwen said.

She beamed a childish grin.

"You don't think I'd do something like that?"

Chapter 60

The old woman was walking down Camelot in a stutter step, paging in a bad lisp what sounded like an Indian name.

"Yabahoo Cooch. Yabahoo Cooch."

No one on second shift had any idea who or what the patient was talking about, except Robin Fielder. "Yabahoo" was a family code word for breasts. "Cooch," was Gwen's term for a woman's lower privates. Gwen had put them together as a screwy nickname for Robin when she wanted to find her in Alpine Manor. Once, she paged her that way on the house public address.

Poor old Ruth, Robin thought. She looked like a caricature of a bellboy in the lobby of a geriatric hotel as she walked along making the page.

"Yabahoo Cooch. Yabahoo Cooch."

Still, she couldn't help but chuckle. Gwen was such a joker. She liked that about her. She always made her laugh. She was always "pickin'," as Gwen called it, or pulling her leg. Most of the time she didn't know when to take her seriously.

Robin also would not argue with what her friends always said. She could easily be had.

"Yes, I was naive and stupid," she later told a friend.

Add to that gullible and trusting. Too many cheerleading practices and not enough reality training, she figured. That was just one more reason she needed to get out of her parents' protective nest and face the world on her own.

And, what a world it was. Robin knew she was falling deeper in love with the girl from Texas with the childlike smile. Spring brought an exhilaration to the affair. While Cathy worked, they snuck out together for midnight drives. While Cathy slept, they visited parks and the Grand Rapids Zoo.

Robin tried to block out the troubling aspects, not only the presence of Cathy, but incidents like the trip to K-Mart Hill. She saw Katherine Brinkman return from the mount, badly beaten. That side of Gwen scared her.

"I can't believe this is happening," Robin had told Lisa Lynch as they waited in the K-Mart parking lot. "I can't believe we're here doing this."

Robin, however, believed Gwen would never harm her. Cathy Wood, she decided, was the source of the violence. The scratches on Gwen's back had disappeared after Gwen asked Cathy to stop, at Robin's urging. But Cathy still has her claws into Gwen, Robin thought. She so easily convinced her to beat up Katherine Brinkman. Gwen was always so ready to please Cathy, to protect her. Afterwards Cathy gloated about the whole affair around Alpine Manor, as though she were saying, "I can get Gwen to do anything I want."

Robin thought, Cathy not only easily involved Gwen, she involved the rest of us as well. I was there. What was I doing there? Cathy's calculating games seem to have an intrigue and magnetism all their own.

Later, Robin felt ashamed she had had any part of it.

Robin wondered what Cathy would do if she ever found out about her liaison with Gwen. Sometimes, she wondered if she already had. There was a rumor going around Alpine Manor that Cathy already knew. Cathy, the story went, had bummed a ride home early from work with another aide and spotted Robin and Gwen speeding away from Effie together in the Luv Truck.

One night in late April, Robin became even more suspicious that Cathy was planning to hurt her. Robin found Gwen waiting for her in the Family Food's parking lot across Four Mile Road. As they sat together in Robin's Mustang, Gwen appeared depressed. Robin could see tears as she looked into her eyes.

"Robin," she said. "I love you."

"I love you too."

"But there's something I *have* to tell you."

A tear ran down Gwen's cheek.

"I killed six people."

"You killed six people?"

Robin found herself repeating the words. She found the proposition so incredible she didn't know what else to say. Robin thought, what did she mean: She *had* to tell me?

"I killed six people. I'm sorry I did it. But I did."

Robin began to cry with her. Somebody in tears always started her own waterworks. They held each other.

"No you didn't," Robin said. "You didn't kill anybody."

Cathy, Robin thought. Yes, Cathy. Who else? She *had* to tell me. Cathy has put her up to this, just like she put Gwen up to Katherine Brinkman. Cathy knows about us and she is making Gwen say this crazy thing for revenge.

"I killed them," Gwen said again.

"No you didn't."

"Yes I did."

"All right, who did you kill?"

Gwen named them. She named six in all. They were former Alpine Manor patients, names Robin Fielder knew quite well. Then Gwen held her face in her hands and said it again.

"Robin, I love you. I really do."

Her wet face was like a cherub's, all puffy and full of an earnest innocence.

My God, Robin thought, is there no end to Cathy's games? This was morbid. This was cruel. She was obviously being forced to tell her this against her will. What kind of twisted game was this? What did Cathy have on Gwen to make her say this?

She would elicit no answers from Gwen, only more of the odd mix of love and confession.

"I love you Robin."

"I know. I love you too."

"I love you, but I did it."

"No you didn't."

"I did."

"Shhhh. No you didn't."

Soon, she was quiet. They sat there for a long time, just holding one another in the car. Cathy is not hurting me, Robin thought. She's hurting Gwen.

On a Friday evening, a couple of weeks later, on May Day, Robin was playing quarters at Lisa Lynch's when she reached for the ringing telephone. It was Gwen, calling from second shift at Alpine Manor to say hello to everyone, as well as to deliver some news.

"Lucille Stoddard is dead," she said.

The seventy-year-old patient had been close to death for days. She had passed away minutes ago, around 8:00 P.M., in the middle of second shift.

"Well, is she one you did in too?" Robin said.

The words came spontaneously. For some time, their talk at Family Foods had been nagging her.

"No," Gwen said, giggling. "You gonna think that now every time somebody dies?"

"No, not now," Robin said.

She was laughing, too. Now she was sure of it. The whole matter had been some kind of sick joke.

Chapter 61

As the days became warmer, Gwen Graham cooled to Cathy Wood, increasingly complaining to Robin and others that she was tiring of her partner's mood swings and destructive vendettas.

One night a half a dozen in the group were at Cathy's house, drinking and spinning 45s into the night. A slew of doubles behind them, everyone was dancing. Inspired by the revelry, one Alpine aide jumped up on a cluttered coffee table, twisting to the music. Everyone circled around her.

Cathy went into hysterics.

"Get out of my house," she screamed. "Get out! And don't ever come back!"

The room was silent, save for the 45 spinning.

"All of you," she screamed again. "All of you out!"

She shooed everyone toward the door like a bunch of chickens. Gwen sat on the couch, red-faced.

"I was too embarrassed to say anything," she later said. "There was no point of arguing with Cathy. She did what she did simply because she wanted to. And I wasn't about to ask her to apologize to anybody, because I knew she would never do that."

Gwen, like others, began to resent Cathy's high-handed behavior at Alpine Manor as well. In early May, despite strong protests from shift supervisor Tish Prescott, Cathy was promoted. She was made "charge tech," a rank just above nurse's aide. Though the nursing home would later deny it, a third shift RN named Sue Davis told one interviewer that Cathy was promoted because of her reputation for verbal abuse. Her new job required less hands-on care.

"Cathy Wood was made charge tech to get her away from patients," Davis said.

The position gave Cathy official clout. She became more demanding. She belittled other aides. She made room checks, piling patient's clothes outside the doors of rooms she decided were not tidy enough. She threw temper tantrums, once flinging a patient's eating tray down the hall. An Alpine RN named Robert Decker later gave a detailed report of her management style.

"She would come over to my station and say, 'What are you doing? I just have to cause some trouble.' And that's the truth, she would. She liked to get things stirred up. She liked to see a lot of people upset, and that would make her day.

"She would come over to somebody else's station and start nagging one of the aides about their not doing their job, and that aide would go to their nurse, their nurse would go to Cathy. It would be a big emotional mess. Everybody's yelling at everybody else. Then she would walk away like that's all she wanted was to stir up a little excitement."

She also knew how to nurture allies. Once, when Decker wrote Cathy up to supervisors for the divisive behavior, a charge nurse tore up the report right in front of him.

"Cathy Wood used to do the charge nurse's work on third shift so she was really tight with her," he later complained.

Superiors were not spared her tirades. One Sunday in late May, when help was short, she refused to give a patient a bedpan simply because the woman wasn't one of her patients. After the woman lay in her own excrement for two hours, Cathy lambasted with profanity the RN who reported her. She told Tish Prescott she would retaliate for the write-up by not showing up for work. By June she had received a warning for chronic absenteeism.

Nurses and supervisors later recalled that Cathy Wood was written up repeatedly for insubordination and inappropriate behavior.

Many of the disciplinary reports, however, mysteriously disappeared or were never included in her employee file.

Cathy was also building a thick personnel record of nursing home "incident reports." She frequently reported accidents: Slips and falls. Back strains. Mysterious bruises and cuts on her hands and wrists. Odd accidents resulting in injured fingers. A patient running over her toe with her chair.

Over a two-year period, she reported seven attacks by patients. One patient scratched her left hand. Another bit her index finger. One kicked her in the chest. Another slugged her in the jaw. One resident reached out of his wheelchair and frantically flailed at her with his fists. One family would protest to the house supervisor that their loved-one was always complaining of Cathy's rough handling.

Cathy Wood's accumulation of patient incidents was well above the typical Alpine aide's. Cathy had ten times as many as Gwen Graham, for example, who had a total of two. Gwen reported suffering a sore left wrist in the deadly days of late February. She offered no explanation for the injury. Earlier, she had strained her shoulder as she caught a falling patient.

Gwen was first depressed, then angry, that she didn't get a charge tech promotion like Cathy's, which also meant a wage increase from $3.40 to $4.00 an hour. She complained to Robin Fielder and others that she deserved the raise. Few would argue she wasn't the harder worker and less divisive among the staff.

In early June, Gwen gave notice to Alpine Manor that she was leaving. Based on a solid recommendation by Margaret Widmaier at Alpine, a temporary service called Portamedic hired Gwen. The agency siphoned a lot of Alpine staff. It paid $2 more an hour than the $3.60 Gwen made at the nursing home. She took the last week of June as vacation. She was scheduled to begin her new assignment on the first of July.

Gwen's vacation was complicated by Cathy's continuing domestic disputes with Ken. Their divorce was finalized on May 1. But the ongoing phone battle between Gwen and Ken had escalated into more insults and crank calls. On a warm June 24 evening it exploded into drunken violence. Ken called Cathy, complaining she was ignoring her daughter. Gwen grabbed the phone from Cathy.

"Look it. If you ever come around here again I'm going to take care of you."

Ken went drinking with a couple of friends at a bar called

Miller's Cave, but he didn't forget the threat. By the end of the night, he was ramming the rear end of Gwen's orange Volkswagen with his car. When the police arrived he had his hand through the screen door, trying to grab Gwen. She had a baseball bat. They cuffed him. He exploded into a drunken hysteria. They booked him on a misdemeanor.

"This isn't over," he vowed, as he was dragged to the cruiser. "This isn't over by a long shot."

After he sobered up in jail, police told Ken that Cathy said she had obtained a court injunction preventing him from even driving on Effie Street. She later boasted at Alpine Manor that she had set him up to be arrested. She boasted she had obtained an injunction. Court records later revealed she had done no such thing.

Turmoil flourished around virtually everything Cathy Wood did. Citing her past experience with Ken, she took over as the manager of the Alpine softball team. The squad practiced or played weekly, then gathered at Cathy's house or Lisa Lynch's. Afterwards, everyone needed a good stiff drink.

Cathy piloted the squad with Machiavellian fervor. During practices, Cathy and Gwen frequently had shouting matches in the middle of the diamond. Gwen wanted to improve play. Cathy was caught up in dishing out childish punishments for those who made mistakes. For example, if an infielder missed a grounder, she had to pirouette while holding her hands on her head.

"C'mon, now do it," she would say. "Turn. Turn. Turn."

Gwen muttered and kicked the dirt. Others obliged.

"Oh, you're so cuuuuute," she would say.

Cathy, however, followed no rules or suggestions. She defiantly walked to first base. She was always thrown out, despite smacking balls into the outfield. Gwen would complain. Then they would bicker some more. Gwen's old partner, Fran Shadden, attended a practice or two.

"She yelled at Gwen a lot," Fran later told a friend. "And when I showed up she kept her eyes glued on her. Even though we had broken up, and were still friends, she wasn't allowed to talk to me very much. It was: You can look, but you can't talk."

After two practices, Fran called it quits.

"Maybe I had pulled away from the lifestyle too much," she later recalled. "I had started going to church and getting my life together. I mean they were adults, but they weren't acting like adults.

They were still trying to be these teenagers. I remember leaving there, and thinking as I left, you know these people are really strange."

Gwen also was having a lot of second thoughts—about softball, about Grand Rapids, about the partner she had pledged to love beyond forever.

"I'm just sick of her hurtin' so many people," she told Robin Fielder. "I'm just sick of people gettin' hurt all the time."

By the games of summer, Gwen was looking for a way out.

Chapter 62

Robin swayed back and forth in the Luv Truck, watching the traffic as Gwen sped east on Four Mile Road toward the Grand River, into Cathy's old haunts in Comstock Park.

"There's Cathy's house," Robin said, as they passed the white farmhouse.

Robin thought they were going on a little joy ride on a windy summer afternoon. But Gwen was brooding. Gwen was speeding.

"Gwen, slow down."

"I've got to find those letters."

"What letters?"

"The letters that Cathy wrote."

Robin told her she was talking in riddles.

Gwen never took her eyes off the road.

"Gwen, what kind of letters?"

"Letters about the murders."

"*Gwen,*" Robin scolded.

She thought, not this mind game again.

"I've just got to find those letters," Gwen said again.

The truck turned up a steep side street off West River Drive and pulled off the berm. Without pausing, Gwen threw the truck in park, jumped out and began climbing a set of ivy-choked steps heading up a wooded hill.

"Gwen, wait."

Robin jogged to catch up.

They were at the old Mill Creek Cemetery, a small, isolated graveyard with pitted stones dating back to the mid 1800s. The graves were staggered up the hill, some choked with poison ivy. Landscaping and shadows from a canopy of oak and sassafras gave the place the atmosphere of a Gustave Doré illustration for Dante's *Inferno.*

"Gwen, please wait."

Robin tried to catch up. She thought, I know this place. Cathy had shown them the graveyard. She told scary stories of being taken there on school outings. She seemed fascinated with the cemetery.

Gwen stopped at the top of the hill, in a clearing bordered by wild briar. Her eyes were on the ground. She paced back and forth like a caged bear in the zoo.

"Gwen, why are we here? What are we doing here?"

"I got to get them letters."

"Why?"

" 'Cause Cathy says she wrote everything down. Everything about the murders. *Everything.* Then she sent it all out in three letters."

Robin asked herself, why must they continue on playing this game? In a cemetery, no less. She decided to play along. Maybe that would stop it.

"Well, why should you care?"

"Cathy threatened me. She said she sent the letters to her post office box, to her sister and to somebody on the softball team. She said, 'If anything ever happens to me, if I'm ever hurt, if I'm ever killed, they'll have letters.' Robin, I *got* to get those letters!"

Gwen's eyebrows nearly met with frustration.

Robin wasn't buying it. This sounds just like Cathy, she thought, something lifted from one of her books. She looked at the old gravestones and thought, if this wasn't so transparent, I could get angry at all this murder bullshit.

A few minutes later they passed Cathy's old house again, then her high school. Gwen drove by the post office. Finally, she parked the truck where they played softball and gazed out at the diamond.

"I wonder who it was," she said. "I wonder who it was on the team. I've got to get those letters."

She seemed to be talking as though Robin wasn't there. That didn't matter. From now on, Robin decided she was going to ignore that kind of talk anyway.

By summer, Robin Fielder was fed up with all the gamesmanship. The most recent mind game she had taken part in she vowed would be her last.

Robin, Gwen, Cathy and another Alpine aide had gone to the beach together. It was the same girl who had danced on Cathy's table at the party. When they returned, Cathy pulled Robin and Gwen aside.

"I'll bet if we leave Gwen alone with her, she'll jump at the chance if Gwen takes her in the bedroom," Cathy said. "We'll go to the store Robin, and Gwen you see if you can do it."

"No, Cathy," Robin said. "Not this time."

"C'mon, it won't hurt anything. Let's see what she does. Let's just see how she reacts."

Finally, Robin and Gwen agreed to the scheme.

"You're both so cuuuute," she said.

Sure enough, when they returned Gwen and the girl were in the bedroom. They were sitting on the bed. Cathy threw a fit. The aide left quickly, humiliated. Cathy was exhilarated. Robin later wondered if it wasn't a payback for stealing the center of attention at one of Cathy's gatherings.

Cathy Wood, Robin decided, played for keeps.

This realization frightened Robin. Cathy *had* to know what was going on between Robin and Gwen.

After one midsummer night of drinking at the Carousel, the insanity appeared to reach its peak.

Brooding over a couple of Jack Daniel's, Gwen then bought a hit of LSD from a lesbian with a large tattoo across her breasts. Her last acid trip had been years ago in high school. She had hallucinated for days. She had tried to hold a friend's little baby. Its head had melted in her hands. She had tried to take a shower. She had melted, and was nearly consumed by the drain.

Robin had no idea Gwen was tripping, but she knew they all had more than their share of drink when the three of them left together. Just a few blocks from downtown, Gwen yelled.

"Stop, let me out!"

She jumped out of Cathy's pickup and began walking down the street.

"C'mon back," Robin said, catching up with her on foot.

"Look it," Gwen yelled. "I'll do what I want."

Cathy screeched to a stop next to them. She sauntered out, grabbed Gwen by the back of her hair like an errant puppy and dragged her back to the truck.

"Don't you *ever* do that again," Cathy said.

Cathy ordered Gwen to sit in the middle.

Fifteen minutes later, they were headed north on Walker Avenue toward Robin's house, when Gwen climbed over Robin and jumped from the truck at an intersection. Cathy jumped out and caught Gwen at the back of the truck. They broke into a full-scale fistfight. Robin heard a guttural scream. She saw hatred in Gwen's eyes. It was the first and last time she ever saw her look like that. Gwen tore into Cathy. Cathy simply picked her up and threw her into the truck bed like a sack of grain. Cathy climbed into the truck bed and yelled to Robin.

"Go. Take off! Take off!"

When the speedometer hit 30 the fighting started again. In the mirror Robin could see the two of them swinging and wrestling. As they rolled around the Luv Truck swayed from side to side.

"Drive," Cathy kept yelling. "Drive."

She was on top of Gwen, beating her. Then Gwen was on her feet.

"Stop," Cathy yelled.

Robin panicked and sped up. She turned to see Gwen hanging on to the side wall with one hand. Her upper body swung out over the road as Robin made a turn. Her shirt was ripped open. Her shirt was off. Her shirt flew away in the night. Her hair was straight back. Her eyes were glazed, staring into the darkness.

Cathy scrambled forward to the cab window on her hands and knees.

"Stop, goddamnit. Stop. Goddamnit, Robin will you stop!"

When she hit the brakes, Gwen leaped from the truck and took off running up a hill.

Robin and Cathy paused to catch their breath.

"Where is she?" Cathy asked.

"Somewhere up there."

Robin pointed at the cemetery. They were in front of Mount Calvary Cemetery.

The two of them searched. Robin probed a thick section of stunted trees and brush north of the grave sites. Halfway up the hill she found her. Gwen was squatting, huddling in a moon shadow, a breast exposed, her fists clenched under her chin. Her eyes were black.

"Go away," she whispered. "Go away. Go away."

Suddenly, Cathy came crashing through the brush. She grabbed Gwen by the hair again, led her to the Luv Truck and pushed her into the seat.

Gwen sat very still, but pled in a small, helpless voice.

"Let me out of here. Let me go. *Please Cathy.* Let me outta here. Oh Cathy, *please* let me go."

A mile up the road, Cathy dropped Robin off at her parents' house. Robin stood in her driveway for a few moments and watched them leave.

Gwen was still pleading as the Luv Truck turned away into the night.

Chapter 63

The argument started at the end of a softball game in late July. The Alpine Manor team had lost every game. Words led to threats and threats led to slaps. Half the team was watching when Gwen slapped Cathy in the face.

"You said you'd never, ever hit me," Cathy said.

She was holding her cheek.

"You're right," Gwen said.

Cathy slapped her back, across the face. Gwen turned to walk away. Cathy grabbed her by the back of the hair and pulled her back.

"Don't you *ever* walk away from me like that."

She marched Gwen over to her Luv Truck.

"Now get in!"

Earlier, Gwen had spoken to Lisa Lynch, who had offered a place to stay if she needed it.

"Cathy was just never going to stop being miserable no matter what," Gwen later recalled. "I tried everything and I was tired of trying. She wouldn't stop fucking with people. It mattered to her. She wouldn't stop. I said, 'Why can't we live our own life and stop fucking with people?' . . . And it was really hard, 'cause I was really in love with Robin and I wanted to leave Cathy but I couldn't."

Cathy also had been talking about suicide. Several times Gwen found her sulking alone in Riverside Park. The night Gwen took the LSD, she found Cathy lying in the back of her own pickup outside the Carousel. She was weeping.

On their way home from the ball diamond, Cathy picked up Jamie. Cathy had three vacation days scheduled. For the first time since Cathy and Gwen were together, she was going to have her daughter spend a couple of nights.

Gwen told Cathy her plans when they got back to the little house on Effie. Then she went into the bedroom and packed.

Ken picked up the phone. Cathy was crying.

"I'm going to have to bring Jamie home. Gwen's leaving, Ken."

"What?"

"She's leaving. Gwen's leaving."

When she dropped off their daughter she told him more. She said Gwen was running off with Robin Fielder, the same girl she had found her with in the closet six months earlier.

"Now I know how you felt, Ken. Now I know how you felt when I left you."

After she drove off, Ken was angry. He thought, how could she even make the comparison? No, you don't know how I felt. You don't know how I felt when you used to come over and tell me about the girls who wanted to marry you. You don't know how I feel now seeing you weep over Gwen. You have shed no tears for us, for our seven years together, for our daughter Jamie.

Cathy's tears, Ken Wood thought, were only for herself.

Chapter 64

A few days later, Robin Fielder joined Gwen by moving into Lisa Lynch's mobile home. She was twenty-one and taking her first step into real independence, but there were few feelings of newfound freedom. Robin couldn't shake the feeling they all were being watched.

"It was as though you could sense her presence, her power all around," Robin later told a friend. "It was like a dark cloud was hanging over Lisa's place."

In fact, Cathy Wood was watching. She parked her black truck on the road that overlooked the mobile home park. She cruised by the trailer at night. She called repeatedly, wanting to talk to Gwen. One day, Gwen complained to everybody, she found Cathy standing silently at the foot of her bed when she awoke.

Gwen was making plans to return to Texas in late August. She had a court date pending. A lawsuit she had filed over her last traffic accident was finally up on the docket. Gwen's Volkswagen had finally given up the ghost. Gwen was driving Robin's Mustang to her job with Portamedic and shuttling Robin to and from Alpine Manor for second shift.

One evening just before midnight, Robin left Alpine to meet Gwen, only to find Cathy's Luv Truck idling outside. Cathy approached slowly as Robin walked toward the parking lot.

"*Robin,*" she said, sweetly drawing out the word. "Can I talk to you a second?"

Robin's stomach jumped.

"Are you going to Texas with Gwen?"

"Yes, I think so."

Cathy's tone changed instantly.

"Robin, what if I tell your parents you're gay?"

Cathy smirked, holding her hands together in front of her.

"Go right ahead. 'Cause they'll find out one day anyway."

"You don't care? That wouldn't bother you?"

"No, but I'll tell them when I think they need to know."

The threat transformed Robin's feelings from fear to anger. She thought, how dare she? How dare she threaten to hurt my parents?

Cathy kept probing.

"What if I told you I could put her away for a long time?"

"Put her where?"

"Put her in prison. What if I did. Would you wait for her?"

"I'd wait for her because she's worth waiting for. Besides, you can't do that anyway."

"Oh, yes I can."

"Cathy, you couldn't."

"What if I told you Gwen and I killed some people?"

Robin was still steaming about her parents. Now this sick mind game. She pointed her finger right in Cathy's face.

"Cathy, I'm sick of your head games. You're not fooling me on this one. This is ridiculous. This is crazy. You're crazy! You're not going to play any more mind games with me. You just want Gwen all to yourself."

"That's right, and what if *I* come to Texas?"

"What?"

"What if *I* came to Texas and found you? I know you know that I'm real smart, and I can find you *anywhere*. What if I come and kill you and Gwen?"

"You wouldn't. You're jealous."

"Just don't be surprised if you see me knocking at your door. I'll kill you. And I'll kill Gwen."

Gwen pulled up in the Mustang. Cathy became matter-of-fact.

"Can I talk to Gwen?"

"I don't own her. I don't own her like you did. She can talk to you if *she* wants."

Robin sat in the Mustang as Gwen joined Cathy in her Luv Truck. When she returned she was crying.

"I love you, and I always will," Gwen said. "But I have to go with Cathy now. I have to go talk with her."

She handed Robin her key ring. The two of them drove off into the night.

Later, she noticed a little purple heart, her key ring charm, was missing. She thought, where could that have gone?

The next day Robin woke to a pounding hangover. She had downed a half bottle of vodka after driving home alone. Drunk, she had called Gwen's sister Corey in Texas, telling her about Cathy's threats. The last thing she remembered was Lisa calming her down as she tucked her into bed.

"It's just a game," Lisa said. "Another stupid mind game by Cathy."

Gwen looked in no better shape when she returned to the trailer in the afternoon. Her eyes were red, her cheeks puffy. Cathy waited in her truck outside. Robin and Lisa watched as she packed her suitcase.

"Where's my gun?" Gwen said. "Give me my gun."

Robin and Lisa had hidden it. They didn't want her to take the rifle. Gwen looked withdrawn and depressed. She demanded the weapon. Gwen left with the suitcase in one hand and the Mann-licher-Carcano rifle in the other.

Later, when Cathy was at work, Gwen called. She called several times over the course of a week. Sometimes Lisa listened as well.

"Why don't you come home?" Robin asked.

"I can't," Gwen said. "Cathy has something on me. She won't let me."

"Is Cathy going to take you to jail?"

"No, she just has something. I can't talk about it."

Over the next few days, Gwen visited a couple of times as well, alone, while Cathy was at work. She looked frightened.

"I want outta there," she said. "And I will come back. I just can't right now. I just can't."

One night Gwen phoned from Cathy's with a series of questions. She didn't seem to be herself.

"When did you have sex with Paul?" she asked.

"Gwen, why are you asking this? You know I didn't."

"You had sex, didn't you? You don't care for me. You just want to break me and Cathy up."

She started saying insensitive things, cruel things. Robin fell to her knees, crying.

"Damn it Gwen," Lisa said, grabbing the phone. "Why are you doing this to her?"

Then, not even a week after she left, Gwen returned to Lisa's. She brought back her gun and her suitcase.

"It's okay," she told Robin. "It's over between me and Cathy. We're just gonna be friends."

Gwen said she planned to appease Cathy with social visits and trips to the movies, until Robin and Gwen could leave for Texas for Gwen's court date and put some miles between the two of them and Cathy.

Later that day, Robin noticed Gwen's back. It was covered with deep scratches, the worst yet. Gwen then told Robin and Lisa some of the details about her stay at Cathy's. She said Cathy was standing over her when she made the phone call to Robin, ordering her to say the cruel things. Cathy was beside herself with jealousy, she said. Cathy tied her up in bed and tried to smother her with a pillow.

"Then she took my gun and stuck it up my cooch," Gwen said.

"She *what?*" Robin said.

"Yep, she stuck it right up there," she said. "It was cold, and I was scared. Sure was."

Robin couldn't believe anyone would do such a thing.

"I thought I was dead for real," Gwen continued. "I'm telling you the girl was upset that I was leaving."

Robin thought, no wonder she was gone for a week.

Chapter 65

Ken Wood received the call from Cathy on a balmy Friday night in early August. Gwen Graham had just tried to move back with her, she said, but she wanted her out of her life.

"Ken," she said. "I just don't want us to be together anymore."

A week ago she was heartsick, he thought. More emotional flip-flopping. What else is new. He listened anyway.

"Ken, we've done things. We've done things I'm ashamed of. Actually, I'm afraid to get back together with her."

"Things? What kind of things?"

"Well, we stole a lawn mower."

And eggs. A mower and eggs. Cathy wouldn't necessarily be ashamed of that. He could sense she wanted to tell him more. He prodded her again. He thought, she's reaching out for help.

"Cathy. Just what things did you guys do?"

"Well, you can't tell anybody."

"Oh c'mon, I want an answer."

"Ken, you have to promise *never* to tell anybody."

"Cathy, you know me. Look it, I promise. I just want to help. I won't tell anybody."

"No matter what?"

"No matter what."

There were several seconds of silence.

"Well, okay. What's the *worst* thing you could think of to do?"

Ken thought for a few moments. Well, murder. Murdering somebody was the worst thing anybody could do, without a doubt. But she doesn't mean *that*.

He told her anyway, just to rule it out.

"Murdering somebody, Cathy. Murder. That's the worst."

There was a pause. Then she said it.

"Well, Ken, try *six* times."

He thought, take it back. Take it back Cathy.

"Cathy, no. You didn't."

"Yes."

And, Lord Jesus, he knew at once it was true.

She continued matter-of-factly.

"Look Ken, I don't want to talk about this on the phone. I want to talk face-to-face."

"Well, come over here. Come over here quick."

He headed for the door. He would meet her outside. He had to get some air.

He paced back and forth in front of his apartment building. Holy shit, he thought. They've been murdering people. They've been murdering people at those crazy parties. He had suspected for months an awful confession like this. He had clues: The bodies around Cathy's bed. The *Phantom* music on her answering machine. Her hints on his couch. Gwen's death threat. The fight! The way they had tried to kill him during the fight.

He saw the black Luv Truck. She already was talking as they

walked toward the door. They had killed patients at Alpine Manor, she said. They had murdered the very ill.

"I told my sister," Cathy said calmly as they walked up the steps to his unit. "I told Barb."

"Did she believe you?"

He couldn't close his door fast enough.

"Well, Ken, I didn't tell her the whole truth."

She sat down on his couch. He plopped down in a chair, stunned again.

"I only told Barb that I knew Gwen was killing people at Alpine Manor. That's not true."

"Why?"

"It wasn't the truth, because I helped."

As she talked she stared into the distance. Her eyes became glassy, and very dark. It was the vacant look Ken knew well. She began talking about a patient Ken would later remember being named Margaret. Gwen had smothered her with washcloths, Cathy said. She put one of them under her chin. The other was rolled and placed over her nose.

Ken looked at the carpet. He couldn't bring himself to look at her face. Murderer, he thought. My wife is a murderer. Or, is she? She only watched. Gwen is the murderer. No, Cathy stood guard. She helped. She was involved. She *is* involved.

One part of him couldn't believe what he was hearing. The other knew it all made sense. Suddenly, he remembered what she had told him years ago: "Ken, I wonder what it's like to stab somebody." Now she knew what it was like to kill.

She explained she was sharing this secret for a reason.

"If I tell you this I know I won't go back."

"What do you mean?"

"I won't go back with Gwen. I know if I tell you I will never go back again with Gwen. Because, I'm afraid I'll go back."

She pointed to her neck, to a hickey.

"Where do you think this came from?"

Gwen was over that very night to pick up some mail, she said. They had sex, she said. She couldn't resist, she added. This way, by telling him, she could free herself. Their secret had been their bond of love.

"Jesus, Cathy."

She continued with more murder details, but he was numb to

shock now. She told him about a supervisor named Tish who almost found out. She told him about stalking the nursing home, marking total care patients for death. They picked people who wouldn't be a threat if they survived. Nobody believed the patients in Alpine Manor anyway, she said.

Then she told him about M-U-R-D-E-R. The name of the first victim, Margaret. That was the letter, M. They were going to spell a homicidal acronym with the victims' names, but they hadn't been able to arrange it.

She talked about people and situations and gave names. She mentioned one patient who was suffering before they killed her, an old woman named Edith.

"That was a mercy killing," Cathy said. "She was in terrible condition."

That's right, Ken thought. They were suffering. A mercy killing. These were mercy killings. They were old. He imagined the victims in comas. Or, they were asleep. They had been killed in their sleep. They never knew what happened to them. Maybe it was for the best.

He found himself negotiating with the truth, trying to make excuses for her.

"Look it Cathy," he said. "This is awful. But you've been through an awful time. You're confused. You haven't killed anybody, either. You felt sorry for these people. You're just messed-up. You need help. All this is because you don't know what kind of life you want to live. You don't know what's going on in your life."

"Oh no," she said, drawing out the word.

She snapped out of her glazed stare and looked at him almost incredulously. She was patronizing, even flippant.

"No, Ken, that's not right," she said. "We did it because it was fun."

He was speechless.

He put her to bed after that. She slept soundly. He was up the entire night. He entertained the idea that she had fabricated the story, but he couldn't make the theory stick. Cathy left the next morning. He was too upset to go to work.

By Saturday night they were on the phone again. She had to get help, he said. She had to see a professional.

"Cathy, there are groups, there are organizations that can help you. You gotta contact somebody. Maybe a psychologist can help you. You gotta get some perspective on this."

Maybe, he thought, perspective will give her courage, so she can go to the police. Somebody had to go to the police.

"Police," Cathy said. "Ken, if you turn me into the police I'll do something. I'll kill myself."

He had given her his word.

Later, he saw a report on CNN about a homosexual nurse's aide in southern Ohio named Donald Harvey, accused of killing more than twenty patients in a Cincinnati hospital. "He builds up tension in his body, so he kills people," a prosecutor said. Ken was enthralled. Gwen killed to "relieve her tension," Cathy had said. Then, the CNN report continued, Harvey began poisoning his enemies and people who posed any threat.

Ken thought, maybe I'm in danger. Only I know the truth. What if Gwen and Cathy get back together. What if they kill me next?

By Sunday, he was crazy with confusion. He had to tell somebody. He had to get some guidance. He was torn between his word to Cathy, his own fears and the civic duty to turn her in to the police.

Dr. Elders, he thought, Dr. Darrell Elders. He would call his old therapist and marriage counselor, the psychologist Cathy had seen once. A psychologist takes an oath of confidentiality. He won't tell anyone, so I won't be breaking my word. He will know what to do. He told the therapist's answering service his call was an emergency. The psychologist called back that night.

Dr. Elders wondered if Cathy might be lying.

Ken thought, yes, she *is* a liar. Cathy has always been a liar. But she's not lying. Cathy only lies to make herself look good. Here, that's not the case. So it has to be true.

"I'm pretty sure they did it," he said.

"Well, make an appointment," he said. "Let's talk more."

Ken was in the psychologist's office early the next day.

"I didn't think you'd be in so soon," the therapist began.

Ken was angry.

"Whatya mean, so soon! I just told you about my wife admitting to killing six people, and Jesus, I wanna talk about it."

When Ken left, he still was confused. The therapist had offered a number of possible scenarios, but given very little advice. He remembered one quite clearly.

"Look it, you told me about her lying all the time," he said. "You have no proof. If you go to the police and that's the case, you might feel pretty foolish. You better have your ducks in order before you go.''

No, he wasn't going to the police, he finally decided, but not because he did not believe her. Cathy will eventually go to the police. If all this doesn't force her to get some professional help, nothing will. One way or the other, he was going to guide her to her own salvation.

That's when the migraine headaches began.

Chapter 66

Lisa Lynch was waking from a nap when Gwen and Robin staggered into her bedroom and plopped on the edge of her bed. She could see and smell where they had been all afternoon.

"You guys," she chided. "You guys just came from the bar."

"Yep, for real," Gwen said.

"What's goin' on?"

Gwen became emotional. She told her she wanted to go back to Texas, but couldn't.

"I'm lookin' for some papers," she said. "Cathy has got some papers on me and she won't let me leave the state."

Lisa rubbed the sleep from her eyes.

"What kind of papers?"

"My brother and I did an armed robbery, and Cathy's got the information. She put it in letters and sent 'em."

Robin interjected.

"Gwen, I thought you said those letters were about killing patients."

Gwen turned and looked at Robin as though she were crazy.

Lisa looked at them both.

"Patients?"

After a year at Alpine Manor, months of keeping her best friend Robin's secrets and an onslaught of mind games from Cathy Wood, little surprised Lisa Lynch anymore, even at the young age of twenty-one. She also knew if Cathy Wood was involved, truth was a relative term.

"Whatya mean, papers?" she asked Gwen again.

"Well, if I leave, Cathy will tell everybody that I was going around killing patients."

"Like who?"

"Like Edith Cook."

Gwen explained Cathy was using the murder of Edith Cook like blackmail. Cathy was threatening to turn her in if she left Michigan.

"Whatya mean you killed her?"

The night she died, Gwen explained, Cathy had stood guard outside her room.

"Then I smothered her with a pillow," she said.

Lisa wanted to know why.

"Because of her gangrene. I couldn't stand listening to her cry at night. I felt bad for her. It was driving me crazy. The gangrene was climbing up her legs."

Lisa looked at Robin.

"You believe this?"

"No, I don't. How *can* you believe it? How can you believe *them?*"

How true, Lisa thought. She knew Cathy Wood too well, and she knew Gwen liked to joke. She remembered how Gwen had joked the day after Lucille Stoddard died, saying that she was putting patients out of their misery. Black humor was common in Alpine, and everyone knew Lucille was a breath away from death.

"Gwen, you are so full of it."

"Yep," Gwen said, swaggering. "Lucille, that's another one I got."

Lisa looked at her two inebriated friends sitting on her mattress. She shook her head. She wished they had let her sleep.

Chapter 67

By mid-August, Robin Fielder could find no reason to remain a nurse's aide at Alpine Manor. The unexpected demise of one of her favorite patients in mid-July hastened her total disillusionment. In that tragic death, Robin again found herself face-to-face with the disturbing presence of Cathy Wood.

The patient was Lois Vanderploeg. Fifty-eight and paralyzed with multiple sclerosis, she was caring, entirely coherent and a committed cigarette smoker. Robin had befriended her by helping her smoke, often taking her own smoking breaks in Lois's room. She was Robin's second mother. Robin decorated her room, threw birthday parties for her and wrote poems about their relationship.

One morning, Robin received a call from Cathy at home, hours before her shift.

"I want to warn you Lois has been sent to the hospital," Cathy said. "They say she's really sick."

Robin rushed to St. Mary's Hospital to be at her bedside in the final hours before she died. Her death was attributed to natural causes, a brain stem infarction. However, there was no autopsy. Robin volunteered to go to Alpine Manor and gather her belongings for the family. She arrived at Alpine just before dawn.

Robin was crying when she found Cathy standing on Abbey Lane.

"Did she die?" Cathy asked.

"Yes. I'm coming to get her stuff."

"Well, you know what *I* heard," Cathy said smugly. "*I* heard she was dropped."

"What?"

Cathy appeared to enjoy furnishing the details.

"Yes, they were taking her to the commode and she was dropped off the commode, and that's what *really* happened."

Robin became hysterical with grief and rage. A supervisor calmed her down. She never was able to confirm Cathy's version of events. But in the following weeks, she nurtured old and new resentments about Alpine Manor as she went about her work.

Robin was just plain fed up with the place always being short on help and long on mind games. She gave Alpine Manor two weeks notice, but she never lasted a week. One day earlier, when they were so short she was doing housekeeping duties, Robin had stormed into the office of Alpine's owner, Ron Westman, when she saw him there on what she considered a rare visit. Westman asked her for her name.

"You know, it would be nice to see your face around here once in a while," she said. "You don't even know who the people are here that work for you. You ought to see how this place is run."

She complained about the turnover and the lousy pay. She complained how aides had no time for real care. She was sick of patients being treated like children. She was tired of rounds being an endless series of boxes to check on care charts. She called the place a "warehouse" and an "assembly line." She was fed up with cliques. She was angry at administrators she never saw. She was sick of eating caffeine pills just to stay awake. She stood up from the chair in front of his desk and pointed in the direction of Abbey Lane, Buckingham, Camelot and Dover.

"Mr. Westman, you don't even know what goes on out there!"

She was not fired for the outburst, but that didn't surprise her. She figured Alpine was in no position to lose the help. A week into her two-week notice she saw the owner walking down the hall on another visit.

"How you doing?" he asked. "By the way, what is your name, anyway?"

"My name is Robin," she said, very calmly. "And I am doing well because I was going to quit one week from now. But I've just decided, I'm not going to quit then. I'm going to quit today."

She was still smiling when she walked out the door.

They packed everything into Robin's 1983 Mustang. They had less than two hundred dollars between the two of them. They were headed for Tyler, Texas and away from Grand Rapids, away from Alpine Manor, away from Cathy and her games.

Robin planned on saying goodbye to her parents, but they were out golfing. She hadn't told them any of her last-minute plans. She was worried she would get questions—about where they were going, about her leaving school, about what they would do. She had always worried they would one day ask her about Gwen.

Their plan was a simple solution to what Robin saw as a situation growing increasingly complex in Cathy's stormy presence. Gwen had been appeasing Cathy with "friendship" dates. Finally, Gwen said Cathy wouldn't make trouble if they left.

They planned to arrive in Texas a few days before August 27, Gwen's court date. They would find a place to live and work. Robin packed clothes, her music tapes, her high school yearbooks and some photo albums.

Gwen insisted on stopping at Cathy's house, just to say goodbye. Gwen went into the little house on Effie and came back outside with her old roommate. They were both in tears. Gwen wrote Cathy a check for under twenty dollars in cash.

Then, Cathy approached Robin and dropped something in her hand. She handled it like a precious souvenir.

"This is yours," Cathy said.

It was Robin's purple plastic heart, from her key chain. Robin thought, how did she ever get that?

Robin had decided earlier not to tell Gwen about Cathy's death threats in the Alpine parking lot. She thought, why stir things up? Still, she didn't understand why they had to stop at Cathy's. She was more miffed by the fact Gwen was weeping as they headed for the freeway. The purpose of the move to Texas was supposed to be to get away from Cathy. Gwen was acting as though she were leaving family. Robin thought, this just doesn't make sense. This is the woman who put a gun up Gwen's vagina. This is the woman who threatened to kill us both.

Robin began crying, too. She cried for her parents, knowing how they would feel when they learned that she was gone. She cried for herself. She thought, what are you doing, you fool? Do you know where you are going? You're in love with another woman. Do you really know her? Do you know what you are doing with your life?

Robin kept driving, pointing the Mustang southwest. She told herself, this is what you must do. This is called growing up.

A couple of hours later they stopped in Chicago, at a White Castle, for lunch. When they returned to the car with a couple of bags of the little hamburgers, clouds of white smoke were pouring from under the car.

"This car is a piece of shit," Robin said.

Together they broke down laughing, soon hysterically. They continued south despite the smoke. The car kept on going. They giggled and joked for miles, cursing the Mustang as they went. Except for one nap, they drove straight on through.

When Robin Fielder saw the sign, "Tyler, Texas—Rose Capital of America," she heaved a sigh of relief not only for the car, but for both herself and Gwen. She felt as if they had finally driven out of the shadow of the big black cloud.

Robin hoped they were done with Cathy Wood for good.

Chapter 68

Several staffers thought Cathy Wood was acting unusually, unreasonably as a matter-of-fact. She would not go near the dead body.

The seventy-seven-year-old patient named Earl Goudzwaard had passed away after dinner, near the middle of second shift. He had only been in Alpine a month, dying of liver cancer. He had been on oxygen before he passed away.

"No, I won't do it," Cathy Wood insisted to a nurse. "I won't clean him up."

Not only wouldn't she clean him up, she refused to go in the room. It was August 15, only a week before Gwen and Robin left.

A beautician named *Maureen Haverhill* had been doing the hair of Lucille Vanderveen for years, even after her customer entered the nursing home named Alpine Manor.

Every week Lucille's son Jim picked her up and brought her to the shop. She suffered from severe arthritis. Sometimes she was a little forgetful, but mostly she was feisty and determined.

Maureen listened attentively as Lucille aired frequent complaints about the nursing home where she stayed. "They," she always said, were stealing her chocolates. "They" were stealing her clothes. "They" were nurse's aides and other patients. "They," Maureen guessed, referred to everything from one person to the facility in general.

One afternoon, in the last quarter of 1987, Maureen could see her eighty-one-year-old customer was quite upset as she helped her to the beauty chair. She started talking when she sat down.

"They tried to kill me last night," she said.

"What did you say Lucy?"

"They tried to kill me last night. They tried to smother me in my bed."

Maureen couldn't believe what she was hearing. It had to be a dream. Maybe Lucy was getting more confused with age.

"Lucy, they wouldn't."

"They put a pillow over my face and tried to smother me."

Her muscles stiffened. She was absolutely serious.

"They pressed, but I fought. I swung and I kicked and I scratched and they couldn't do it."

Maureen stopped primping her customer's hair and said soothingly: "Now, Lucy no one would do that there. No one tried to kill you."

Lucy's head spun toward her. The customer glared, looking her in the eyes.

"They did too!"

Maureen Haverhill dropped the subject. She'd heard a lot of crazy things over the years through sets and perms. She sometimes wondered where old people came up with crazy stories like that.

Lucille Vanderveen was admitted to Alpine Manor on July 31, 1987. She died early in 1988 of natural causes after being discharged to Butterworth Hospital. Her admission date was most significant.

Lucy Vanderveen was admitted to the nursing home five full weeks after Gwendolyn Gail Graham had left.

PART
THREE

1988-89

Chapter 69

The dispatcher called Tom Freeman during dinner, proving what the Walker detective had known for years. Nobody needs a vacation more than somebody who just came back from one. The International Police Association junket to West Germany was a rousing week of global police brotherhood in Bavarian beer halls, but it was no way to prepare for overtime on his first day back.

The dispatcher had a message: "Call Wyoming PD." Freeman picked up the phone and listened to what a sergeant from the southwest suburb had to say.

"I don't know. I gotta guy down here and he's talking about homicides, about some murders. He lives here, but it's in your city. I'm not gonna even touch it."

The drive took less than fifteen minutes. The route was lined with trees yellow and red with autumn. The amber light of a setting sun transformed the colors into surreal shades. It was October 6, a Thursday evening.

The man waiting for Tom Freeman at Wyoming PD was polite, earnest and quite troubled.

His name was Ken Wood.

Freeman listened for only a few minutes, then decided that he had better take him back to Walker PD. He didn't want to give Wood the chance to have any second thoughts. He didn't want Wood to get lost.

"The Walker Police Department sits right on Remembrance Road, right next to a great big cornfield," Freeman liked to tell everyone. And damn if it wasn't true.

Freeman figured the farm fields contributed to Walker's low crime rate as much as anything. Walker cops employed traffic expertise more than investigative technique. In his twelve years as an officer, eight as a detective, Freeman had worked on only five homicides. The eighteen thousand good folks of Walker read about a local murder maybe every two years. There were less than two dozen armed robberies annually. There were less than ten rapes.

Tom Freeman headed a detective bureau of two. He included himself in the count. Neither police work nor his thirty-four years had robbed him of his affable nature. He left his ties in the closet every day he could. His grin was boyish, sometimes mischievous. His slim six-foot frame and dark mustache created an impression of authority, but his ability to blush deep red betrayed him more often than he liked to admit.

"With Tom Freeman," one fellow cop said, "what you see is exactly what you get."

Back at Walker PD, Freeman offered a chair to Ken Wood and pulled a recorder out of his desk. From what he had heard so far, he wanted this story on tape.

"In the room with me at the Walker Police Department on the sixth of October 1988 is Kenneth Gordon Wood, white male, DOB 10-21-58."

Freeman positioned the microphone.

"Kenneth, would you give me the information you told me earlier, involving a situation at Alpine Manor, in the city of Walker. Why don't you start from what information your wife has told you, and we'll go from there?"

Ken Wood began.

"She told me that starting in February 1987, that she and her girlfriend Gwen Graham, had murdered or suffocated a woman. I believe her name was Margaret Mead. I know for sure it was Margaret, or am pretty sure it was Margaret, and that between February and April of 1987, that they had suffocated six different patients at Alpine Manor."

"How did she tell you this?" Freeman asked.

Wood detailed the circumstances of his ex-wife's confession that Friday night in August of 1987.

"Now, why did you come to the Wyoming Police Department to report this?" Freeman asked.

"They were the closest police station, only four blocks from my house. If I had to drive all the way over here, I would have changed my mind before I got here."

Freeman was happy he had driven Wood to Walker, but troubled by the dates. Jesus Christ, he thought, his ex-wife supposedly told him this fourteen months ago. She's a lesbian. Maybe he's got a grudge. Maybe he's full of shit. He asked another question.

"Why tonight, I mean, why . . ."

"There was a lot of different nights. I mean there have been times that I've been very close to calling the police and reporting her. I took her to Las Vegas for a weekend, back Valentine's weekend, this last February, and we were gone for three nights. I spent seven hundred dollars on her, taking her to Vegas, and two of the three nights, she pissed me off."

Okay, Freeman thought, that's seven months ago.

But Wood was just getting started. His answer would take two pages of an eighteen-page transcript. Freeman soon realized just how badly Ken Wood needed to talk.

"The first night she was drinking and she got obnoxious at the gambling table," he continued. "She started laughing when the dealer would win, and it was like she was into watching other people lose. I got upset with her. I was one of them losing too. You don't openly cheer the dealer on, and upset other people when they're losing money.

"Then, on Sunday, we were out to dinner and I got in an argument with her 'cause I told her I didn't approve of her life-style. I didn't approve of the fact that she didn't see our daughter. I didn't think she had been a good mother. She was being irresponsible, and she got real pissed off at me then and wouldn't talk to me . . . When she gets mad, she can be very cold, I mean scary cold.

"I guess going to Vegas was kind of my way of finding out what Cathy was still really like . . . I knew at that time that she had killed, or that she had told me that she had killed these people. I asked her to get help, and I knew she didn't, and then I wondered whether, you know . . . is Cathy dangerous? . . . When I got back I felt Cathy was still a very dangerous person. I thought that especially on Sunday, when she got really mad at me. I mean, sometimes you can see when somebody's got a lot of hate inside, especially when you've been around them for a long time . . ."

For fifteen minutes Wood groped for reasons.

"The crime was one where the people really didn't suffer . . . The police aren't looking for her, they are not looking for a murder. The families aren't tormented by the fact that a family member has been murdered. They thought they just died.

"I felt like if she wasn't a threat, to do it again, I didn't want to destroy my life, and I didn't want to destroy her life by turning her in, but I felt like I should find out if Cathy was dangerous. I know she can hate with the best of them."

Wood digressed into stories about his ex-wife's parents, her all-night parties and the bodies she saw at the foot of her bed.

This ex-wife of his, Freeman decided, sure has him swimming in one big sea of shit. The bottom line appeared to be that he had finally had his fill.

"I can't be worrying about what is going on with Cathy all of the time," he finally said.

"Do you think Cathy has some mental problems?"

Wood took a deep breath, and gave a one-word answer.

"Yeah."

Wood, meanwhile, admitted he had been seeing a psychologist himself. When Freeman heard him say that the therapist had advised him against talking to the police, the detective wondered if the whole night wasn't going to yield much more than a few more bucks on his check.

The detective kept asking questions anyway. Wood appeared more bent on psychoanalyzing his ex-wife than providing forensic evidence. He kept painting a sympathetic portrait.

"I think Cathy had several tragedies, a couple of them with her mother and father, very cold people. I think her mother's idea of a husband is somebody to pay the bills and put a roof over her head. That's it, and then you sleep with him every once in a while to keep him happy and keep him around."

Freeman wanted dates, places, locations of people. They were hard to find in all the extraneous subplots. Wood spun narratives about Cathy's weight, her lesbian affairs and troubles with her daughter. He heard about David/Debbie and Dawn Male. Wood provided Cathy's version of the Alpine Manor soap opera.

However, Freeman found the information concerning Gwen Graham and the murders intriguing. Graham had a violent streak and self-inflicted burn marks on her arms, Ken said. The two lesbians stalked the nursing home for weeks picking their victims out.

They planned to kill fellow employees as well. Cathy also had told her sister some of these details, Wood said.

Freeman wondered about Cathy's credibility.

"In the years you've been married with Cathy, how often have you caught her in lies?"

"Well, she used to lie all of the time, that would be the one thing I'd really get pissed off about . . ."

"What things have you caught her in lies about?"

"It's been two or three years since we've been together, since we've been split up, I caught her in a lot of lies. But while we were married, that's hard to say. A lot of little things, and those are the things that bothered me the most. Why lie about the little things? It doesn't make any sense. It's lying to be lying. It's lying to say: You don't need to know the truth about anything . . ."

This whole thing could be a big ruse, Freeman decided. He would begin in the morning with background checks, including getting a copy of the couple's divorce papers from the county clerk.

After Freeman dropped Ken Wood off back at his car in Wyoming, he went home to jet lag and the eleven o'clock news. The stories were dull compared to what he had heard over the last three hours.

In fact, the story from Wood's ex-wife seemed scripted. As he pondered the details, one sensational element stood out: Wood had said his ex-wife told him that their victims were chosen by the initials of their names.

"She told me that they tried to spell out M-U-R-D-E-R," he'd said.

Chapter 70

As he drove away from the police station, Ken Wood found no catharsis. He felt as if he had betrayed an old friend. This made no sense, and he knew it, considering all the havoc Cathy and her secret had wreaked in his life.

Plagued by headaches and numbed by auto work, he had taken a buy-out from General Motors. The spoils had financed their trip to Las Vegas. He had hoped the weekend might inspire renewal. It did no such thing. He would never forget the sight of Cathy in the new dress he bought for her. She was wearing it at the blackjack table, cheering the dealer on as he lost.

He had been rationalizing the murders for months. They had talked about the killings one more time, about a month after her first confession. When her water was turned off for a delinquent bill, Cathy spent the night. They lay together in bed, talking.

"I must have really loved Gwen to do that with her," she said.

He was miffed.

"How can you relate love to killing somebody?"

"Well, those people were probably better off dead."

She started to talk about the patients' conditions.

"No," he said, stopping her. "You said you did it because it was fun. You played God. You decided when these people would go. You played God."

She didn't respond. The conversation was over. She slept soundly. He spent another night pacing.

Ken was ashamed that she had been involved. Now he was involved, too. Ken knew the detective had been dissatisfied with his answers. But how could he explain it? It had taken so many months for him to sort the mess out.

In the beginning, he had often found himself thinking like her. The victims were vegetables anyway. Their deaths would have been blessings under normal circumstances. Why not let their families think that they had passed away peacefully? The truth only would create pain, for everyone, he rationalized. What would this do to Jamie? What would it do to our lives?

Ken also decided Cathy was no threat in Alpine Manor. Gwen was the mastermind. Gwen was the instigator. That's the way Cathy had portrayed it. Without Gwen there would be no more murders. Still, he sometimes turned to the obituary page, looking for Alpine's name, looking for a rash of deaths.

In time, he realized he had been a fool for thinking she would ever get help. For a while, she claimed to be attending a self-help group. He knew that was a lie. Whenever he brought up therapy, she accused him of wanting to change her sexual preference. He couldn't seem to make her understand that was not the issue. He thought, why doesn't she realize the gravity of what she and Gwen have done?

Her indifference only continued. She began nursing school, while other parts of her life hit new lows. Her girlfriends became less attractive. She ran with alcoholics and questionable company from South Division. Her mother evicted her from Effie Place. She moved in with her father and grandmother. She was living in the basement.

By the summer, he felt Cathy was deliberately trying to irritate him. She played more mind games. She made more turmoil out of scheduled visitations and phone calls with Jamie. Sometimes he wondered if she was trying to make him angry enough so that he would go to the police.

He knew she was toying with him. He knew she always had. He thought, she thinks she has got me where I don't know whether I am coming or going. And he was questioning his own motives. She had always been so good at inspiring that. He wondered if turning her into the police would really be an act of jealousy.

By autumn, his own plans to chart a new life had fallen apart. He had hoped to purchase a convenience store with his GM buy-out, but the deal had fallen through. He felt overwhelmed. Balancing single parenthood, a new business and Cathy's turmoil would have been an impossible juggling act. He took a job delivering auto parts. As he shuttled mufflers and brakes, Cathy's secret gnawed at him on long stretches of highway.

The final obstacle was their own credibility. He wondered if anyone would believe him, if anyone would believe her. He revealed what Cathy had told him to his sister and brother-in-law, and listened to the anticipated responses. Cathy was playing games with him, they said.

He decided to investigate a bit on his own. He talked to the husband of a barmaid he knew. This man worked for the Kent County medical examiner. Ken approached him one day over a beer at the tavern.

"This is going to sound like a strange question," he began. "But when people die is it easy to tell the cause of death after they've been dead for a while?"

"Well, it's hard. But it can be done."

"What if they're really old people that are really sick and stuff like that?"

"Well, that's even harder. But it still can be done."

The turning point came when he called Florida and talked to Cathy's sister Barb. Shortly after Cathy first confessed in August, they had talked. The subject of murder never came up, but Barb seemed worried about the course of Cathy's life.

"Cathy's going to end up in prison one day," she said.

Recently, Ken had called her again. He brought up the killings point-blank. Cathy apparently had told Barb more than Cathy had led Ken to believe. Barb said her husband thought Cathy was making it all up. Barb said she was worried about her sister, but could do little from twelve hundred miles away.

That did it. Ken told her he was going to go to the police. Cathy needed help, and he couldn't carry the burden anymore alone.

"Well, Ken," she said, "if you need me to talk to them, I will."

Ken was glad he had Cathy's sister as a backup. As he headed for home, he had no way of knowing whether the detective from Walker believed him or not.

Chapter 71

Day House Supervisor Marty Slocum knew the routine. Since the charge tech had switched to first shift, she had come to know Cathy Wood as well as any manager could.

"Mom," Cathy said. "Cookie wants to talk."

She approached her in the hall, in tears.

"Cookie" was the name Cathy had given herself. "Mom" was the role Marty Slocum knew all too well. For many of her fifteen years as an Alpine Manor RN, she had assumed the position of surrogate staff mother, serving as confidant and intercessor as the need arose. The role seemed especially important to Cathy.

When Cathy reached Marty's office, she sat in the chair, facing her. This was an important distinction. Sometimes Cathy liked to face the wall, folding her hands and putting her back to Marty.

"Mom, Cookie has been a naughty girl," she would say then.

On those occasions she would make Marty extract the story, like the time she had picked up a seedy stranger on South Division and cruised all night around Grand Rapids.

"Cathy, you mean you picked up a strange man—down there?"

"Cookie was naughty."

She said it in a tiny, childish voice. Then, they would have a talk. Cathy always left with the same farewell.

"Toodle do," she said.

Marty believed the routine was for attention. Cathy Wood loved attention—lots of it. Marty would never forget the time Cathy complained how hurt she was that someone had forgotten her twenty-sixth birthday. Then, two days later she totally ignored Marty's fiftieth.

That sort of thing bothered Marty. The fact that Cathy was a lesbian, or that others on the staff were gay, did not. She was concerned with their work, not their private lives.

How entangled those lives could be. Marty was surprised Cathy wasn't more upset over Gwen's departure more than a year ago. They had seemed so inseparable. She remembered what Gwen always used to say when she asked her to work a double. "Gotta check with my woman first," she always drawled.

After Gwen left, Cathy did seem to suffer from anxiety. She kept asking Marty if her employment records were up to date.

"I want you to know who to contact if something happens to me," she said.

She was also concerned about Robin Fielder.

"You know, Marty, something is going to happen to Robin, and nobody is going to know," she told her once. "She's gonna end up dead in a ditch down there, and nobody up here is going to know about it."

What in God's name was she talking about, Marty wondered. However, it wouldn't be the first time Cathy Wood had ever talked in riddles.

"Cathy, do you think Gwen is ever going to come back?" she asked her not too long ago.

"Who knows, *could be,*" she said, drawing out the words.

She acted confident of it, in a smirking kind of way.

Lately, however, Cathy had been bragging about making some kind of change in her life.

"Mom, I'm trying to be a good girl," she kept saying. "I'm trying to be good."

Marty assumed she meant less carousing and more schoolwork. With her quick mind well-directed, she thought, Cathy Wood could make quite a splash in life.

Sometimes Cathy talked about having two lives, the one she had in Alpine Manor, the other on the outside. One was secure and safe; the other was troubled and unpredictable. In Alpine she had control. People were dependant on her. Her life outside had only become worse. She had lost her house. Marty had always felt that alone had attracted a lot of her friends. She had the place to party. Now she only had her Luv Truck.

"Mom, when I'm in here at work I know exactly what I'm supposed to do," Cathy once confessed to Marty. "I have my head on straight. But when I leave here, I fall apart."

As Cathy came into her office in tears this first week in October, she confided a new crisis.

"I'm pregnant," Cathy said.

Marty calmly talked about her options. Cathy thought abortion was probably best. She cited her weight and her failure as a mother to Jamie. However, that meant money, she said. She hinted about a loan. Marty suggested she talk to her grandmother about that.

The next day Cathy was upbeat. She said she had the money, she had an abortion scheduled for the following Monday.

"Thanks, Mom," she said. "Toodle do."

Later, Marty discovered the pregnancy was a lie to raise quick cash for a security deposit on an apartment. It was the first time she had ever caught Cathy Wood lying. It wouldn't be the last.

Cathy indeed was about to give birth, but not to a baby.

It all started on October 7, three days before her supposed Monday appointment with the abortionist. Marty would remember that Friday clearly. It was Cathy Wood's last day at Alpine Manor.

She didn't say "toodle do," not when she walked out the door with the police.

Chapter 72

Tom Freeman had never seen anything like it in police work. He was transporting Cathy Wood from Alpine Manor to Walker PD, a ten-minute ride. Her hands folded, she was sitting next to him in the front seat—and she wasn't saying a word.

He found the silence unnerving. Goddamnit, he thought, something is wrong here.

Freeman had met her inside the front door of the nursing home, after she was paged. He had introduced himself as a Walker detective, forcing himself not to react to the commanding presence of the giant platinum blonde who quietly appeared in the vestibule.

"I wanna talk to you," he said.

She looked at him blankly.

"Okay. Where are we going?"

"To the police department."

"I have to tell my supervisors."

"They know already."

She had one request. She wanted her coat.

And then nothing. Not one question. Not one comment. Not one goddamn thing. He thought, isn't she even curious why she's being hauled to Walker PD? Both the guilty and the innocent always wanted to know. They usually chatted the miles away.

It was not the first surprise of the early afternoon of Friday, October 7. With Ken Wood's statement, Freeman had secured a search warrant for the nursing home. The warrant called for Catherine May Wood's employment record and the medical records of all patients who had died during her employment. For help, he had brought along Roger Kaliniak, Walker's other detective, a former patrolman new to the bureau.

Freeman had already met Jackie Cromwell, who had recently been promoted from nursing director to administrator. Eight months earlier an insane patient had crushed another patient's skull with a fatal assault with a cane. Cromwell and her assistant Margaret Widmaier appeared stunned both by Ken Wood's allegations and the warrant request.

"Do you have any idea how long this is going to take?" the administrator said. "We're talking about a lot of records."

As Widmaier began accumulating the records, Kaliniak made wisecracks and swiped candies from a bowl on the administrator's desk. Freeman asked routine questions. They waited nearly an hour for the first set.

"What do you know about Cathy Wood?"

"Well, she's a big woman," Cromwell had said. "A very big woman. She's working today, as a matter-of-fact."

As Freeman provided more details, Cromwell suggested that the "Margaret" Ken Wood was talking about might be Marguerite, a Marguerite Chambers, in fact. She died in January. They narrowed down the period for patient deaths from January to June of 1987.

Even then, Freeman was overwhelmed when he began probing the boxes of files arriving in Cromwell's office. There were thousands of pages of daily aide charts, nurse's notes, prescriptions,

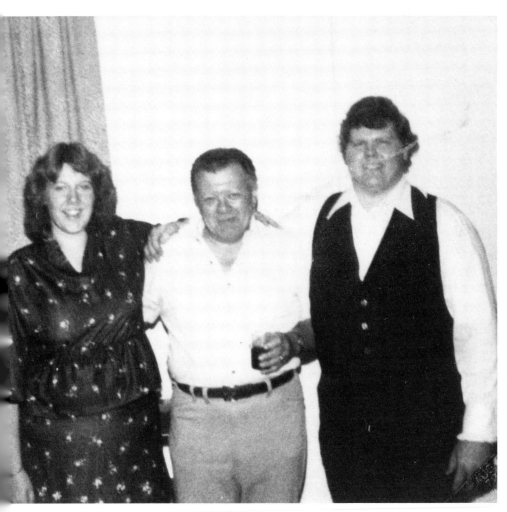

Cathy and Ken Wood with Ken's father on the night of their wedding.

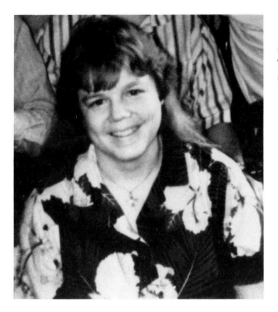

Gwen Graham in Tyler, Texas before she moved to Grand Rapids.

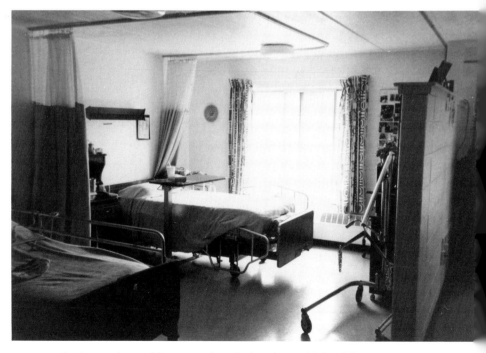

Bed one, the position near the window in an Alpine Manor room.

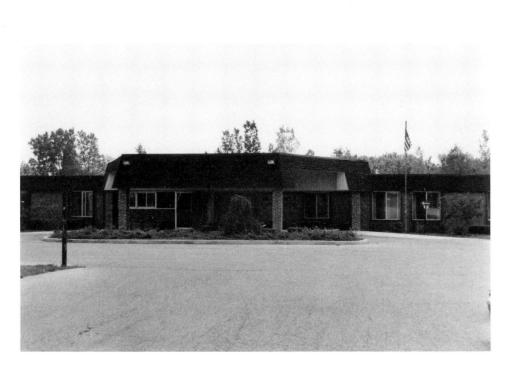

The exterior of Alpine Manor.

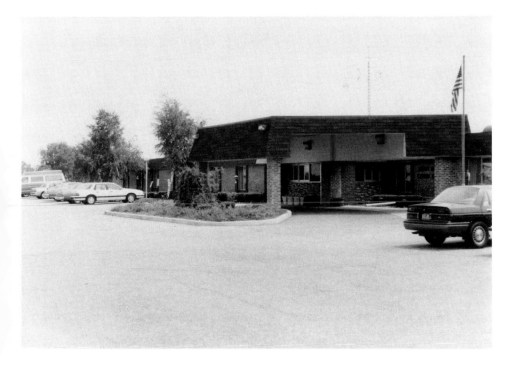

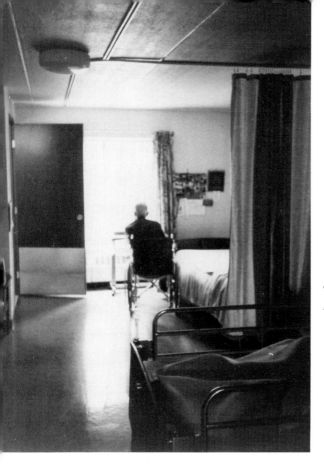

The interior of a typical
Alpine Manor patient room.

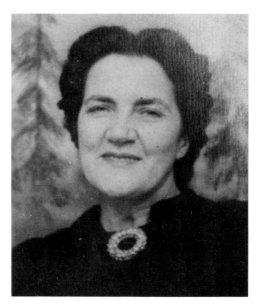

Myrtle Luce, victim.

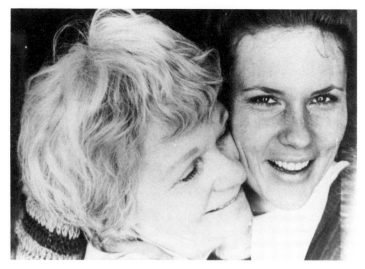

Mae "Maisy" Mason, victim, with her daughter Linda.

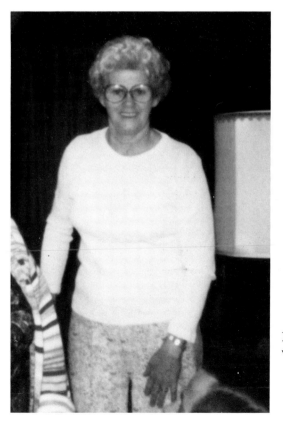

Marguerite Chambers,
victim, in healthier days.

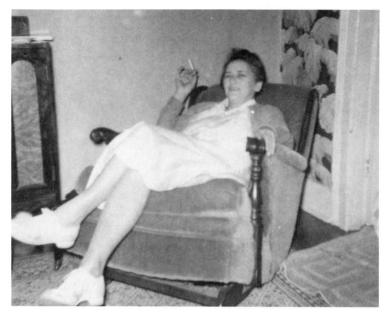

Bell Burkhard, victim.

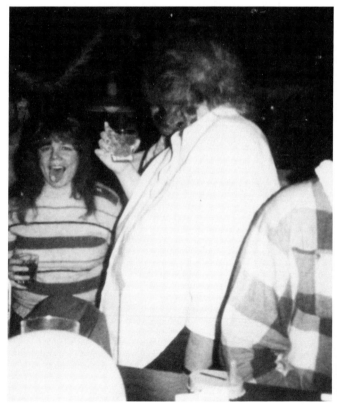

Gwen Graham and
Cathy Wood partying
at the Carousel before
all the madness began.

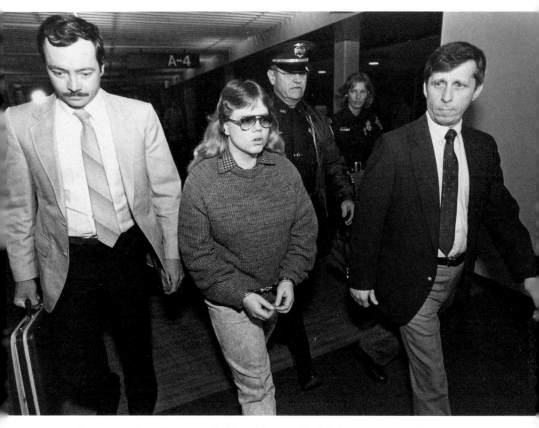

Detectives Tom Freeman (left) and Roger Kaliniak accompany Gwen Graham through Kent County Airport after she waived extradition in Tyler, Texas. *(Courtesy of Grand Rapids Press/Rex D. Larson)*

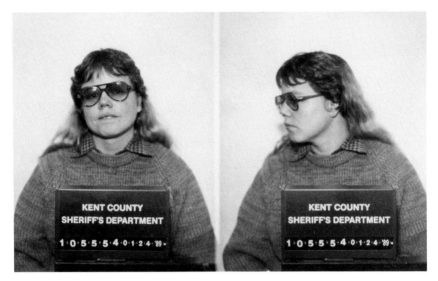

Gwen Graham at her booking.

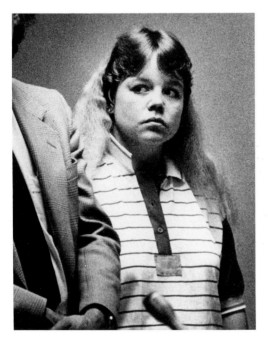

Gwen Graham at her arraignment on murder
charges in March 1989.   *(Courtesy of Grand
Rapids Press)*

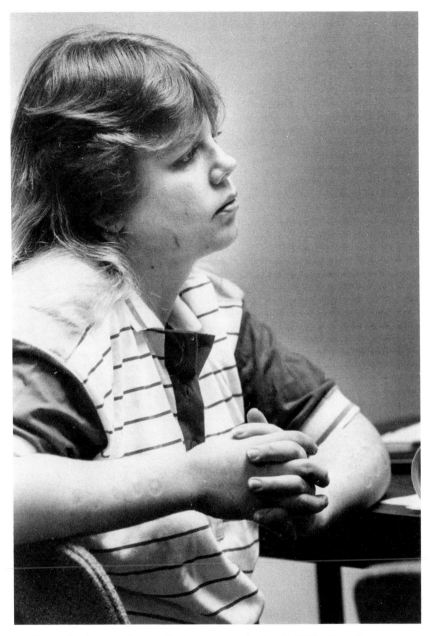

Gwen Graham at her preliminary exam in April 1989. She often wore short-sleeved blouses to display her scars. *(Courtesy of Grand Rapids Press/Noel Webley II)*

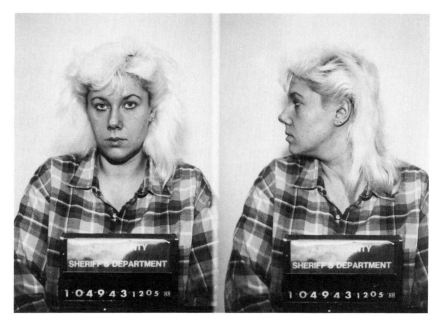

Cathy Wood at her booking.

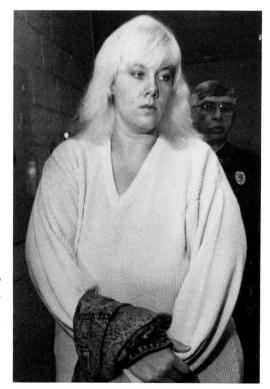

Cathy Wood on her way to her preliminary examination in January 1989. *(Courtesy of Grand Rapids/John Kringas)*

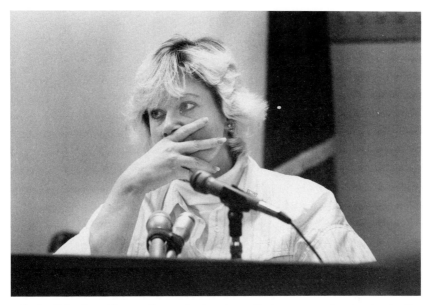

Cathy Wood testifies at Gwen Graham's preliminary examination in April 1989. *(Courtesy of Grand Rapids Press/Noel Webley II)*

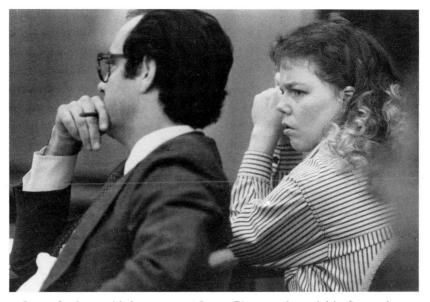

Gwen Graham with her attorney James Piazza at her trial in September 1989. *(Courtesy of Grand Rapids Press/Anna Moore Butzner)*

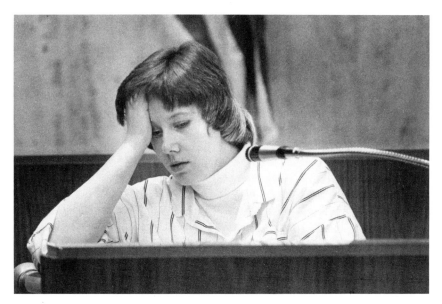

Cathy Wood during her tearful, drama-laced testimony at Gwen Graham's trial. *(Courtesy of Grand Rapids Press/Anna Moore Butzner)*

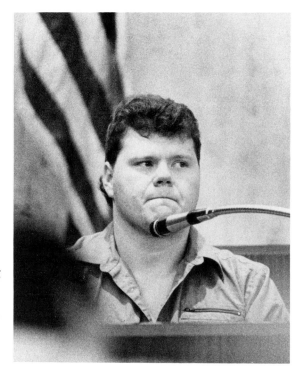

Ken Wood testifying at Gwen Graham's trial. *(Courtesy of Grand Rapids Press)*

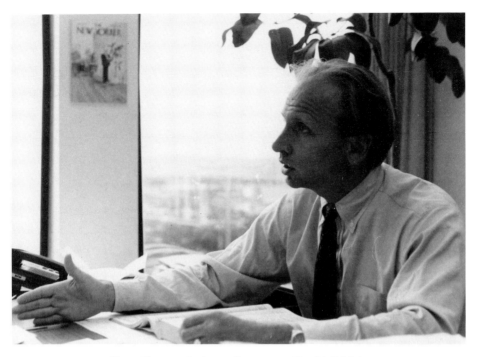

Kent County Assistant Prosecutor David Schieber.

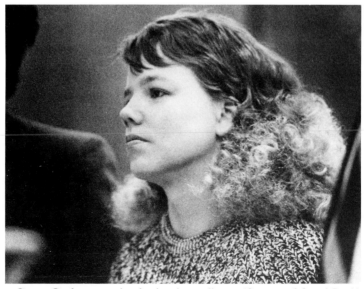

Gwen Graham awaits the jury's verdict. *(Courtesy of Grand Rapids Press/Anna Moore Butzner)*

Gwen Graham's jailhouse tracings and artwork for Robin Fielder.

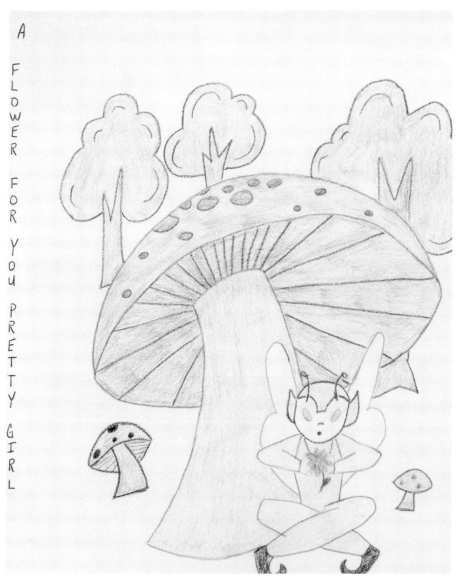

"A Flower for You Pretty Girl"

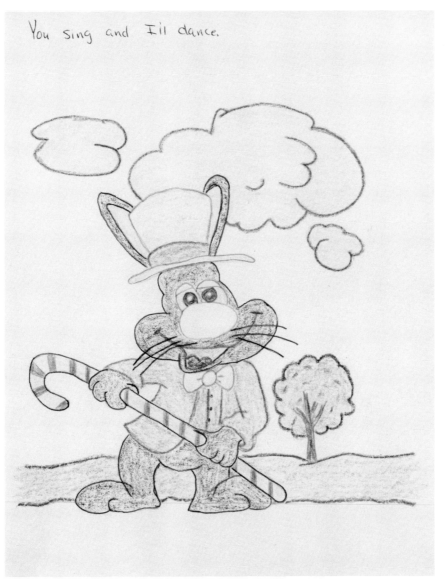

"You Sing and I'll Dance"

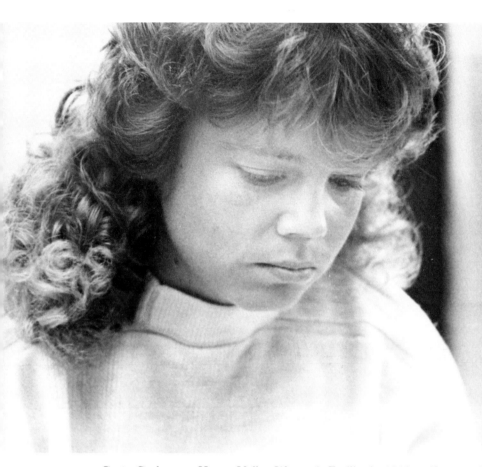

Gwen Graham at Huron Valley Women's Facility in 1991. *(Courtesy of Michelle Andonian)*

family histories, recreation schedules and more. After more than an hour of this he turned to Kaliniak.

"Rog, you stay here till they're done and get these down to the department. I'm gonna talk to Cathy Wood. What have we got to lose anyway?"

By 4:00 p.m., Tom Freeman and Cathy Wood were sitting across from one another in an interview room at the department on Remembrance Road. He asked if he could use a tape recorder.

"Oh no," she said, sighing. "I can't stand it. I did that once. And, I can't stand the sound of my voice."

"Well, I'll take notes then, okay?"

She nodded. Then he read her her rights. She still was willing to talk. She signed a card acknowledging that she knew her options under the law.

He began with fifteen minutes of basics about her work and marriage, then served up the central question.

"Your ex-husband came in here last night," he began. "And he has informed us that you and a Gwen Graham are involved in the homicide of a person named Margaret."

Cathy's head went back about three inches, as though she were viewing an object with disbelief.

"Oh," she said, sighing. "That's made up. He's just mad. He just wants to get even with me."

Freeman came right back.

"Well, I don't think he's making this up."

"Right," she said, sighing again. "It was a big joke. A big practical joke."

Shit, Freeman thought, now what? She wasn't rattled. In fact, she was flippant. He went for a reliable interrogation ploy. He executed the perfectly accurate bluff.

He looked at her dead seriously.

"Well, Cathy. I don't think it is a big joke. I have my partner at Alpine Manor right now. We have obtained all the information with a search warrant. And what we've seen in the medical records is not a practical joke."

Her comeback was instantaneous, without reflection. Again, she was almost flippant.

"Okay," she said. "I'll tell you the truth."

She began by correcting him.

"Her name was not *Margaret.* It was *Marguerite.* Marguerite Chambers. I walked in on her and she was holding a washcloth on her chin and nose."

Freeman felt his diaphragm tug at his lungs as she began providing a slew of details. Her tone was as light as if she were chatting about the latest office gossip.

There were several victims, she said. Gwen had killed them all in the winter of 1987. Cathy pinpointed the station where she had been working. She remembered which shift. She dropped the names of those who had cleaned up the victims.

Freeman struggled to catch up. Just minutes ago, he thought, she was saying we were all full of shit. Now she is racing ahead of my questions. He tried to slow her down.

"Wait a minute, Cathy. Now let's stick with Marguerite Chambers. You're not being truthful with me. You told Ken you were there when she was smothered."

She continued without a stutter, making it sound like the contradiction was in his mind, not in her story. She was there, watching Gwen from the doorway of her room.

"And Marguerite was making lots of noise," she said. "She was grunting and her body was having spasms."

"When are we talking about?"

"Oh, January eighth That date sticks out in my mind. Yes, January eighth I know something happened on January eighth."

She couldn't remember the name of the aide who prepared the body for the funeral home. Gwen, however, was one of the ones who helped.

"Riiiiiight," she said, as though she finally had a secure hold on the memory.

Then, her demeanor switched instantly to confidently matter-of-fact.

"Yep. Gwen thought it was funny."

She kept right on going. She named four names at first, four victims: Marguerite Chambers, Mae Mason, Belle Burkhard and Edith Cook. There were more, but she couldn't remember their names. Freeman slid a list of the deceased from the Alpine Manor records across the interview table.

"Oh, riiight," she said. "Myrtle Luce. I remember her because of her daughter. Her daughter used to come in and make sure she was well taken care of."

Freeman tried to structure the interview with questions on each victim. But not even an hour into their talk he realized he could not keep order to her train of thought. She was scattered. She leaped from day to day, month to month. She instantly switched locations and subject matter. She went from patient to patient.

Damn it, he thought, I need that tape recorder.

"Slow down, Cathy," he said more than once.

As he scribbled, she would switch subjects again. She talked about her latest girlfriend, her family, back to Alpine and then her Luv Truck.

Jesus Christ, Freeman told himself, she's being interrogated about multiple murder and she's talking about her fucking Luv Truck!

An hour into the interview, he felt as though she were giving him answers to a crossword puzzle and expecting him to put it together without the grid. The interview became exasperating at times. He tried to keep her focussed on Marguerite Chambers.

"Well, how did you know she was suffocating her?" he asked. "All you've told me is that she had a washcloth under her chin. She could have been wiping off vomit."

"I just knew."

"How?"

"I just did."

Common sense told him the only way she would know Marguerite Chambers was smothered was if she was involved.

"Cathy, look it, I could go talk to Gwen Graham and she could tell me this is all bullshit, that maybe you did the smothering here. If you are involved, you know, it's the first one who comes to the window that gets the break."

She looked at him, but was silent.

He decided not to push. He didn't want to piss her off. He didn't want to lose her, not yet.

He tried another angle, but she dodged his questions. She and Gwen were roommates, he said. They were lovers, for Chrissakes.

"What about that?" Freeman asked.

"Well, she threatened to kill me with a gun if I told anyone," Cathy finally said.

Gwen also tried to smother her, she added. After Marguerite

Chambers was killed, she said, Gwen tied her up in her own bed with restraints. She thought they were going to have sex. But Gwen took a pair of socks from the dresser, slid them over her hands and tried to smother her.

"You see," Cathy said. "I don't know if that was that night, or the next day. But it was the week of January eighth."

That's another one of her irritating habits, he decided. *I don't know.* She used the phrase repeatedly. But instead of saying simply "I don't know," she linked it with a compelling fact, often as a surprise.

"Now Edith Cook. I don't know if Gwen took a souvenir that time or not. I don't know if it was piece a jewelry or not."

When Freeman tried to explore such revelations he found himself more confused.

"You see, Mr. Freeman, I don't know," she would say. "I don't know if the souvenir was that time, or if it was with Marguerite."

He thought, we're talking about murder here, not a trip to the goddamn supermarket. Her recall of detail makes no sense. She remembered shifts, dates, times, but then drew major blanks on more important facts.

How did it all start?

"Well, I don't know how. I don't know if Gwen brought the subject of murder up, or what. You see, I don't know that."

He could see one puzzle grid taking shape. She was distancing herself from the act of murder.

"Well, why did Gwen do this?" he asked.

She said Gwen always felt greatly relieved after killing. It appeared to ease her frustrations in life.

"She said it relieved her tension," Cathy said.

The story became more surreal than Ken Wood's version. Freeman found himself more captivated. After more than two hours, she had provided some detail on three more killings besides Marguerite Chambers and Myrtle Luce.

Mae Mason: Cathy and Gwen were probably working different stations. "Something funny happened about Mae Mason's death. I don't know if it was the aide's reaction, or not."

Belle Burkhard: Cathy said Gwen walked up to her station and placed a washcloth on the counter. "Gwen always had a washcloth in her back pocket." Gwen took a sock for a souvenir. An aide named Pat Ritter found her dead. Gwen said Belle was so strong that she had to put her knee on her arm. "The administration thought Pat Ritter failed to turn Belle and that's why her arm was discolored."

Edith Cook: She had gangrene. She was a mercy killing. Jewelry was the souvenir.

Gwen Graham, Cathy said, had told her in advance that she was going to kill all these patients.

Freeman wanted to know about spelling M-U-R-D-E-R, as Ken Wood had explained the day before. They went over the names of the patients. He looked at the initials of the first and last names.

"That doesn't spell murder, Cathy," he said. "How does that spell murder?"

Instead of answering, she came back on another track, as though she were running two or three subjects ahead of him, as though he were thinking in a vacuum.

"Are you gonna put me in jail?" she asked, studying his face.

"No," he said. "Right now I'm interested in Gwen Graham."

He wanted to know how long they lived together. She provided the exact dates.

"Look, I'm interested in Gwen," he said again. "But Cathy, you're gonna have to help us."

Tom Freeman had decided to play along with the role Cathy Wood had fashioned for herself. He was going to treat her like a witness. She had defined the game. He would play it on her terms, for a while. Besides, at this point she was all he had.

Freeman excused himself and walked the twenty feet to the office of his chief, Walter Sprenger. The detective felt both exhilarated and psychologically spent. He felt Cathy Wood had good reason to distance herself from the deaths. Already, he felt her story had elements of the truth. He wondered what would have been more taxing, all those medical records or another couple of hours with the mercurial thinking patterns of Catherine May Wood.

Chief Sprenger looked up at him from a pile of papers.

"Walter, you're not going to believe this. She's admitting to some of this shit."

For a few moments Freeman was overcome with anxiety. Six homicides, he thought.

"Goddamn," he muttered, looking out the window. "I wish this was across the street."

The street was the line of Kent County's jurisdiction. On the other side the sheriff's department would have the case. Freeman already had one homicide working, another oddball case involving a guy named O'Brien who gunned down his uncle in the middle of his golf game.

Freeman shook off the apprehension. Shit, he thought, no. This Alpine Manor thing could be a case of a lifetime.

"Walter, I'm gonna need some help on this. I need some help on just the transport alone."

Freeman didn't want to be in a car alone again with Cathy Wood. The practice had been drilled into him, into all police officers. You don't get in the car alone with a woman suspect. If you do, you radio in your miles. You don't give her the opportunity to make accusations later.

Another cop had strolled into Sprenger's office. Bill Brown was Walker's assistant police chief. He had preceded Freeman in the detective bureau and had been his tutor on the job. Brown listened to some of the details. He was skeptical.

"I don't know, Tom. There's a real possibility it all could be just a lot of bullshit."

"I know, I know. But, you know, I've been sitting in the room with her for nearly three hours. And, damn it, something tells me she's telling the truth."

Brown said he would help with the transport. Freeman joked.

"You never know," he said. "After all, she might be the psycho in the case."

Chapter 73

Back in the interview room, Cathy Wood offered up another tantalizing possibility. She had letters, she told Freeman, from Gwen Graham. There might be something in those letters about the murders. She had them, she said, back at her grandmother's house.

Freeman phoned the Kent County Prosecutor's Office, specifically Dave Schieber, the assistant prosecutor who helped prepare the Alpine Manor search warrant. Freeman wondered if he needed a warrant for those letters. He didn't want to give a judge a chance to throw out good evidence.

"Bring her down here," Schieber said. "Let's talk about this, and see what we have."

Freeman was afraid of something like that. The prosecutor's office had a policy: Somebody from the office made all homicide scenes. Here, there was no scene. So, take the interviewee *to* the prosecutor. This is a first, Freeman bitched to himself. When Cathy Wood sees the Hall of Justice she'll turn into a deaf-mute.

The detective expected nothing less from Dave Schieber. For years, the two of them had nurtured a professional relationship that ranged from backslaps to damn near outright hate. More than one Walker cop considered the attorney arrogant and ambitious. They endured condescending remarks and his habit of giving orders to cops simply because in a courtroom he knew his trade.

Freeman and Roger Kaliniak found a way to retaliate. They pronounced the attorney's last name *Schiebers,* always put an "s" where none belonged. They knew he hated that.

"Schiebers wants her downtown," Freeman told Bill Brown.

It was past dinnertime. Freeman and Brown offered to stop at a Burger King on Pearl Street, near the Hall of Justice. In the drive-thru Cathy Wood listed a large order, one that included a Whaler and a large fries.

"Oh, but give me a Diet Coke," she said.

The regular office staff had gone home by the time the three of them walked into the prosecutor's office complex, their Burger King bags in hand. They spread the food and drinks out on the conference table in the impressive personal office of Prosecutor William A. Forsyth, who also had left for the day. The fourth-floor windows provided a panoramic view of the setting sun and the rapids of the Grand River as the brown water raced by below.

The setting was lofty for anyone, let alone a low-paid charge tech still wearing her Alpine whites. Cathy Wood was so relaxed she was serene.

"Cathy," Freeman said. "This is Kent County Prosecutor Dave Schiebers."

Cathy gazed up at the young attorney. He extended his hand,

later using it to push back a gathering of his blond hair. He was tall and slim. He was dressed in a suit, his collar sparkling white under the fluorescent light.

Cathy's eyes brightened.

"Wow," she said. "You must be somebody really important."

He smiled.

They hit it off right away. They began to banter. Cathy, Freeman later decided, almost appeared to be flirting.

"Has Tom informed you of your rights," Schieber said, getting down to business.

Cathy nodded.

"Well, you want to tell me what happened?"

Cathy sketched out the Alpine Manor story for the assistant prosecutor. There were some new details, but the narrative was basically the same.

"Cathy, how do I know you're telling the truth," Schieber said when she finished. "Do you have anything to confirm this?"

She told him about the letters.

"But there's private things in those," she said, sighing.

"Cathy," Tom said. "You know we're not interested in that."

Then she had a question.

"Should I get a lawyer?"

Schieber turned to her.

"That's your decision, naturally."

Cathy half smiled.

"Well, I want to help."

"Look Cathy," the attorney continued. "I'm not sure what I should do. What *I* do depends on what you're going to do."

He turned to Freeman.

"Tom," he said, motioning with his hand. "Read Cathy her rights again."

She listened as Freeman read them. Then she signed her second index card acknowledging as much. She appeared more concerned about proving her story than her own legal vulnerability. Cathy wanted to go get the letters.

"Tom, we don't need a search warrant," Schieber said. "As long as she's providing these letters with her consent."

Cathy nodded again.

Soon, Tom Freeman, Bill Brown and Cathy Wood were on the

down elevator. Schieber said he would meet them later that night, there at the Hall of Justice.

Freeman listened to Cathy's plan as his department Oldsmobile Cutless idled in front of her grandmother's apartment in Comstock Park.

"My father lives with my grandmother, and he likes to argue," she said, "Especially when he's been drinking. I don't want him to know you're the police."

Freeman said he would be the only one going inside with her.

"I got it, we'll pretend you're a friend," she said. "In fact, I'm gonna pretend you're my boyfriend. They'll probably be happy because they never see me with boys anyway."

"Well, okay," he said.

"Oh, you're so cuuuute."

It wasn't the first time he had heard that line.

Freeman dismissed the masquerade as undercover work. Yes, he would go into the house on her terms. He just wanted those letters.

Freeman planned to make small talk while Cathy went into her basement bedroom. Inside, he started doing just that with John Carpenter and his mother. They were having a couple of beers at the kitchen table.

"C'mon Tom," Cathy said.

She turned to her family.

"Tom's coming down to the bedroom with me."

Freeman felt his face warm as he descended the steps. Shit, how does this look, he thought.

At the bottom of the stairs he could see her queen-sized bed. It was unmade. The entire room, in fact, was in disarray. He could see books, lots of books. Stephen King and other horror titles were everywhere.

Cathy reached under a dresser and pulled out a red and blue shoe box. She cradled it between her two hands gingerly, setting it down and carefully lifting off the top. She began confirming the contents, but then started sorting out other materials. She produced a checkbook for a joint account she had shared with Gwen Graham.

"You don't want this," she said.

"Keep it together, Cathy. We can sort through it later."

He wanted out of that bedroom. He wanted out of the house. He didn't like the situation at all, especially with her family upstairs.

She handed him the box.

"Oh," Cathy sighed. "You know I want to change. I want to get out of these whites."

Freeman looked up from the box. He started to go up the stairs.

"No, my dad," Cathy said. "Wait here. I'll change here."

Change. Where? How? Freeman could feel heat radiating from his cheeks.

Cathy stood still, her hands folded in front of her. She lifted her index finger shoulder-high and motioned.

"Around," she said. "Turn around."

"Cathy, no . . ."

"Turn, c'mon. It will only take fifteen seconds. Turn. Turn. Turn."

He found himself pivoting with her finger.

His back to her, he held the shoe box in his hands. His face felt like a blast furnace. It must have been as red as a lake in hell. He could hear her nylon uniform hissing as she pulled it off her large frame. He had never felt so vulnerable as a cop.

He thought, Tom, goddamnit, she's a suspect, for Chrissake!

The first fear was immediate. A knife in the back. He could get a knife in the back. If I'm gonna be stabbed by a three-hundred-pound homicidal fucking dike, he thought, I want it in the god-damn front. Wouldn't I look good. A back wound from a suspect. Wouldn't I look like an asshole!

A deeper apprehension gripped him when he no longer could hear her clothes rustle. She was standing there, stark baby-ass naked. *A police officer does not put himself in a compromising position that could later damage his case.* You log your miles. You transported females with a partner. You don't go into the bedroom with a woman and *let her get fucking naked!*

Freeman couldn't believe he had let her go that far. He thought, but I have the letters. I have the fucking letters.

Then she said she was done.

"C'mon, let's go," she said.

He lingered for a second, relishing the fact that it was over, for now, at least. She had changed into stone-washed jeans, a loose blouse and dark flats. She was as upbeat as ever.

He hoped his face was getting back to normal as they ascended the stairs.

"Toodle do," Cathy said, as they walked out the door.

Back at the conference table in the Hall of Justice the four of them went through the letters. They took turns reading them out loud.

Cathy seemed embarrassed by some of the material. Several times she grabbed letters off the top of the pile.

"Oh, no, I don't want you to read that one!"

She held them close to her, eyeing everyone.

"Cathy," Tom told her. "This is our profession. We've seen all types of things. There's nothing to be embarrassed about typical love letters."

But, Freeman thought to himself, they weren't typical love letters. These women were in their mid-twenties, and the stuff read like what he remembered in fourth and fifth grade. The content was maudlin. There were poems, correspondences on nurse's notepaper and letters from Gwen Graham postmarked Tyler, Texas.

There was nothing that corroborated her story.

Shit, Freeman thought, I went through all that for nothing.

As Cathy packed the letters back in the box, Schieber and Freeman stepped into another office for a conference. Freeman wondered about an arrest warrant for Gwen Graham.

"No, I'm not writing any warrant."

"But Dave, I do think she's telling the truth."

The assistant prosecutor was condescending.

"Tom, a couple of lesbians. Love letters. This looks like something more suited for the pages of the *National Enquirer* than the office of the Kent County Prosecutor."

Goddamn *Schiebers*, Freeman thought.

Already the attorney had switched the subject. Schieber wanted Freeman to concentrate on the O'Brien case, the golf course killing they had going together.

"Damn it Dave, what if she is telling the truth?"

The attorney paused for a couple of seconds, reflecting.

"This is the end of it—for now, at least. Just release her. Send her home."

* * *

Freeman dropped Bill Brown off before Cathy. He didn't call in
the mileage. He figured he'd already blown it so bad down in her
bedroom, what the hell difference did it make.

He drove Cathy to the Alpine Manor parking lot. One of Cathy's
friends had her Luv Truck, and she was going to pick her up there
at the end of second shift. She still was beaming about the ruse she
had pulled on her father and grandmother.

"Tom, that's so *cool,*" she said, drawing out the word. "They
think I have a boyfriend."

"Right, Cathy."

"Tom, you're so cuuuute."

He laughed. He was humoring her. She was one very odd crea-
ture, but he couldn't shake the feeling that at least some of what he
had heard that day was the truth. He had no plans to drop the
investigation. He suggested she drop by Walker PD the next day.

"We can talk some more," he said.

Cathy agreed, but she wanted to squeeze everything she could
out of the boyfriend ruse. Her friend was waiting for her at Alpine.

"Watch this," she said, before getting out of the car.

She walked to the driver's window, bent over and said it loudly
so her friend could hear her.

"Thanks Tom," she said. "Oh Tom, I had a great time."

Christ, he thought, she's still making this look like a date. She's
still playing a game.

Tom Freeman's mind was churning. It was nearly 11:00 P.M. It
had been a long day, maybe his longest ever. He would not sleep at
all that night.

He watched her black truck speed away, disappearing into the
darkness so only its taillights glared back in red. Okay, he thought,
as he pointed the department Olds toward home. We can play
games.

Already, Tom Freeman was planning a few of his own.

Chapter 74

By October, Robin Fielder had finally shaken the feeling that Cathy Wood was hovering over her life again.

Just before Gwen's twenty-fifth birthday, in August, a card arrived in the mail, postmarked Grand Rapids. It pictured a hummingbird suspended over a flower. The words "I love you" were scrawled on the back. It was unsigned, but Robin knew who had sent it.

The card was the first correspondence in eight months. Gwen and Cathy had written each other frequently after they moved. Robin didn't understand the lingering bond. Gwen sometimes broke into tears when they first moved to Texas.

"Hold me, Robin."

"Gwen, why are you crying."

"I just miss Cathy. I just miss her, I do."

In Grand Rapids, she might have stormed out, hurt. In Tyler, she felt she no longer had that choice. She was a thousand miles from home.

When Gwen's lawsuit was dismissed a year ago, they had decided to stay in Tyler anyway. They spent their first two months with Gwen's sister, Corey, in the rural farmhouse where Gwen was raised. It had peeled wood siding, a sagging porch and chickens in the yard. It was a long way from Robin's pool parties behind her parents' ranch home in Walker.

The old house troubled Gwen far more than Robin. Gwen was besieged by old fears. The house made her physically sick. She was constipated their first two weeks there. She wouldn't shower or use the toilet unless she was accompanied by Robin or Corey.

Robin finally asked her why.

"When I was little my head was flushed in the toilet."

Robin decided Gwen's childhood was spent in hell. Every time she saw Gwen break into another sweat, unable to use the bathroom, she felt increasingly sorry for her.

One day, she met Gwen's mother, Linda. The woman seemed pleasant, but Robin sensed a chill between the two of them. They appeared to be going through the motions for Robin's benefit. Gwen said they had never gotten along. She told her how she had once almost choked her to death in a fight.

"Do you love your mom?" Robin asked.

"I try to like her," Gwen said. "But I don't have to love her."

Gwen also claimed the old house had a ghost, that it walked the halls at night. Already, Robin had decided Gwen was afflicted with a morbid sense of humor. The joke about the dead patients at Alpine was continuing.

One day they were chatting with Gwen's sister Corey and an aunt when the sight of a spider running across the floor inspired stories about Cathy and her mind games. Corey asked about the call Robin had made after Cathy threatened her in the Alpine Manor parking lot. Robin told them she was still afraid of Cathy, that she would make good on her threats.

"Well, did you kill six people?" Corey asked.

Gwen looked at her incredulously.

"For real? No. I'm sure."

From that day on, Gwen made the Alpine deaths a running joke. In the middle of a conversation, she would blurt it out, often on an unrelated matter.

"Do you think we'll see some rain, Gwen?" someone would ask.

"No. But how should I know? I killed six people."

They both had found work in the health field again, as aides in Mother Francis Hospital. They worked wards catering to orthopedics, ophthalmology and neurosurgery. Gwen said she liked walking through the hospital nursery. She liked the little babies. She loved being around the small ones in her family as well. One day Gwen joked with Corey about the hospital.

"Wouldn't it be funny if when the mother came to visit the baby, you smashed it up against the window?" Gwen said.

"Whatya mean?" Corey asked.

"You know, if you pushed their faces up against the window, shmooshing their lips up," Gwen said.

"Gwen, you're crazy," Robin said. "That's sick."

Robin wondered in the early months if Cathy was the source

behind the morbid humor. Not only were they writing, Cathy was calling at Corey's house. One night Gwen appeared shaken after she phoned.

"Cathy says she's done it again," she said.

Gwen explained Cathy said she had killed more patients in Alpine Manor.

"Gwen, would you guys stop that," Robin said. "It's sick."

Robin was concerned about the serious side of their calls and correspondences. For a while, she worried about losing Gwen to Cathy. She found a bunch of love letters, one in which it appeared that Gwen was leading Cathy on. Robin confronted Gwen and asked her to put an end to it. The letters stopped in January, after they moved out of Corey's house and into a trailer park. "I thought you didn't really love me," Gwen apologized. "I thought you were just using me to get away from your parents."

By the summer, Robin could say she and Gwen were reasonably happy. The nights of partying at the Carousel in Grand Rapids had been replaced by a simple life in their mobile home. Robin tossed her caffeine pills. They went treasure hunting in thrift shops and took long drives in the country. Gwen worked on her motorcycle. Most nights they were content to just watch TV. Since moving to Texas they had been to a bar only once. Gwen's drinking had decreased dramatically. She smoked pot instead.

A couple of times when Gwen was high she brought up the Alpine deaths again. Robin figured she was trying to scare her, as the story had only become more elaborate. Cathy, Gwen said, had devised the plan to murder patients while they were doing crossword puzzles one day back in the little house on Effie.

"For real. Right while she was workin' on that crossword in the *Star*."

Cathy had marked not only patients for death, but Alpine aides as well, Gwen said. She wanted to lure Angie Brozak down to the Fish Ladder and stab her in the back, then throw her into the raging current. She planned to kill Lisa Lynch that way.

"She even wanted to kill you, Robin."

"No, c'mon."

"But I said no, you were too nice."

"That's sick."

"Well whatya expect? I did kill six people."

And that's why Robin could never take her seriously. Everything that was supposed to happen never did. She thought, Lisa wasn't killed. Neither was Angie. As for the six patients, where was the prison term Cathy threatened? It's been fourteen months. Where are the cops?

"I wish you would quit that murder stuff," Robin complained. "It's not even funny anymore."

It was one of Robin's few complaints. Since they had moved to Texas, she looked to Gwen for guidance about most everything. She was comfortable having Gwen in charge, but Gwen wasn't.

"Robin, I can't make all your decisions for you," she complained. "You've got to start deciding things on your own."

They had differences when it came to sex as well. Robin saw her more as a friend than a lover. And Gwen spent more time in bed tossing and turning than sleeping or making love. Like the constipation, her insomnia began when they moved. Often she stayed up for two days at a time, until exhaustion and a half dozen joints finally knocked her out.

"Why can't you sleep Gwen?" she asked once.

"I'm afraid if I go to sleep I'll never wake up."

Robin struggled with her own ghosts, too. Her mother was crushed not only by her departure, but by the way she left. They still wrote and talked, but her father refused to speak with her. She suspected they both had figured out her relationship with Gwen.

After the card with the hummingbird arrived, Cathy's presence seemed to regenerate in their lives for a while. In late August, Gwen renewed an old friendship with a Texas chum named Deborah Kidder. They had worked together in convenience stores. Debbie now was in the Navy. The three of them went to Lake Tyler and returned to the trailer to grill steaks and drink a lot of beer. The subject of Cathy came up at the kitchen table. They talked about her mind games.

"Well, I sure wish I could see what she looked like," Debbie said.

Gwen produced a photo. Robin had snapped the picture of Cathy. She was in shorts, sunglasses and a big hat, standing next to her parents' pool.

Debbie put a lighter to the corner.

"Bye-bye Cathy."

Gwen protested, but she was too late. The flame almost scorched Debbie's fingertips as she dropped it into the ashtray.

"Shall I tell her?" Gwen said after dinner.

Gwen was rocking back and forth in the living room recliner. She had just smoked a joint. Debbie was lying on the couch.

"Tell her what?" asked Robin.

"You know, about the patients."

"I don't care. You know how I feel about that."

Robin rose to clean up the dishes. She wanted no part of the sick joke.

When she came back into the living room Gwen was finishing up the story. They had suffocated six patients with pillows, she said. With the patient named Marguerite, Cathy stood watch in the doorway.

"Do you believe this?" Debbie said, turning to Robin.

"No, I don't believe it. Are you kidding?"

Then Gwen added a twist Robin hadn't heard before.

"We took souvenirs. From one patient we got a sock."

Debbie sat up on the couch. Her face wore a curious half-smile.

"Okay, Gwen," she said. "Then why did you kill them? Euthanasia?"

"Whatya mean."

"Mercy killing?"

Gwen took another swig of beer, rocking back and forth in her chair.

"Well, at first I felt sorry for 'em. But then, it was fun."

"That's ridiculous," Debbie half shouted.

"That's morbid," Robin added.

By coincidence, two weeks later, Debbie Kidder went to Grand Rapids to visit family there. She stopped at the Carousel and played a game of pool with a woman who turned out to be none other than Cathy Wood. She told Cathy she was an old friend of Gwen Graham's. Debbie called Robin and Gwen with news of the contact.

"She's huge," Debbie said, excitedly. "She's big and evil-looking."

That was in September. It was the last Robin had heard about Cathy Wood and the murder nonsense. Robin was infuriated by Gwen's chat with Debbie. She told her so after Gwen sobered up.

"Gwen, I just don't want to hear that anymore. You shouldn't say stuff like that to people. Why are you even telling Debbie things like that?"

Gwen looked down at her shoes.

"You're right," she said. "Maybe telling Debbie that was a big mistake. Maybe it was a big mistake for real."

Chapter 75

On Saturday morning, the day after his interview with Cathy, Tom Freeman enlisted more help in the form of a polygraph operator with the Michigan State Police named John Hulsing.

Freeman knew sooner or later somebody in the prosecutor's office would ask for a poly on Cathy Wood. He figured he might as well start the process in motion.

They met for coffee. Freeman explained what he had so far.

"Well John, what do you make of this shit?"

Hulsing was relaxed, but pensive. He had a master's degree in psychology as well as twenty-five years as a cop.

"Well, it's awfully bizarre. It doesn't add up. Sounds like, you know, she could be making all this up."

Hulsing offered some theories about Cathy Wood's motivation for undressing in her basement bedroom with Freeman present on Friday night.

"Well, Tom," he concluded, chiding. "Do you think she's in love with you?"

"Shit."

"Be careful."

"Look it, we may need to run her."

"How big did you say she was?"

Freeman guessed 240, 260 maybe.

"Jesus, Tom, she's fat. Probably too fat. I always have problems running fat people."

Freeman put little stock in the tests anyway. He wished the attorneys in the prosecutor's office thought the same. Ever since he'd had two suspects pass polygraphs, but later confess, he considered the charts largely worthless. The results couldn't be used in court, and sometimes they created more problems at the investigative level than solutions.

"Look it, I wouldn't wire my dog up to one," Freeman often said.

However, Freeman also knew he didn't have to believe in the polygraph. Only the suspect did. That's when the confessions came. Plus, he respected the interrogating talents of Hulsing. Over the years the lieutenant and his charts had helped close a half dozen of his cases.

Before they left, Hulsing made a prediction.

"Well, if it pans out this is a very big case, Tom. This is not only big for you, but it will get national attention."

"John," Freeman said, "I'm fully aware of that."

Back at his office later that day, Freeman did a double take. Through the window he could see a woman in a black motorcycle jacket and leather cap wandering around among the police vehicles in the Walker PD parking lot.

"Jesus Christ, who in the hell is that?"

"Oh, that's Nancy," said Cathy Wood.

Cathy had shown up early Saturday afternoon, as promised. She had parked her Luv Truck in front of the station and left her friend, a former Alpine aide named Nancy Harris, to wander the grounds.

"Well, Jesus, let's invite her in," Freeman said.

He sent his partner Roger Kaliniak. Rog could keep her company.

"So you brought a friend?"

Cathy was as matter-of-fact as she had been the night before.

"I don't want to lose my truck. She can drive it away. She'll hide it from the finance company. I'm behind on my payments."

"Well, why can't you hide it?"

She answered earnestly.

"Well, I know one of these days you're going to take me to jail."

There was an uncomfortable silence.

The comment confirmed what Freeman already suspected. She wasn't as naive as she appeared nor as innocent as she acted. Cathy Wood had to have figured she was vulnerable, after signing two Miranda cards on Friday.

Freeman asked her to detail her story again. The request yielded another display of her random recall. She added new details, including the news that Gwen had been inspired to more killing after a wrestling match in the bathroom with a patient named Maurice

Spanogle. This time Freeman asked her to write her story down. She agreed to sign it. Finally, he had a signed statement.

It read:

In the fall of 1986 I was roommates with Dawn Male and we both worked at Alpine Manor Nursing Home. In September I met her best friend Gwen Graham. Dawn and I couldn't get along so she moved out and, needing a roommate, Gwen moved in the last week of September.

We both worked at Alpine Manor also. We worked it seemed all the time different shifts and double shifts. In January of 1987, we both were working second shift and I went over to Dover to see what lunch break we were taking.

After looking for her for a few minutes and not finding her, I started going into rooms with the curtains drawn. Marguerite's door was shut so I opened it and it hit the curtain. I looked and saw Gwen on the far side of the bed holding a washcloth under her chin and over her nose. Marguerite was making noises. I couldn't believe Gwen was doing that. I backed out of the room and went back to Camelot.

I believe it was the next day we talked about it. She said she'd shoot me if I said anything. And, not wanting to be hurt or to lose her, I didn't say anything.

Later that week she tied me up, and me, thinking we were just playing, I went along with it. Then she went to the dresser and got out a pair of socks and held me almost the same way she did Marguerite . . .

She said killing eased her frustrations.

I thought about saying something to someone then, but still didn't want her taken from me.

When Maurice died, she came over to Abbey to tell me what happened, that she and Jim Shooter had been very rough with him and then he died. The nurse over there thought he had a heart attack straining to have a BM. She thought that was funny.

I can't remember the sequence of the rest but she'd either tell me ahead of time of one, or after. Not always beforehand did that resident die.

I think that on most of them I was in the building or even on the same station. We were short of help and few times I think we were the only two on a station, and when Myrtle Luce died as I remember she was on my hall and Gwen was on the other.

When Mae Mason died I was on Camelot. I don't remember where Gwen was and a new girl found Mae.

Marguerite was on Gwen's station and the boy that had her couldn't clean her up and so she thought it was exciting that she had to.

Belle Burkhard was on my station, A. I was sitting at the desk and Gwen came up and put a rolled up washcloth on the desk. I watched her walk down the hall with another washcloth in her back pocket. I thought that was another way to scare me. She was always leaving those where I could find them. On my car. Even at home on the shower.

Well, Pat [Ritter] went to do rounds and Belle had died. Pat was accused of not turning Belle because her arm was funny in some way, bruised or red, I can't really remember. Anyway I knew that Gwen had did that and felt so afraid. Later she told me Belle's arm was like that because she fought so bad that she had to put her knee on it.

Edith Cook was real sick, had gangrene real bad. Gwen took her teeth because she hadn't taken them out first. She didn't want any bite marks on her lips.

I wasn't working on the night Lisa [Lynch] and Robin [Fielder] and I were playing quarters at Lisa's with some neighbors. I don't know when she told me, but she was working a double and told me she did Lucy [Stoddard].

Around this time she had her father send her a rifle in the mail. And she put it together and made me fire it out the back door to see how it would sound when she shot me. If it came to that.

Summer of 1987. We started fighting a lot and Gwen moved in with Robin at Lisa's. Then I received a letter from Texas saying that her trial date was due. So I gave it to her and she told me she and Robin were going. I told her that if she left I would tell. I was worrying about this continuing. I thought I could make her quit.

I realized she was really leaving and thought she was going to kill me so I told my sister Barbara, my ex-husband Ken Wood and my friend Shawn Thatcher how afraid I was and that if anything ever happened to me this is what happened and why.

She left for Texas and we wrote to each other till about December, then mainly just phone calls where she told me she was coming back up here to get me and make me go away with her.

After May, all correspondence quit except I sent her one

card and she had a friend come up to me in the bar and talk to me.

I never suffocated anybody.

Freeman decided to make a confirmation.

"You said you told your sister. What's her phone number?"

Cathy recited her number in Florida. He went to an adjacent room to make the call. He asked Barbara if indeed Cathy had told her about the murders.

"Well, why didn't you go to the police?"

"I thought she was under emotional stress," the voice on the phone explained. "I thought she had made it up."

When he returned to his office Cathy was crying.

"I've lost my best friend," she said.

"What do you mean?"

"My sister was my best friend."

She had heard the conversation through the door. Up until then she had been matter-of-fact, even flippant. Her first show of real emotion surprised him. She had big puppy dog eyes.

Freeman decided he had better start backing up Cathy's story with something more than her goodwill. He planned to chat with Shawn Thatcher, the Alpine aide she mentioned. Meanwhile, Kaliniak already was taking a statement from Nancy Harris.

As Cathy wiped her tears, Assistant Prosecutor David Schieber strolled through the door. He was in Walker talking to the victim's family in the O'Brien murder case. He handed Freeman a list of checks he wanted done on the case.

"You remember Dave Schiebers?" Freeman said, snatching the list from the assistant prosecutor.

"Cathy, what's wrong?"

Freeman answered for her.

"She's upset. I just talked to her sister. She heard about the murders, too."

The attorney straddled an office chair. Freeman could hear them talking as he ran an errand in another room. He thought, Schiebers get off my turf. You're in my office now, goddamnit!

Later Kaliniak and Nancy Harris joined them in the small bureau office. Schieber began asking her questions about sex between women, about the nature of lesbian relationships.

"I just want to understand how it is," he said. "How was it with Gwen?"

Kaliniak and Harris piped up. They talked about roles of domi-nance and submission in sex. Who was the butch? Who was the femme? What was a bull dike? Who was in charge in the relation-ship? Who was in charge in bed?

Schieber happened to say he was getting married soon.

"Hey," Nancy said, "you wanna do something that will really turn on your wife. Rub yourself with Vick's Vapor Rub before you do it, you know."

Kaliniak laughed. Cathy appeared embarrassed.

Freeman thought, what does all this shit have to do with my case? This is a circus.

A few minutes later, he met with Schieber privately. Freeman wanted to brainstorm about Alpine Manor. There were other ele-ments needed before anyone could be charged with murder: A body or two, for starters. Some hard evidence from an autopsy. Circum-stantial evidence.

The assistant prosecutor was disinterested.

"Look, concentrate on the O'Brien case."

"Goddamn *Schiebers,*" Freeman cursed under his breath.

Before she and Nancy Harris sped off in her Luv Truck, Freeman told Cathy Wood to keep in touch.

Chapter 76

The search warrant and murder allegations inspired a common reaction among Alpine Manor's upper management. They thought the story was a ruse, an act of revenge by Ken Wood.

Margaret Widmaier gleaned an anecdote making the rumor circuit. Recently, the story went, Ken had followed Cathy back from lunch and had an argument with her in the parking lot. There were harsh words. He called her a bitch.

"If I can't have you," he reportedly said, "nobody else will."

Ken later denied the account, speculating it was more fiction from Cathy. But in Alpine Manor, the story fit the disparaging profile Cathy had been drawing of Ken throughout the three years and two months she had worked in the nursing home.

Those who ran Alpine Manor simply didn't see their facility as the kind of place where killers stalked the halls. When Walker detectives showed up with the warrant, Jackie Cromwell and others were feeling good about a rave review Alpine had just received from the government agency that certified the nursing home for Medicaid. Besides, Cathy Wood and Gwen Graham were considered two of Alpine's very best aides.

The idea that murder had occurred was entertained only briefly by Jackie Cromwell and Margaret Widmaier. After the Walker police came up with a list of five possible victims, Widmaier checked nursing files with detective Roger Kaliniak, comparing daily work records with patient deaths. Everyone was expecting a major discrepancy, a death while they were off. There was none.

Widmaier turned to Cromwell.

"Oh my God, Jackie. I think it's true."

Ronald Westman, Alpine's owner, was informed about the allegations over the weekend. Soon, an official posture was formulated by Alpine Manor that would not change for more than two years: The nursing home would cooperate fully with police. However, until proven otherwise, Alpine management found it difficult to believe there were any actual killings.

On Monday, October 9, Cathy Wood was not accorded the same benefit of doubt. She called the nursing home, inquiring about her work status.

"You're suspended until further investigation," Widmaier said.

Cathy took it calmly.

Several days later, Cathy inquired about her vacation pay. She talked to Marty Slocum. Slocum was taken back by her voice. She did not sound like Cathy. The supervisor guessed it was stress or something. She sounded several tones higher in pitch.

"I don't know about vacation, Cathy," she told her. "I'll have to check into it."

Soon, Cathy's mother Pat was involved. Her daughter was due

that pay, she told Alpine Manor, police investigation or not. She gave administrators a choice.

"Do you want to mail it. Or, do you want me to come in there and pick it up?"

The check was mailed. It would be her last.

Chapter 77

Before the Walker police had a second pot of coffee brewing Monday morning, Russell Shawn Thatcher was in the interview room with detectives Tom Freeman and Roger Kaliniak.

Over the past year, Thatcher said, he had become Cathy Wood's friend and confidant. He was twenty-one, slim and good-looking. He had worked as an Alpine aide from February to late August of 1987.

Early on, Freeman wanted to know if Cathy had spoken to him about the ongoing investigation.

"Have you ever talked to Cathy, in the past week?"

"No, I haven't," he said.

Freeman would find out two months later that he had lied. In fact, Thatcher had talked to Cathy about the ongoing investigation at length the day before.

Thatcher confirmed Cathy had told him in the summer of 1987 that Gwen Graham had smothered patients. She told him while they lunched at a restaurant called the West Side Deli. Apparently, it was just after Gwen left for Texas.

"How did this come up?" asked Freeman.

"I think it had built up so long, and she just needed to feel she had to tell somebody, somebody she felt she could trust at that time. I knew that after she had told me that it was just a great relief for her to get it out."

"What was your reaction when she told you this? What did you tell her?"

"I was really shocked and, I don't know what I told her first off. I don't know what I exactly said. I remember her saying that she didn't want to go to the police and I had said, I don't think that's a good idea . . . You shouldn't put yourself in this spot. You don't have Gwen here. You're just going to cause a problem. What if Gwen comes back to town? Then there is going to be something on it. Then she is really gonna be angered if nothing develops out of it."

Freeman wanted to confirm the menacing profile Cathy had been drawing of Gwen Graham.

"Was she scared of Gwen?" he asked.

"Yeah."

Earlier, Freeman had made mental notes of the two women's vast differences in size.

"Why?" he asked Thatcher.

"The thought that Gwen could do *this,* and Gwen was a tough girl. Cathy is big, but she is not strong, and she's not a fighter like Gwen would be . . ."

Freeman zeroed in on Cathy's credibility.

"Do you think Cathy would make something like this up?"

"No, she's never lied to me."

Thatcher said he didn't think Cathy was involved.

"Knowing her, she could never do that. There is just no way. So I just don't question it one bit."

Thatcher's observations were consistent with the description Cathy had provided of her relationship with Gwen. Gwen was the feared, dominant partner. Cathy was a troubled follower who would do anything for love.

Thatcher described the day he met Cathy. He, too, had looked into her big, sad eyes.

"I met her at a bar," he explained. "She was the first one there. She just sat there lonely, and I went over and started talking to her."

He praised her as a nurse's aide, but added she had been treated badly by her ex-husband. He had caused her to put on all the weight.

"She loves her daughter Jamie," Thatcher added.

He presented quite a different picture of Gwen, though he admitted he had not spent much time getting to know her.

". . .Every time I talked to her she was real nice to me and there were no problems, so she seems nice, but I don't think she is as nice as it appears on the outside."

He told Freeman and Kaliniak about Gwen's beating of Katherine Brinkman on K-Mart Hill, minus the fact that Cathy had set it up.

"I never realized Gwen's strength until I knew that happened and seen Katherine afterwards."

Thatcher also appeared to know about the circumstances of patient Maurice Spanogle's death. He had heard how Gwen struggled with the patient in the bathroom. Spanogle's wife, who was also a resident, had told Thatcher she heard her husband say "get your cotton pickin' hands off me" from the bathroom before he died.

He was asked, was Gwen capable of killing patients?

"Yes."

"Is Robin afraid of Gwen?" Kaliniak asked.

"That I don't know, obviously not. They've been together for over a year. But that's nothing either. Maybe Robin right now is living in fear of her. We don't know. But Cathy was with Gwen for a while, too. But now, I find out that she was very scared of Gwen."

Freeman saw problems with the story: Why hadn't Thatcher come to the police more than a year ago? He would explore that later. For now, however, the detective decided he had three confirmations of Cathy Wood's story. He had signed statements from Thatcher, Ken Wood and her friend Nancy Harris.

Kaliniak's interview with Harris fit the continuing theme of Gwen Graham as mastermind and perpetrator, though, like the others, Harris's version was based solely on her conversations with Cathy Wood. Harris said just one month ago, at the fish ladder on the Grand River, Cathy told her she feared for her life because of Gwen. She told her Gwen had smothered a patient at Alpine Manor.

There was something else. Kaliniak pointed it out when he handed the statement to Freeman.

"Shit, Tom. Says here she even got her kicks killing the family dog."

Harris's statement concluded:

". . . Cathy mentioned to me was that Gwen enjoyed killing and that her family, her father, were very sick people. Cathy told me Gwen mentioned one time that her father got angry at the dog and told Gwen to go shoot it. Gwen did this, but only took half of the head off the dog the first shot. But she enjoyed it so much she let the dog suffer and watched. I have no doubt that Cathy has been numb from fear and guilt since meeting this woman."

Tom Freeman decided, for now, that it would be counterproductive to interview anybody else. He wanted to keep the lid on the investigation. More interviews meant more risk the media would sniff it out. The last thing he wanted was to lose control of the case.

By Monday afternoon, Freeman and his old boss Bill Brown were on their way to the Hall of Justice. It was time to have another chat with not only David Schieber, but Prosecutor William Forsyth himself.

Freeman wanted to talk about the emerging portrait of Gwen Graham. The detective already had decided that the nurse's aide from Texas looked like a brooding, self-mutilating psycho who loved pain, and liked to dish it out.

As far as Tom Freeman was concerned, it was the picture of a cold killer.

Chapter 78

They had spent the first part of Thursday chauffeuring Gwen's stepbrother around Tyler so he could fill out applications. He was out of work and had a baby on the way. Gwen wanted to help him find a job.

Late in the afternoon, Gwen wrenched her bike, while Robin fixed everyone dinner. Robin was balancing her plate in her lap in front of the TV when someone gave Gwen the opening. Gwen had downed a few beers. Robin hadn't heard the line in weeks.

"Well, how would I know. I killed six people."

Robin thought, Gwen, just shut up. One of these times you are going to say that once too often.

The screech of tire rubber outside punctuated her thought.

Gwen stood straight up, looking out the window.

"I don't live here!"

She bolted toward the bathroom.

Robin looked out. There were police cars, coming in all directions, sliding to a stop in front of their trailer.

Suddenly, there were three knocks—three rapid, hard knocks. Robin opened the door to three men in suits, then others in uniforms. At first, she could only answer with one word.

"Are you Robin Fielder?"

"No."

"Do you know Gwen Graham?"

"No."

"Do you live here?"

"No."

"Well, what's your name?"

"Robin Fielder."

One man began reading a piece of paper, a search warrant. Two others headed to the back of the trailer. Uniformed officers began rummaging through the mobile home.

"What do you want?" Robin said.

She could feel herself coming apart. Gwen's last words repeated in her head. Six people. Six people. *Six people.* She has said that stupid line too many times, and now, by God, they're here. They're here for Gwen. They're here for me.

She began to stammer, then cry, then shout.

"What do you want?"

"We've got her," somebody said.

Robin turned to see one man leading Gwen by the arm from the hallway. She saw a pair of handcuffs.

"What do you want?" Robin screamed. "What do you want?"

"Get her out of here," somebody said, pointing to Robin.

"No, this is my trailer," Robin screamed. "I won't. What do you want?"

"Goddamnit, get her out!" Tom Freeman tried to pull the hysterical young woman from the mobile home. She clutched the doorknob with her hands, while the rest of her body collapsed on the steps.

"C'mon, Robin."

She sobbed, clutching the door tighter. Then she screamed again.

"What do you want?"

"It's okay, c'mon."

She screamed at the top of her lungs.

"What do you want?"

Finally, he pulled her away with an assertive jerk, and walked her to the back seat of a squad car.

Jesus Christ, Freeman thought. She must know something. She was a West Catholic grad with no criminal record, the background check showed. There had been no hint she would go absolutely berserk at the sight of cops.

It was October 12, six days after Ken Wood had walked into Wyoming PD with his story. The Monday meeting at the prosecutor's office had resulted in Freeman and Deputy Chief Bill Brown flying to Tyler. They had secured a search warrant from a Texas judge for letters from Cathy Wood to Gwen Graham and any property that might have belonged to Alpine patients. They were in Texas looking for souvenirs.

"Look it, beyond that, we simply cannot do anything more," Schieber had advised. "Plus, you've got to talk to Gwen Graham."

Everyone knew that questioning Graham might very well backfire. In the best-case scenario she would confess. The worst case was not outright denial.

"We could go down there and she says, 'I didn't kill anybody, but Cathy told me she did,' " Freeman told Schieber. "Then we have the word of one against the other. Then we don't have shit."

The case couldn't hold together without some credible testimony by one of them. If they told similar stories about one another in a vacuum of hard evidence, who would a jury believe?

Freeman was less apprehensive about the trip after contacting the Tyler police. One of the department's homicide detectives was married to a cousin of Gwen Graham's. His name was Danny Alexander. In Texas they talked about Gwen over dinner.

"After she came back from California, she wasn't the same girl," Alexander told them. "That's what my wife said."

Not only did Alexander know where Gwen lived, but he found out she had an outstanding misdemeanor warrant for writing $611 in bad checks in 1985. The money was for rent and motorcycle parts. The plan was to execute the search warrant, then book Graham at Tyler PD on the Texas misdemeanor. The arrest might soften her up for Freeman's interview.

First, however, Freeman had to get Robin Fielder under control.

She became hysterical again as a patrolmen led Gwen Graham to a squad car for transport to Tyler PD. As the cruiser sped off, she looked as if she was ready to pass out.

"Look, Robin, you need a drink of water?"

She nodded. He walked her to a garden hose.

Back in the car, he tried to make small talk about Grand Rapids. They had both gone to some of the same Catholic schools.

"Now Robin, I'm going to tell you why I'm here."

She nodded.

"You see, Cathy Wood told us . . ."

He never finished the sentence.

"She's making it up. She's making it up. She's making it up."

She started sobbing again. He thought, I never said anything, and already she's covering. He calmed her again.

"Cathy is making this up," she said again, sniffling.

"Making what up?"

She told him how Cathy Wood had confronted her in the Alpine Manor parking lot, threatening to turn Gwen in for murder.

"But it's a mind game. Cathy is crazy. She's evil, don't you understand. It was like she had Gwen hypnotized for a long time."

Inside, the search warrant had turned up a brown paper bag full of letters from Cathy Wood. Robin agreed to go to Tyler PD with Freeman, Bill Brown and Danny Alexander. When they arrived, Freeman put her in an interview room.

"Will you write down what you told me in the car?" he asked, handing her paper and pen.

She nodded.

A few minutes later Freeman joined Gwen Graham and Danny Alexander. She was dressed in sweat pants and a T-shirt with the logo of Mother Francis Hospital. Her hair was unkempt and greasy. She had seen the search warrant. She knew they were there on a murder investigation. She waived her rights and was ready to talk.

"Would you agree to take a polygraph about what we're going to talk about today," Freeman asked.

She agreed.

Freeman began with banter about Alpine Manor, how it was understaffed, how schizophrenics there sometimes caused problems.

"Yep, sure do," she said, nodding.

She seemed so agreeable, he expected her to unload allegations against Cathy at any time.

"What do you think of euthanasia, Gwen?"

"Don't believe in it, no sir."

"Why?"

"Well, every patient has got the right to live."

He asked her about dealing with patients. Was she ever rough with them? Did she see any abuse? Finally, he cut to the central question.

"Well, Cathy has told us that you have killed patients at Alpine Manor."

Gwen chuckled.

"That was a game. That was a joke. You all came down here all this way for that?"

Freeman didn't smile.

"If it is a joke, it's one hell of a joke to have lasted now for almost two years."

"Look, I never killed anyone. You don't need to spend more than five minutes with Cathy to realize she's a fruitcake. She played jokes, mind games, all the time, for real."

Freeman decided to become specific.

"Well, let's talk about just one patient then. Let's talk about Marguerite Chambers."

Gwen's mouth dropped open. He let silence work on her for a few seconds. Finally, she spoke.

"I don't want to talk. I don't want to talk anymore. I want a lawyer."

Freeman rose and excused himself. Gwen looked up and added something before he left.

"Look, Cathy's just not happy. She's trying to get even with me 'cause we had a relationship. She's trying to get even 'cause I left with Robin, and she's still in love."

"She still wants a lawyer," Alexander said, emerging a few minutes later. "Tom, did you see her face drop?"

Freeman nodded. Gwen still wanted to take the polygraph, Alexander said. Meanwhile, Tyler could book her on the check charges.

Freeman had an idea.

"Look it, let's put Robin in there with her and see what happens."

They watched from the one-way glass as Robin was escorted to the doorway of the room. Inside, alone, she dropped to her knees in front of Gwen, putting her face in her lap. She was crying. Gwen patted her on the head.

"You're a good puppy," she said. "You're a real good puppy. Everything is going to be all right."

Robin calmed.

"Danny, look at that," Freeman said.

Damn, he thought. He wished he had that kind of power, the kind of power Gwen had over Robin Fielder. He didn't have a confession, but he had another confirmation. Cathy was right. Gwen was the manipulator.

Robin Fielder, Freeman decided, would probably do anything for Gwen Graham as well.

Chapter 79

Robin couldn't believe how far Cathy had gone this time.

"This is just a head game Cathy is playing," Gwen whispered to her when her head was in her lap. "You don't have to say a thing."

Gwen said police were probably watching through the mirror on the wall. Robin didn't tell Gwen she had already given them a written statement.

Later, with a bail bondsman, Gwen posted bail on the bad check misdemeanor, just in time for them to report for their late shift at Mother Francis Hospital. Gwen also talked to an attorney, her uncle. He recommended she go ahead with the polygraph.

The next day, as they drove to downtown Tyler for the examination, Gwen appeared nervous. She wondered out loud what kind of questions they would ask. There was no joking about dead patients this time. Robin wished there never had been.

"I wonder if I'll pass it."

"Of course you will."

Gwen nodded her head.

"Yep, I sure will. I know how to pass a lie detector. You do it by thinking of something good."

Gwen looked at Robin, lovingly.

"When they ask the questions, I'll just think of you."

After dropping Gwen off at the police department, Robin went back to their trailer to wait for her call. Alone, she felt engulfed by Cathy's treachery. She worried about losing Gwen. She thought, Gwen is all I have. My father has disowned me. I can't go back to Grand Rapids. Not now. My family would never accept me for what I am, for what I've become.

Robin Fielder felt as if she were dead inside and everything around her were in chaos. The trailer was still in a shambles from the police search. We should have never burned Cathy's picture, she thought. Debbie Kidder should never have looked up Cathy in Grand Rapids. Look what that has done.

Robin began picking up. She hung their clothes back in the closets and put books back in the boxes where they belonged. That's when she thought of it.

My God, the diary. Did they get the diary!

She had kept one through all of 1987, her Virginia Slims Book of Days. It detailed everything.

She searched frantically from room to room. She rooted through boxed collections of memorabilia and rifled through dresser drawers. She pulled piles of junk from closet corners. She opened suitcases and duffel bags. She found the diary tucked in the liner pocket of an old purse.

Burn it, she thought. I'll burn everything that has to do with Cathy and Gwen. I'll burn their entire sick past.

She rounded up old bills from Effie and other paperwork. She found letters the police had missed. She put everything in a big pile outside in the trash. As she put a match to the paper, some of the entries in her book of days flashed through her mind. There was the conversation about the patients in the Family Foods parking lot. The trip to the graveyard. The talk with Lisa Lynch. The jokes Gwen made with her family.

No one knows the truth, she thought. No one knows how clever

Cathy is at twisting and distorting the facts. I'm not going to give her any ammunition for her sick game.

The police would never understand, she thought as she watched the flames. She already knew by the way they talked, the police didn't know Cathy Wood at all.

Tom Freeman listened to the analysis of the polygraph examiner named Ray Lewis. The retired Dallas policeman, now in private business, arrived at Tyler PD meticulously dressed in a suit and carrying a portable polygraph unit at his side.

He ran Gwen Graham several times. There were four questions:

1. January, 1987, at the Alpine Manor Nursing Home, did you yourself cause the death of Marguerite Chambers?

2. Did you place your hand or any object over Marguerite Chambers' mouth and nose and cause her to suffocate?

3. Did you ever tell Cathy you killed or caused the death of anyone?

4. Did you kill Marguerite Chambers?

Lewis was troubled with the results. Graham didn't even show a response in some areas where even a normal, truthful subject would. Lewis elaborated on the technical details of his scoring system, then gave Freeman his bottom line.

"Well, it's inconclusive."

Freeman told himself: Yes, and that's exactly why I wouldn't run my dog on one.

"But do you want my personal opinion, apart from the charts?"

"Sure."

"She's a cold-blooded killer."

Freeman made another try at interviewing Graham. He bluffed with the results, telling her she was deceptive. She stuck to her story. This was all a joke, a mind game by Cathy Wood.

Freeman and Bill Brown would be returning to Grand Rapids with not much more than a handful of love letters. They found no souvenirs. Ahead, back home, was another polygraph. Freeman had scheduled Cathy Wood for one with John Hulsing of the state police.

A week since the investigation began, Freeman was convinced he had been face-to-face with a serial killer. He wondered what she was up to in Mother Francis Hospital. He wondered if there were more bodies at the nursing homes where she worked as a temporary after leaving Alpine Manor.

He wasn't the only one concerned. As the polygraph examiner prepared to head to his next stop, they chatted more about the case. The Texan wanted to know more details.

"So tell me, what's this little gal do now?" Lewis asked.

"She works at Mother Francis Hospital in Tyler. She's a nurse's aide."

He looked off to the horizon.

"Lord," he said, "my mother's a patient there right now."

Chapter 80

Before she ever arrived for testing, State Police Lieutenant John Hulsing had some thoughts about the twenty-six-year-old nurse's aide named Catherine May Wood.

From the details already provided by Tom Freeman, he suspected she was manipulative. Freeman was worried about the police ethics of being in her basement bedroom. Hulsing believed the detective's anxiety had less to do with procedure and more to do with his suppressed fears of being her pawn.

"At that point she had the psychological hook into him," Hulsing later told another investigator. "I told him I thought she had fallen in love with him. It was a facetious comment, but there was some truth in it."

The woman who arrived for her polygraph examination on Monday, October 24 exceeded Hulsing's expectations. He felt she was trying to stroke him at the start. She looked him in the eyes, smiling during their pre-exam interview. She began with her own question.

"Are you a psychologist?"

"I am a psychologist, but I'm not practicing psychology right now."

"I thought so. Your voice is so *nice.*"

She was cordial, upbeat, almost effervescent.

"She was extremely smooth," he later recalled. "Someone trying to compliment me—that sort of thing is extremely rare in that setting."

Hulsing believed that twenty-five years with the state police and a year of clinical training in psychology with federal and state prisoners had equipped him with his own set of detectors apart from those that came with the polygraph. In twelve years as an examiner he had worked on more than one hundred-twenty homicides. He was fifty-one and planned to retire from police work within the year. He wanted to practice psychology full-time.

As for the polygraph, Hulsing knew the procedure had been analyzed and debated for years. The theory of its operation was a simple one: When a person being tested fears detection, that fear produces a measurable physiological reaction when the subject responds deceptively. Specifically, the machine measured changes in respiration, blood pressure, heartbeat and galvanic skin response.

Reams of studies basically concluded its reliability varied with the operator, the person being examined and the circumstances surrounding the test. Hulsing also knew that twelve state police examiners across Michigan, in doing some 3500 exams a year, averaged 800 felony confessions as a result of the instrument.

"These were confessions or admissions that the initial investigator either could not, would not or was unable to obtain," he explained. "So it is a very useful tool. The state police consider it a very useful investigative aid, and that's all they consider it as."

Like most state police examiners, Hulsing began with a general interview of forty-five minutes or so, without employing the machine. It helped relax the subject, but also provided insight into memory, personality, medical conditions and powers of concentration. Meanwhile, Freeman, or any other investigator, could eavesdrop on video from another room. Most took notes or made a tape with a provided VCR.

Two of Hulsing's stock questions often yielded revealing answers.

"What is the best thing that ever happened to you?" he asked Cathy.

"Well, my daughter," she said at first.

Then she changed it.

"Gwen. Having Gwen was the best thing that ever happened to me."

"The worst?"

"Losing Gwen. Losing Gwen was the worst."

Hulsing found the answers compelling. In murder cases, invariably suspects or witnesses were trying to come to grips with the case. He would have expected responses like "seeing Gwen kill those people" or "being dragged into all this."

Freeman had asked Hulsing to ask her about spelling M-U-R-D-E-R.

"I understand you were going to kill someone whose last names corresponded to those letters?"

"Yes, I said that," she said. "But that's not true."

When they took a break before the formal exam, he approached Freeman privately. He found him not with the eavesdropping monitor, but in the waiting room.

"Tom, did you hear her response in there?"

He was stunned by Freeman's answer.

"No, I've been out here talking to the girlfriend that drove her here."

Not only hadn't the detective watched or taken notes, he hadn't loaded the VCR with a tape. In a dozen years of exams he had only seen that happen once or twice. In fact, he thought, Freeman had always paid close attention in a dozen previous exams.

"Tom, why? Why weren't you watching?"

"John, I want to remain objective. I don't wanna hear anything."

It simply didn't make any sense. Most detectives were fixed on the monitor on far less important cases. This could pan out into the biggest case of his career. He thought, doesn't Freeman want to know the truth?

Hulsing returned to the examining room for the formal part of the test. Setting them among a grouping of others used for comparative purposes, he focused the exam on three questions:

1. Are you lying about Gwen to get her in trouble?
2. Did you see Gwen smother Marguerite?
3. Are you giving Detective Freeman a false story about Gwen causing deaths?

He would run the questions three times.

In the first round, Hulsing decided she was trying to manipulate the results. Three years ago, he had wired the subject's chair with a motion sensor. It was helpful in detecting people who tried to tamper with results using techniques passed along on the streets. Some tensed their legs. Others squeezed their buttocks. The more subtle simply pressed a single large toe into the floor. Hulsing's sensor picked it up.

It picked up Cathy's toe, while there wasn't a hint of stress in her voice or her face.

Such tactics produced misleading readings on the charts. It didn't matter. The fact that Cathy Wood was doing it was more telling than the chart. Studies showed that only the deceptive employ such techniques.

On the second round of questions, Hulsing detected another pattern. As they went through the questions again he asked her to answer first with the truth, then a lie. She changed the pitch in her voice and the response time to questions and answers she apparently wanted to affect. He thought, she's shaping herself into different personalities for each question. She also was using her toe again.

After the third round of questions he had seen enough.

"There was absolutely no question in my mind from experience that she was playing a game," he said later. "She was playing a very subtle, intelligent game. A cognitive game."

She had all the behaviors of a chronic liar, Hulsing decided. She revealed in test questions unrelated to the murder that she had made false statements to get others in trouble. She included among her marks the name of her ex-husband Ken, her friend Nancy, a girl named Brinkman and somebody called Slocum.

Hulsing first gave the test results to Cathy Wood.

"Cathy, you're not being truthful."

He noticed an immediate change in her demeanor. Her face was blank. There were no more compliments or enthusiastic smiles.

She began to offer an explanation.

"Well, I didn't really see Gwen suffocate Marguerite Chambers," she said, coldly. "Gwen only told me she suffocated Marguerite."

Hulsing explained she had many opportunities during the two-hour exam to amend the questions. He had asked her repeatedly if they accurately reflected her statements.

He took Freeman aside privately.

"Tom, without any question this gal is not telling me the truth. She's lying."

He told him about her manipulations. Freeman was disturbed, angry even. Hulsing found himself trying to sell the detective on the test's results.

"Well, I believe her," Freeman said.

Then Hulsing told him again, in front of Cathy Wood.

"Tom, she's just not being truthful."

Freeman turned to Cathy, then Hulsing.

"Well, Cathy, I believe you."

Hulsing wasn't shocked at such disagreement in front of a suspect. He knew all the roles detectives played. Empathy was a proven investigative technique. If Freeman didn't keep feeding Cathy the attention, she just might cut him off. Hulsing considered Tom Freeman to be a good cop. He just hoped he wasn't getting sucked in too far by his own methods.

From what he had seen so far, John Hulsing had already worked up his own, private psychological profile of Cathy Wood. She had textbook manifestations of antisocial and narcissistic personality disorders. Some might call Cathy Wood a psychopath, a manipulative troublemaker void of real empathy or conscience.

The state police lieutenant had seen people like her before. They were more predictable than they thought. If one ruse didn't work, they often tried another. After Freeman and Cathy Wood, Hulsing made the prediction to his colleagues in the district headquarters.

"She'll be back," he said. "She'll be back with another story."

Chapter 81

On the way out the door of the Michigan State Police District Headquarters, Tom Freeman started a strategic spat. He figured he had nothing to lose. Without something more solid from Cathy Wood, his case was finished.

"Here you go, Cathy."

He handed her a couple of his business cards.

"I'm sick of this shit," he said. "You're holding out on me."

She looked at him with hurt eyes.

"I mean it. I can't do anything more. You're involved, and you know more than you're telling me. I'm all done. You're the one who's gonna have to clear this up—for you, and for me."

He walked quickly to his car, looking back once.

"You've got my card," he said.

Freeman predicted to himself she would call. He believed she wanted to please him. People had been shitting on her all her life, he decided. He had shown her some respect, some decency. She would respond to that.

Also, while Cathy was with Hulsing, he had told her friend Nancy Harris something he was sure she would relay to Cathy. If autopsies were done on the nursing home victims, there would be evidence of suffocation, he told her. Bodies might be exhumed. He thought, let Cathy Wood sit at home and give that some thought.

People *were* murdered. He could feel it.

Tom Freeman also knew he had convinced no one but himself. His old mentor Bill Brown was suspicious of the case. David Schieber was shitting on the case. His partner Roger Kaliniak was shooting him strange looks. Now, John Hulsing had joined the chorus.

Freeman thought, but I'm the one who talks to her. I'm the one who looks her in the eyes. There's truth there, goddamnit! Some-where in all her bullshit there is truth.

The call came three days later, in the midafternoon of October 27. She wanted to clear everything up. She had been lying, she said.

"Tom, meet me at work."

She was waitressing at a fast-food restaurant called Chick-a-dees in Eastbrook Mall.

No, he thought. No more games. On my terms, my territory now. He felt he had earned the offensive with three days of nerves, and he wasn't about to give it back easily.

"Cathy, you have to come to the department."

"I'm not coming to the police department, cause you're gonna put me in jail this time."

She was whining.

"That might be true. But you have to come here."

"Well, *all right,*" she said, sighing the word. "I just can't live with myself. I gotta talk to you."

They agreed to meet at 10:00 P.M., after her shift. Ten minutes later she called back. She was crying.

"I have to talk to you now," she said.

After Freeman hung up he pulled a large file folder out of his desk and punched small holes in the top. Inside he slid a small cassette recorder. He was sick of trying to keep up with fractured logic. He would tape her whether she liked it or not.

The Luv Truck arrived at Walker PD a few minutes later, at 4:00 P.M. They sat down in the interview room and began to talk. She wasn't crying anymore.

"Don't you have your tape recorder on?" she began.

"You never wanted a tape recorder, Cathy."

"Well, let's get one on."

"I'll tell you what, Cath, let's move to another room."

He placed her in an interview room, then came back with the recorder, minus the folder and half chuckling to himself. The woman is goddamn telepathic, he thought.

He walked casually, but inside he was electric. The goddamn ploy, he thought, the calculated fucking gamble *worked!* It was the kind of moment that flipped a switch in every cop, every investigator. He read Cathy her rights.

"Do you understand those rights, Cathy?"

She was formal.

"Yes, sir."

"Okay. Okay, you contacted me by phone this afternoon and asked to see me in reference to this case, and the reason why you came in here was to, what? Explain that to me."

She began slowly.

"Well, you know the whole thing already and I, I know that I'm in a lot of trouble, and I might as well tell you exactly how, exactly how it is, or how I remember it to be. So that a year or two years down the line it doesn't come up again, I want it done right now, and over with. And, I feel, I don't know why I did it. I might as well, I might as well pay for what I did, *because I helped.*"

Yes ma'm, Freeman thought. He glanced at the spinning cassette.

"Okay, tell me from the beginning as far as what you told me earlier as what you and Gwen Graham talked about."

"We talked about killing people in the nursing home and just decided that we were going to do it and . . ."

"What was your reason for it? Was there any reason that came up?"

"No."

She elaborated on some basics, but continued to avoid motive. The discussion was in the house on Effie. It was in the beginning of January 1987. Freeman asked again about spelling M-U-R-D-E-R.

"Was that brought up during that conversation with Gwen?"

"No, not the initials, I think."

"Was it ever brought up?"

"Yes."

"Okay."

"There, there was a book they keep at the nursing home with all the names on it as they die or are discharged to a hospital, and we were going to try to make it spell M-U-R-D-E-R going down."

"Did you succeed in doing that?"

"No."

"Did you try using Marguerite Chambers as the first patient, is that why?"

"I don't think so, I don't think she was included in that, no."

"Why was Marguerite Chambers the first to die?"

"I don't know. I don't know how they were decided on. I can't remember that."

Bullshit, Freeman thought. This is goddamn murder.

"Do you recall the date you discussed this with Gwen?"

"I think it was the first week in January."

"You mentioned earlier to me January the eighth you thought . . ."

She finished for him.

"Something happened January 8th. I don't know because Marguerite was suffocated two different times, and the first time she just didn't die. So maybe that was the eighth."

Freeman thought, January the eighth, *again*. She had mentioned it a half dozen times, but it fit nothing in the records.

He wanted to get back to Marguerite.

"Well how do you know that [she was suffocated twice] if you weren't present in the room?"

"I don't know."

"Tell me what happened on Marguerite Chambers' death."

"There were two different times though I'm not sure if I'm mixing them together or not."

"There were two different dates too?"

"Uh huh. Her husband would—her husband would come and see her, so Gwen went in there. One time I was in the hallway, I don't know—I'm mixing them together. One time I was in the hallway and I walked in the room and I saw what she was doing. She was jerking like that, and Gwen was holding her on the far side of the bed. And I went back out and I was in the hallway. The night she died I went to Camelot, but this was the second time, I know this. I went to Camelot and then all the rest I told you was accurate. But the first time I don't remember where I was or what I was doing, but I know that, see I don't know those two are too mixed up together for me. But in between those two, she acted real weird and she was, she was sick all the time, and had a high temp, and it might have been a week maybe a few days."

Freeman thought, the information has changed, but Cathy Wood's manner of delivery had not. She was jumping all over the place on him again. She was employing her favorite phrase: "I don't know." There was a pattern. She remembered circumstances and conversations three different ways, delivered simultaneously: *Gwen*

*might have said or did it. She might have said or did it. "I don't know"
who said or did it.*

Tom Freeman would never get accustomed to that. But at least
now they were making some progress. Cathy Wood certainly was no
longer merely a witness, he thought.

The interview continued for two days, lasting well past the dinner
hour on October 27 and resuming just before lunch for several
hours the following day.

The number of potential victims increased from six to eight,
Cathy adding the names of Ruth Van Dyke and a ninety-year-old
retired bookkeeper named Wanda Urbanski, who had died on
March 2, 1977. Urbanski's name surfaced as Cathy looked at a list
Freeman had of the Alpine dead. She was trying to explain M-U-R-
D-E-R, but she appeared to only be speculating.

"I must have assumed that was the "U" when I looked at the
list," she said. "And Ruth Van Dyke," I'm not really sure about. I'm
really not sure about that one, but I remember [Gwen] holding her
. . ."

Cathy was evasive about the M-U-R-D-E-R plan. She said the
"M" was for Marguerite, but later she would say it began with Mae
Mason. She was consistent about one thing. They had abandoned
the homicidal spelling bee because the logistics of picking the right
victims at the right time became too difficult.

Freeman probed the spelling plan extensively because so far
Cathy had provided very little motive. After two days of interviewing,
however, Cathy's version of the story now had a beginning, middle
and an end.

The idea for the killings was brought up by Gwen one night in
bed. "And then we kind of dropped it. And then it came up again
and we just decided we were going to do it."

Freeman asked, ". . . As far as planning the deaths of patients,
what did you talk about, exactly, what was your conversation?"

"We talked about that we would get caught, and she said, no, we
wouldn't because just the two of us would know. And then she said
that—no, and then I think I said it. I don't remember how it came
up. It might have been me that said it, that if we did this, then we
could never be separated from each other. She liked that because we
would have each other *forever,* and that's how the conversation went.

Not how we were going to do it, or what we were going to do, or just that it was something that would bind us together forever."

She eyed Freeman. She seemed embarrassed.

"Oh God," she said. "That's silly, but that's what it was."

He asked her to speculate about psychological motivation.

"Why did Gwen do it?"

"I am only guessing, but she liked pain and painful things. So I don't know. She has had a lot of pain in her life. I don't know if she wanted to make other people feel the same, I don't really know. I did it because I felt a lot of rejection all my life, and I did not want to lose her and I thought that helping her do whatever she wanted, no matter what, was the right thing. That's how *I* felt."

With the M-U-R-D-E-R motive apparently just a passing fancy, Freeman tried to determine how and why the victims were chosen.

"Do you have any idea why Marguerite? There are two hundred patients in there."

Cathy shook her head.

"I don't know that."

"Why all white females? Why females?"

Cathy quickly came up with an exception. There was a man. She said Gwen had unsuccessfully tried to kill the patient she would later name as Donald Randall. His jaw was too strong. Gwen had told him, "I'm going to kill you tonight," but failed.

Freeman tried it another way. He went after the details on every death.

"How did you plan, and Gwen, Marguerite Chambers' death?"

"I don't remember how it was that we picked her out. I don't remember if it was me or if it was her. We had talked about it. We decided it was going to be her. I don't know why. Then I fed her dinner. See I don't know if it was the first time or the second time because those two are so confusing for me."

With a couple more questions, she finally firmed up a version. She stood outside of Marguerite Chambers' room as a lookout, she said, briefly entering the room as Gwen was suffocating the patient. Gwen, she said had smothered her into unconsciousness a first time, but as they waited for a supervisor to be called to the room, the page on the public address never came.

"I remember her telling me she was dead, and we were waiting, and then nothing happened," she explained. "So she went back by there, and she goes, she was really shocked, she said, Marguerite is still alive. I said, how can she be? And she said I don't know she must have took a breath or something happened or she convulsed or something . . . So then we kind of decided that we had to do it again, and Gwen was going to hold her longer."

The victim had to be held several minutes after she appeared to be dead, Cathy said.

Again, Freeman went after motive. *Why was Marguerite the first?*

"I think you know that," he said.

"Yes I do," Cathy said.

Finally, Freeman thought.

"Why?"

"I don't know."

He threw up his hands.

"Now, I don't understand that," he said.

"I don't know. I don't know how we picked them, I really don't."

A few minutes later she reiterated the point.

". . . There was no specific reason. I mean we didn't pick out people because of certain things."

While Cathy Wood's memory for specifics seemed to go off and on like a slow strobe, certain consistent themes unfolded in the two late October interviews and subsequent talks with Freeman. They would not change for the duration of the Alpine Manor murder case.

First, the method of death was consistent. Washcloths were used to avoid fingerprints and trauma to the face. Gwen, Cathy said, also employed rolled washcloths to keep Cathy in a state of submissive terror. She left them as calling cards in the rooms. She draped them over the shower in Cathy's basement. She let them flap out of her back pocket.

Second, Gwen Graham was a domineering psychopath. Gwen enjoyed a macabre mix of sex and death. Some patients aroused her sexually. Gwen first proposed the killing. Gwen proposed the method. Gwen did the hands-on killing. At first, Gwen had promised to stop killing after Marguerite. But then Gwen saw Maurice Spanogle's heart attack as "a sign" that the killing must continue. Gwen was rough with patients. Gwen was a brawler on the job and off. Gwen obtained a certain "release" through murder. From what Tom Freeman had seen of the scarred-up Texan, he didn't doubt the portrayal.

Third, while Cathy admitted taking part in the choice of victims,

she did so reluctantly. Her role was largely as a lookout and con-
spirator in the cover-up. The role matched her personality, Freeman
decided. Though large, she seemed so fragile. He thought, being
that big must truly be a sonovabitch. She needed attention. Gwen
gave it to her. He couldn't get out of his head that picture of Robin
Fielder falling to her knees for Graham. He told Cathy what he saw.

"That's just how I was with her, too," she said.

Cathy provided more detail in the two late October interviews.
She pinpointed their whereabouts on most of the deaths. She drew
blanks on important conversations, but remembered patient room
numbers, shifts, breaks and stations. Though nearly two years has
passed, all checked out with Alpine Manor records.

In her new version of events, she admitted playing an important
part in most of the homicides.

Belle Burkhard: Cathy said she sat at Abbey Lane station, listening with the intercom switched to the victim's room. As Gwen
smothered her, she listened to sheets rustling and groans of the
life-and-death struggle. Also, Cathy watched Gwen leave the room
and return to her assignment on Dover. She remembered her washcloth flapping in her back pocket. She also clearly remembered Pat
Ritter screaming and running up the hall after finding Belle's body.

"She was real upset, Pat was," Cathy said.

Mae Mason: Cathy said that while Gwen was smothering her in
Abbey Lane, she intercepted Night House Supervisor Marty Slocum
and kept her occupied in Camelot.

"I know Mrs. Slocum likes gossip, she gets off on that big-time,"
she explained. "So I was making up stuff to keep her on Camelot,
while this was going on in Abbey Lane."

Lucille Stoddard: Cathy said she wasn't working that night.
Cathy wasn't sure whether Gwen had killed Stoddard or not.

Ruth Van Dyke: Cathy was evasive, or unsure. She did name her
in a list of victims on her station.

"But earlier, you said that you weren't sure whether or not Ruth
was killed," Freeman pointed out.

"Ruth Van Dyke, right, but I was in the hall at one time she was
holding her."

"How do you know that, did you see her?"

"No, I don't think so, but I don't know."

"I don't understand."

She seemed eager to please him.

"I don't know what you want me to say," Cathy said.

Freeman thought, Damn it! You either saw her, or you didn't. She continued.

"I don't know if I went in the room or not, but see, I know most of them I didn't see."

Myrtle Luce: Cathy hinted at some additional criteria for killing.

"Myrtle was decided on because she was hard to care for too," Cathy said. "So maybe that had something to do with it. They [all] were real hard to care for."

Edith Cook: Cathy remembered handling her false teeth. The detail came up when Freeman proposed exhuming Cook's body. There might be abrasions caused by teeth during smothering. Cathy said she was a lookout from Abbey station, but hinted she became more involved after the homicide.

"Because Gwen said she thought she made a mistake," she explained. "She thought she might have done it with her teeth in, and so I don't know if I took them out or she did. Then I wrapped them in an Attend and threw them in the [garbage]. But I don't know if I took them out. I can't remember that."

Then there was the matter of souvenirs. She had mentioned them in earlier talks. He asked her again about Marguerite's MOTHER balloon.

"Who took the souvenir?"

". . . I don't know who took it, I, I don't remember that."

"Where did these souvenirs go? They went to the Effie street residence, is that correct?"

"Second shelf in the bedroom."

"Where could they possibly be now?"

"They were thrown away a long time ago. Gwen went over there to throw them away."

"How long did she keep the souvenirs?"

"Till she left."

She detailed a souvenir taken from Mae Mason. It was a little white house, with a working front door. She drew him a picture. It was the size for a key chain token.

"Gwen brought it to me like it was a prize, and she gave it to me. And I brought it home and I put it on the shelf."

Cathy also recanted some earlier statements.

"Gwen never threatened to kill me," she said. "But when she left [for Texas] I thought she might."

Gwen left for Texas more than three months after the last homicide. Freeman went to the question that begged to be asked.

"How come it stopped?"

She was matter-of-fact.

"I didn't want to do it anymore."

The answer was in conflict with her portrait of herself as the reluctant accomplice. Freeman came back quickly.

"She agreed to stop? Was it you?"

She offered more.

"I don't, I just wouldn't help anymore. I didn't really want to help after the first one, but she wanted to take turns. She wanted to do one and she wanted me to do one, and I couldn't do that."

"Why?"

"I couldn't kill anybody. I know I helped. I know I helped pick them out, but for me to actually, I couldn't. Those people in there were, uh, they were, they were, a lot of those people in there were like family to me and I couldn't do that to them. That's real bad to say that, I know. I *couldn't.*"

Freeman wanted to know if Gwen ever talked about killing after leaving Alpine. Cathy said she had talked to her on the phone in Texas. Cathy said Gwen wanted to kill a hitchhiker. She had also mentioned the nursery at Mother Francis in Tyler.

"She said she wanted to take a baby and smash it up against the window."

At the end of the first interview, Cathy told Freeman she had been playing an evasive game with him in previous interviews. She was no longer, she said. The next day, she indicated she could pass a polygraph, if the questions were accurate.

She also said she knew that confirmation of her story might mean a prison term for her. She had been told earlier that fabricating a story could mean time behind bars for filing a false police report.

"If I'm going to go to prison I might as well go for what I did," she said.

Freeman sensed she had a big need to be believed. She said prison was the worst thing that could happen to Gwen Graham, but "that's not what I'm most afraid of."

She momentarily stepped out of the unwilling accomplice mode.

"I'm really sorry these things happened and I need to pay for it now. I didn't kill them, but I had just as much input into it as she did."

The next day Freeman probed the area more.

"What's the worst thing that could happen to you today?"

"Gwen could be out there waiting to kill me."

The best?

"That I could go with Jamie someplace and no one would ever bother me again, or know where I was or anything like that."

"But yet you told me that you really did not have any maternal instincts toward your daughter."

No, now she wanted her daughter. She could be a better parent than Ken.

"I know, that has changed a lot in the last week," she said. "And I don't know why."

She's not the only thing that's changed, Tom Freeman thought. Now he had something for Bill Brown, David Schieber and all the rest of the doubting Thomases to ponder. She was implicating herself. *That* had to carry some weight. Sure she still was evasive. But she had a *need* to get it off her chest, even to pay for the crime.

He would send her home before conferring with the prosecutor's office. The last thing she would do was run, he decided.

Tom Freeman had found a new ploy. He was going to continue challenging Cathy Wood to *prove* she was telling the truth. Later, she would say her worst fear was being considered "crazy." She said she feared a sanitarium more than prison.

Before the interview ended, he asked her if she had given any thought to that date she kept bringing up.

"Did you ever recall why January eighth meant something to you?"

"I don't know if that's the first time we talked about [murder] or not. I don't know that. I kept Marguerite's obituary on my bulletin board for a real long time . . . I thought that it said January. I recall it saying January eighth, so maybe I messed that up somehow."

She looked perplexed.

"January eighth, though, I think it means something, but I don't remember what."

Chapter 82

After the police from Michigan left Tyler they talked about what might happen next.

"They may be back," Gwen said.

They were lying on the bed.

"What for?" said Robin. "You didn't do it."

Gwen gazed at the ceiling.

"They will be back."

"But you didn't do it. What can we do?"

"There's nothing we can do. We're just gonna get ready for work."

Six days after her polygraph, Gwen told Robin that Mother Francis Hospital no longer wanted her on the job. The Walker police had informed the hospital of the nature of the investigation.

"They don't even want me in the building. They told me to have you pick up my check."

Robin thought, more surprises. My life already has changed so much.

She wondered what would have happened if she would have never hired in at Alpine Manor. She wondered what would have happened if she never embraced Gwen Graham for the first time.

She would always remember that night, the way Cathy Wood stormed out of the apartment after catching them together. Robin and Gwen considered it their anniversary. The date was in her diary, the one she had burned.

The date was January 8.

Chapter 83

Roger Kaliniak figured his role during his first year as a detective was to watch, learn and investigate where he was told. However, thirteen years in a squad car also had provided some pretty good training in the ways of the human beast, he figured. He knew a con artist when he saw one.

Her name was Catherine May Wood.

Kaliniak was somewhat concerned about his good friend and boss, Tom Freeman. He could see Tom was pushing hard. He hoped Tom wasn't pushing himself right into the hands of the big platinum blond.

Forty-seven years of life alone had made Kaliniak awfully skeptical. He took nothing at face value, especially a suspect's statement. What do you expect to gain out of this? That was the key question. From what he had seen, Cathy Wood didn't strike him as someone who much gave a shit about a clear conscience. That removed, what did she want? Revenge, against Graham? He considered that as important as the central question: Was she even telling the truth?

Sometimes Kaliniak threw in his two cents.

"But Rog, when you're talking to someone one-on-one, sometimes you can develop a relationship," Tom would say. "You can really tell whether they're telling the truth, because you're dealing with them on a daily basis."

Maybe Tom was too decent for her, Kaliniak thought. Despite his foul mouth and swagger, Tom cared about people more than most cops, and more than he liked to admit.

"I think he felt sympathy for her," Kaliniak later said.

Kaliniak did not. Every time he talked to her he couldn't shake the feeling she was interviewing him, though she rarely asked a question. He felt on the defensive. At the gut level, he never felt any feedback.

Roger Kaliniak found Cathy Wood unnerving.

"When you talked with her, you felt as though you were talking to a shadow," he later said.

Chapter 84

Walker Deputy Chief Bill Brown glanced at Tom Freeman behind the wheel of the department Oldsmobile as they headed toward Lansing. He knew he was frustrated.

"Tom, I know how you feel. Chances are these things could have happened in Alpine, but I'm just not convinced."

Freeman's jaw muscles flexed. The five years they worked together in the detective bureau had forged a strong friendship. Brown knew Tom would not misinterpret his difference of opinion as a stop sign from a superior.

"You're the one that's in the middle of this," he always reminded him. "You're the one that has the benefits of the feelings, the belief."

Since day one, Cathy Wood's story had seemed too contrived for the deputy chief. The tale would have reminded him of a plot from her Stephen King collection, had it not been so riddled with holes. If she can't get the little things right, Brown thought, how can we believe the major material? Cathy's two new statements certainly commanded everyone's attention. But by early November, the prosecutor's office was treating the case as fodder for insults.

"Find something to blow this out of the water," one assistant told them. "Don't you guys have anything better to do out there in Walker?"

By mid-November, the case was limbo. Tom talked with Cathy on almost a daily basis by telephone. He provided regular updates from their chats. Often he popped into Brown's office shaking his head.

"Jesus Christ, Bill, you're not going to believe what she told me today."

Cathy was sharing intimate details. She told Tom about her childhood, her parents and the girl David/Debbie. She told him how she had gained weight, how she was entirely dependant on Ken. Gwen had been her salvation. For the first time in her life she was a "pretty girl," she said.

Cathy increasingly steeped her story in S&M and lesbian sex. It was beyond bizarre. She told him of their euphoric orgasms during lovemaking sessions in the days after Marguerite Chambers was killed. Murder had become their aphrodisiac.

Beyond the jokes generated in Walker PD, Brown had to admit the lesbian element was unfamiliar territory for everyone. Even Walker's most jaded cops had been taken aback by her stories of bed-hopping, group sex and fistfights between women.

The unfamiliar territory was one reason they were driving to Lansing, the state capital. They had made an appointment with the director of the state police behavioral science section, Dr. Gary Kaufmann. They wanted to see if Cathy Wood and Gwen Graham matched up to psychological criminal profiles.

Cathy kept calling being a lesbian a "life-style." Brown in executing the search warrant at Gwen Graham's trailer, expected to find lesbian literature, sexual paraphernalia, dildos and such. There was none of that. It inspired one of the first questions Brown asked Kaufmann, after they arrived in the police psychologist's office.

"There was nothing like that in the trailer. Why?"

"Well, they are true lesbians," Kaufmann said. "Things like dildos represent males. That's not what they're after. Being a lesbian constitutes more than a sexual act. They are in a true relationship, one that involves two people, two beings, just like heterosexuals."

Kaufmann, who had been doing criminal profiling for nearly ten years, was more than intrigued by the Alpine Manor story. He was animated.

"It lit him right up," Brown later recalled.

The psychologist delved into the prevailing thought in police psychology. He was less concerned with sexual orientation and more attentive to basic personality problems. He mentioned borderline, narcissistic and antisocial personality disorders. He explained how criminal paring often occurs among such types.

Usually, he explained, one of the perpetrators was dominant, a manipulative antisocial or narcissistic personality. The other was passive, a follower. Borderline types fell into this role. Borderlines had intense personal relationships and often undertook frantic efforts to avoid real or imagined abandonment.

"We're talking about a dynamic duo here," Kaufmann said. "In this case, a deadly duo, so to speak."

Freeman related Cathy's oral history about her dependence on others. In fact, virtually everything they had to offer Kaufmann had come from Cathy Wood. So far, Brown would later observe, the entire production had been Cathy Wood's show.

"Well, don't be surprised if Cathy is more involved," Kaufmann said. "She can be manipulative too, but in a more passive kind of way."

Freeman told him about Graham's fights, her smoldering violent streak. He told her about the scars on her arms. Kaufmann speculated the burns could indicate an antisocial personality. Gwen Graham might be a psychopath, he said.

"Well, one theory behind psychopathy is that the psychopath requires greater amounts of stimulation to achieve greater amounts of gratification. The burns could be evidence of that."

Freeman detailed what he thought was Graham's hypnotic power over Robin Fielder.

"All this is a matter of power," Kaufmann said. "The ultimate power is having the power of life and death over an individual. Gwen Graham could very well be a killing machine."

They talked for two hours.

"Well," Freeman finally said. "Then these things could have happened. We're not just dealing with a fruitcake here."

Kaufmann looked at them both pensively.

"Of course they could have happened."

Brown and Freeman wanted some advise on a new course for the investigation. They told Kaufmann about the polygraph Cathy had flunked. Kaufmann suggested a new test. They could test her not as a witness, as John Hulsing had, but as a suspect.

"We'll just repolygraph Cathy," he said.

Brown wondered about the protocol. Hulsing would not run her again. In fact, he had retired. Most state police examiners would not examine a subject formerly tested by a colleague.

"I've got the examiner for you," Kaufmann said. "Right here in Lansing. We work together all the time."

His name was John Palmatier. Kaufmann picked up the phone and made the call.

"No problem," Kaufmann said. "In fact, he's intrigued himself by the dynamics of the case."

They set the date for November 23.

The police psychologist had been fascinating, Brown told Freeman as they drove back to Grand Rapids. But as far as the deputy chief was concerned, Kaufmann had not shaken the uncomfortable feeling he had about Cathy Wood. Brown planned to attend the new polygraph.

"I'd like to see this gal in action," Brown said.

Gary Kaufmann said he planned to be there as well. He wanted to observe before making further analysis.

They could all eavesdrop on a monitor.

She still had little credibility, but nearly two months into the investigation, Cathy Wood was drawing quite a crowd.

Chapter 85

"I'm a silly girl sometimes. I go off and I start talking and then before I realize what I've even said I've said everything you want to know.

—Cathy Wood, October 24, 1990.

She was looking again for an edge, Tom Freeman figured. Or, she's just plain fucking with me. Why else would Cathy Wood drive all the way to Walker PD, when she could have picked up the phone?

"Tom, I'm not going," she said.

It was the evening of November 23. Freeman and Bill Brown were waiting to drive Cathy to the state capital. Her hair was styled and her makeup on. But she was reneging on her agreement to take the second polygraph.

The night was already steeped in anxiety. Everyone connected with the investigation knew the exam was pivotal. If Cathy Wood didn't pass, let alone take, the new polygraph, the Alpine Manor murder investigation was finished. There was nothing left to do but exhume the bodies of possible victims for autopsy, but nobody was going to traumatize families and stir public interest without some certainty of an arrest.

Freeman sometimes wondered who was playing whom. He felt he had detected many of Cathy's moves over the many weeks. In all his years as a cop, no suspect had frustrated him more. Some days he felt sorry for her. Other times he cursed the bitch. She could make him laugh one minute and squint in disgust the next. At times she was telepathic. Often she guessed what he was thinking. Often she knew his darker side. She also had the troubling ability to make him doubt his own words, his own memory.

"No Tom," she would say. "You didn't say *that.*"

She drew out the word, sounding so damn innocently miffed.

Lately, he was doubting himself. Lately, she was getting to him. He didn't like that.

Tom Freeman wanted to arrest her. And, he wanted to make it stick.

But he wasn't going to beg. He decided to make her feel like a giant pain in the ass. He suspected her fragile ego couldn't handle that. She's not as smart as she thinks, he thought, or she wouldn't be here in the first place.

"Hey, it's up to you Cath," he began, seemingly indifferent at first.

Then he displayed irritation.

"You know, I wish you would have called me earlier. You know, you've screwed up our plans. This polygraph operator is making a special trip to Lansing for you."

She made him wait a few seconds.

"Well," she sighed. "Okay."

During the one-hour trip to the capital she became quite talkative. The subject of drunk drivers came up in the banter.

"They should be home instead of out killing someone," she said.

The irony of the statement didn't escape Cathy, either.
"Listen to *me,*" she said.

An hour later, the department Oldsmobile from Walker turned
into the sprawling Michigan State Police complex in Lansing. They
were greeted by a couple dozen blue state police cruisers, parked so
uniformly, for use by the state academy, that they looked as though
they had fallen in at attention like troops.

The polygraph examiner that introduced himself inside the First
District headquarters stood six-foot-five, had penetrating brown
eyes and bore a resemblance to William Powell with his thin mustache and a dark widow's peak.

As a district examiner, John Palmatier, at only thirty-eight, was
already one of the more colorful and sometimes controversial, characters in the Michigan State Police. He was a helicopter pilot with
the National Guard and a former MP who had served in Japan and
Thailand. His style in the examiner's room was clearly antimacho.
His technique was a hybrid of the personal confessor and the all-
seeing orb. He brought to his craft studies in experimental psychology and Eastern religion.

"The polygraph exam is an art as well as a science," Palmatier
liked to say. "And the more a polygraph examiner combines the
two, the more proficient he becomes."

Some colleagues didn't like the mix. His lengthy pre-exam interviews were laced with personal philosophy as he probed in a near-
hypnotic voice. Later, in one highly publicized murder case, he
obtained a confession from a father who drove the family station
wagon into the Detroit River, drowning his four children. The Michigan Court of Appeals upheld a ruling dismissing the confession. It
agreed with a lower court that said Palmatier's marathon interview
was the equivalent of an Oriental POW interrogation. Palmatier
later made light of the ruling with new visitors.

"Welcome to the brainwashing section," he said.

The small room where he conducted his exams offered a subject
both star status and subtle hints that here began the path to full
serenity. The room was lined with acoustic tile and lit with fluorescent light. The "client," as he liked to call a subject, settled into a
big black executive's chair next to the polygraph instrument. Palmatier sat in the corner, in a small chair which helped diminish his size.

During the pre-exam interview, the subject faced Palmatier and a glass case with three shelves. On the top shelf sat three ivory figurines. They were the Chinese figurines representing 'See,' 'speak' and 'hear' no evil. On the middle shelf, Palmatier's polygraph license. On the bottom, there was more ivory—the serene figure of two doves perched in a lotus blossom tree.

Hidden in darkness behind the figurines were camera lenses. Freeman, Brown and, later, police psychologist Gary Kaufmann would monitor from a nearby room. They watched her for a few minutes after she was shown into the exam room. One section of the screen showed her body, the other her face. She wore dark flats, stone-washed jeans and a loose-fitting blouse with stripes. She sat, running her fingernail across her bared teeth, waiting.

Finally, John Palmatier sat down in the small chair, pushing himself back into the corner. A hole was worn in the wainscotting from the back rest. Cathy Wood was his 1,244th exam, number 291 that year.

Palmatier opened with pleasantries, then a casual mention of his extensive polygraph training.

"Do you have to be a police officer?" she asked.

"No, but it helps."

The police officer often saw people in their own element, he said. Police officers had special insight.

"Doctors, lawyers, psychologists. When those people see us, it's in a controlled environment. And we're all actors on a stage, and we behave as we believe it is appropriate for the situation."

After he explained her rights under both Miranda and Michigan's polygraph statute, he asked if she had any questions. She wondered about a statement on the Michigan list: "No promises or threats have been made to me or no pressure of any kind has been used against me." She was worried she alone would be charged for the murders.

"Tom tells me that . . . in my mind I think if I pass the lie detector test people will have to believe that at least I think this happened. If I fail, then they'll think I'm a loon for making this up or that I did it myself. And *he* says that would never happen."

She paused, then apologized.

"I'm getting nervous here."

She looked away, then tears began to flow.

"That's okay," he said in a calming voice. "Don't be upset about it, because I understand where you are coming from."

In time, he would hand her a paper towel.

"They're kind of rough, but it's all I have."

She would clutch the towel through much of the pre-exam interview, repeatedly dabbing her eyes. She cried when she talked about her own psyche, her childhood, her current predicament. All her tears were for herself.

She reiterated Freeman had made a promise.

". . . He tells me that there's no way that anybody could ever think that I did this, and I don't believe that."

Palmatier employed a standard loftier than the law.

"Well, what we are looking for is the truth. Whether you did, or didn't, only you know . . ."

He applied some psychological balm.

"I've talked to many people who have been in situations like this. And even if they killed one person themselves, it doesn't necessarily make them a bad person. Because there are other things going on that might mitigate what is going on. That's why here I first look for what happened, then I'm interested in *why*—and that many times changes completely what really did happen."

He offered her a solution, then switched subjects in one breath.

"If a person demonstrated an interest in getting their lives straightened around, then I have to respect that. You're how old now?"

"Twenty-six."

Palmatier started to say she had three-quarters of the rest of her life before her, but she answered his point before he made it.

"Yeah," she interrupted. "But a twenty-six-year-old who is going to spend the rest of her life in prison."

He said in her kind of case he had seen sentences ranging from life to under two years.

"I tell people, don't worry about that. You probably can't directly change what's going to happen, whether you talk or don't talk. It's like a snowball rolling down a big hill. It's moving. If you want to jump on it and break it up . . ."

She was ahead of him again.

"I know, those little snowballs are going to become big snowballs."

"Right, and if you sit on the bottom of the hill, it's going to be hell to try and stop that sucker. And you're not going to have a chance. And that's one of the reasons Tom brought you down here, so he could find out where he really stands, and then he will talk [to you]."

Then, Palmatier, in a calm, but exceptionally earnest tone, put himself in a league of his own.

"You see, I don't promise anybody anything in here. The one thing I will not do, is I will not lie to you. I help people talk more freely than they ever have."

Cathy had another question. She was worried about her long record of lies.

"Will things that I've done—that I've never told anybody about, that I'm nervous about—affect this? Things that have nothing to do with this?"

"I will clear some of that up for you."

She didn't understand. She continued, sounding like an expert herself.

"People who have to lie a long time in their lives, it's just as easy for them to tell a lie as tell the truth."

He explained that even pathological liars knew they were lying. She continued.

"Sometimes a lie comes out. And I don't even think about it. It's no effort at all . . . 'Cause I've had to hide myself so long it's not a problem anymore."

Palmatier said he possessed skills not connected with the polygraph instrument.

"It's like the poets said, many, many years ago. The eyes are a window to a person's soul. And when you get to look into as many pairs of eyes as I do, you learn to read them."

Tom Freeman sat watching the eavesdropping monitor. He still hated polygraphs, but the situation was certainly ironic. Everything was reversed. Cathy Wood was taking a polygraph to prove she had committed a crime. They were testing a pathological liar, hoping to catch her in the truth.

Finally, Freeman thought, she's met her match with the chopper pilot. Palmatier seemed to have as much bullshit going for him as she did. Cathy was studying him intently as he talked. He had all of her attention.

"Bill, can you believe this guy?" Freeman said to the deputy chief.

He nodded.

"Yeah, he's something else."

As Palmatier took basic information about her physical and mental health, he applied flattery. Cathy Wood in recent months had lost considerable weight.

"How much do you weigh?"

"Two eighty three."

"You don't look that large."

She studied his face.

They talked about her visits to a psychologist. She said her therapist had only made her feel silly. She said she tried to manipulate a written personality test one gave her to make herself appear more normal. She told the therapist she thought she was ugly, but the psychologist only laughed at her.

"He probably wasn't laughing at you, as much as he was laughing with you," Palmatier tried to explain. "Because, seriously, you have a pretty face."

"No, I don't," she snapped.

"Well, it's a perception."

"Yeah."

She was crying again. He used their difference of opinion as another lesson in *truth*.

"What is the truth? Is it what I see, or what you see?"

Then she revealed what only a handful of people already knew about Catherine May Wood. Most importantly, she knew it.

"The only thing I know about the way I look is that I can get things if I want to. That's the only thing I know about it."

When Palmatier asked her father's occupation, she unloaded on her dad, shedding more tears.

"He was never there. He worked second shift. It was awful when he was at home anyway, because he was always drunk when he was there."

"Physically abusive?"

"Yes."

"Sexual abuse?"

"No."

"He just liked to beat up on everybody?" Palmatier offered.

"He doesn't remember it now, though."

Palmatier moved to a couple of his stock questions. She stayed with the parental theme.

"In your whole life who is the one person you most respected?"

She was silent for ten seconds.

"There isn't anybody," she said.

"On the other hand, who is the one person you most disrespect."

She answered immediately.

"My mom."

"Why?"

"Well, it's really a tie between my mom and my dad, oh . . ."

She cried again. Her delivery sounded more tragic than the substance of her story. She married Ken, she said, just to get away. Her mother gave her too much sense of responsibility, first to her younger siblings, then to herself, she said.

"It used to be if there was a movie at five o'clock, I'd have to be there at 4:15, because you couldn't be late."

And, seconds later, "She wasn't a good mom, I don't think. I don't think she really loved us. I *know* she didn't."

Palmatier tried to sooth.

"All she did was the discipline side," he said. "None of the love side, the caring, the nurturing."

She contradicted him.

"No, we didn't get any discipline from her. She'd tell my dad."

In fact, she said, one time the kids told their father they thought their mother was crazy. She did crazy things.

"Like what?"

"She wanted to play with us when friends were over. She got real mad if there was a cookie gone. She had to have money. Money was her thing."

Later, he asked her another set of best/worst questions.

"What is the worst thing that ever happened to you emotionally?"

She waited ten seconds before answering.

"When Gwen left."

"The best?"

"Losing weight."

She continued portraying herself as one of life's unfortunate victims.

He tried to put her at ease. The interview process was "a little scary for people, because they feel naked," he said. "But I don't do it without feeling."

She cried more.

"Yeah, but as long as I smile on the outside, no one can see how much I hurt on the inside."

For nearly ninety minutes, Palmatier talked with her. He commented on psychology, human physiology, her birth order, personality tests, macho cops, child-rearing, denial and repression and the states where she was born and raised. There was no subject on which he did not appear to be an expert.

"See, I've lived all over halfway across the world," he said at one point.

It all was polished interrogative technique. He first set himself up as a gentle, but infallible confessor. Only then did he ask her for her version of events on the Alpine Manor murders. He added that he didn't care what she had already told the Walker police.

"My only interest is getting you through this thing. So I ask you to tell me everything you remember. I don't care what it is. I just want to get you through this thing."

Through her entire narrative about the murders she looked down at her knees. Unlike the waterworks for her own troubles, she did not shed one tear in talking about the murders, the victims, their families. There was no longer the strong eye contact she had maintained with him earlier.

Right off, for the first—and only—time in the Alpine Manor investigation, she admitted that she had marked Marguerite Chambers for death.

"I think it was, the first one, we were just going to kill somebody. So we decided on, I think I decided it *actually*. I don't know if it was both of us, or if it was just me. I keep thinking most of it was me."

She couldn't recall whether she had witnessed the first attempt on Marguerite, but she detailed what had transpired.

"The first time it didn't work and she came in and told me. She said, 'Marguerite is still alive.' And I said, 'How can she be?' She goes, 'I don't know, she must have breathed or something like that.' Oh no!"

Cathy half chuckled and rolled her eyes into her head, replaying her surprise when Gwen had delivered the macabre news.

On the second, successful attempt, she said she was outside the door. She also said—for the first, and only time—that victims were picked based upon which aides were caring for them. In Marguerite's case, it was a new aide who knew little about nursing. He had worked at Alpine only a few weeks.

"Gwen was in the room and the door was shut and the curtains were drawn . . . and we were gonna, I think we were gonna pick people on who was assigned to them. And this young boy had her that night . . . And I went in the room and she was on the far side of the bed and she was holding Marguerite with . . . making noises. I could hear it in the hallway too."

Her tone switched to an earnest Shirley Temple-like pouting.

"And I didn't want to be there anymore, so I told Gwen I was leaving. It was a long time."

Cathy said she had almost inadvertently revealed to Tish Prescott outside her office that she knew Marguerite was dead.

Gwen helped clean up the body, she said. "And Gwen liked that."

She talked about the funeral home where Marguerite's body was sent. She called the staffer from the funeral home the "coroner," the same incorrect term used by the mysterious caller to the Hunderman family in the minutes after Marguerite's death.

". . . and the coroner guy helped put Marguerite on the stretcher. Now you know, I can't think, Marguerite went to Reyer's Funeral Home, and I don't know if that had something to do with it beforehand because that was right around the corner from where we lived. 'Cause we were talking about going to see her there, but we never did."

There was another revelation. They were supposed to take turns killing. Her turn was next, she said.

"And we'd go around and we'd hold other people's noses and their mouths to see how they acted."

She rolled her eyes, and half smiled.

"How *awful.*"

Then she continued. She picked a victim for herself named Madeline Young.

"She couldn't move. She had contractions, I think they call them. She was so stiff. I gave her juice all the time and she'd look at me. I knew she could hear me. I knew when I talked to her, I knew she'd be an easy one to do. I thought, it's my turn. She won't fight at all. But I just couldn't when I looked at her. I couldn't."

So then, she said, it was Gwen's turn again, even though she had failed to follow through.

Cathy basically told Palmatier the same versions of the other deaths as she had told Walker police. She was unsure about Ruth Van Dyke. As previously, she could offer no details on Wanda Urbanski. Edith Cook was very sick with gangrene, she said.

Palmatier wanted to know about the victims.

"You think you maybe felt sorry for them?"

She answered by talking not only about her relationship with the victims, but about relationships between mothers and daughters.

"Not Belle, I didn't. I really didn't like Belle. She was so hard to take care of. But Marguerite I felt bad for because she was such a young, pretty lady, and she had Alzheimer's so bad. And Myrtle, we were both there that night. And she did Myrtle . . . and they called the daughter and she was wired-out about it. 'Cause she loved her mom *so much*, and she was in there all the time giving them a hand."

She turned and looked at Palmatier.

"It was almost exciting, you know."

Palmatier didn't react.

"It is," he agreed. "Because what it is, at that moment, there's not a greater power on earth, than the power of life and death."

She almost interrupted him.

"How come I couldn't do it?"

"Is it possible, that you did do it, at least once?"

She was very calm, rational. She looked him right in the eyes.

"No."

"And you're just frightened about what the consequences might be?"

"No . . . They think I did one?"

She was incredulous, that the Walker police might think that. She had a half-smile.

"They don't know," said Palmatier.

"Oh, I see. No, I never did that."

He told her killing and planning or facilitating killing were treated similarly in the eyes of the law.

"The bottom line is that a person could be charged just as though they did the crime themselves."

"I know that. I know that. I know that."

"So that's the reason why here . . ."

She interrupted him.

"I was hoping that this, that this whole thing would come out and I could go to prison and not have to worry about bills, not have to worry about being responsible. But I don't want to go anymore. For some reason, I don't want to go anymore. Maybe it's the reality that I could go."

Palmatier brought up Gwen Graham leaving her, then probed the possibility he had already discussed with the Walker police. Cathy might be fabricating the story simply for revenge, and was willing to endure prison herself for that end.

"There's a part of you that said, get even!" Palmatier said. "That's normal. We want the other person to hurt too."

Cathy was matter-of-fact.

"But I did get even. When she was living with Robin, I still slept with her. I felt: Ha, ha, Robin. And she told me things that her and Robin did."

"Like what?"

"Sexual things. She was so fascinated with Robin because she couldn't get her to have an orgasm."

Cathy switched subjects instantly, back to the taking of turns on killing, the Walker police, then the polygraph.

"You know when she left she still wanted me to do this . . . but I never did. Oh my gosh! They think I did one."

She smiled broadly, then continued like an adolescent confident she had all the right answers.

"I'll pass. I'll pass."

Palmatier redirected her back to Gwen. He reminded her she had started telling confidants like Ken about the murders after Gwen dumped her. She was setting her up for revenge.

No, he had it wrong. Gwen, Cathy said, kept promising she would come back to her, even after moving to Texas.

"You see, she was supposed to . . . she was supposed to be with me forever . . . And then she really left. Maybe I did tell people that so she wouldn't go, but I didn't make it up."

In a special way, she also said, each murder added to their eternal bond. They had secrets to share and keep.

Cathy digressed into her past relationships. She told him about David/Debbie. She told him she couldn't stand being touched by Ken. He had used the information about the murders to control her for months, she claimed. Ken had been urging her to seek a psychologist, but she didn't need one, "not for being gay," she said. Palmatier brought her back around to the killings.

"What kind of time period are we talking about? January?"

"They tell me it's the eighteenth. But I keep wanting to think it was the eighth . . . to May I think it was."

"And how many people died in between then?"

She was still unclear on the numbers.

Palmatier tried to trip her up with modus operandi.

"You say you would hold the people, but then you couldn't follow through?"

She contradicted herself.

"You see, I never used the washcloth and towel. I would just use my fingers to see what they would do. So maybe I did use a washcloth and towel on them, but when they would move or struggle, I couldn't hold them."

He told her there were three great crime laboratories in the world, the FBI, Scotland Yard and the Michigan State Police. They had lasers now. They could lift fingerprints off the dead.

"Even if she used a washcloth?" she asked quickly.

Palmatier gambled with a bluff. He had no idea he was talking to the reader of scores of crime books. He hesitated, then answered affirmatively.

"How could it go through?" she asked, again quickly.

"What happens is you get so much pressure . . ."

She never let him finish. She had her answer.

"Cool. Oh that's *cool.*"

"There's a very good possibility . . ." he tried to interject.

"That's *cool,*" she said, cutting him off again. She was ecstatic. " 'Cause my fingerprints wouldn't be on *any* of them."

He wanted to know the ones she did hold.

"Stephen Farkus," she said.

"That's a hell of a name."

"He couldn't move, and I pinched his nose one time and he said, 'Let go of my goddamn nose!' Real loud. So he was definitely out."

"Who else?"

"Madeline. She was. If I would have done one, it would have

been Madeline . . . I couldn't. I couldn't. I couldn't, for some reason. I don't know why I kept saying: I'll take my turn. I'll take my turn. I didn't want [Gwen] maybe to . . . I don't know why. I'm not going to guess."

Palmatier returned once more to the possibility that her story was fabricated. This time he employed the proven interview technique of detached speculation. It allowed a subject to speak about himself, while avoiding direct incrimination.

"If a person would want to make up a story like this, what kind of person would it take?"

"To make up a story like this?" Cathy asked back. "Anybody could."

"What do you think would push them far enough to make them want to do something like that?"

She didn't answer for eighteen seconds, the most thought she'd given to any question in the interview.

"I don't know," she said.

Palmatier said fabrication of such a story was a crime. A judge could order anything from jail to probation to psychotherapy.

"What do you think should happen to a person who would make something up like this?"

She weighed each possibility as she answered.

"For someone to make this up to the point where they went to the police and they said all this stuff. They're awfully unhappy. Awfully lonely. In fact, that's where they get their attention from. And maybe they even want to go [to prison] like I did because then they won't have to worry about anything. But they don't care about prison, but they can still be lonely."

Without pause she switched into the first person. She was talking about herself.

"I really don't know how counseling would help. I know it would. Everybody tells me it would. But, when I was there, it just seems like you listened to the doctor babble for an hour on how you should do this or do that . . ."

Inside the room with the monitor, police psychologist Gary Kaufmann was animated. Her answers to the speculative question made it appear that Cathy was likening herself to a fake witness.

"Look at this," he said. "See, she's not being truthful."

He predicted Palmatier would never pass her in the formal part of the exam.

Bill Brown had been watching as well. He leaned back deeply in his chair.

"I keep thinking this is all bullshit," he kept saying.

Tom Freeman couldn't stand the comments anymore. He'd had enough. He had to step outside. He lit a cigarette and paced back and forth in front of the district headquarters. The wind was blowing, but he was too pissed to be cold. He heard a hollow clanging of steel against aluminum. He looked up. He watched the November wind flying the American flag across the Michigan night.

"Goddamnit," he said to himself.

He said it out loud, between the clanging.

"All this work hasn't been for nothing. She's gotta pass this goddamn thing."

Chapter 86

As he began to formulate the actual polygraph examination, John Palmatier asked Cathy Wood if there were any questions in particular on which she would like to be tested.

"If I made it up," she said.

Palmatier caught himself, as though he had forgotten.

"Oh, there was something your husband said about the word M-U-R-D-E-R."

She indicated she was the first to see the book of dead and discharged patients. In contrast to her previous testimony, she didn't say Gwen was with her at the time.

"I remember sitting there with the supervisor one night and trying to look at it, and we were going to try to kill them in order to spell that."

"Trying to give people a clue, like a mystery?" Palmatier asked.

"No, I don't know what it was. That was deranged. I don't know, but—we tried that. We didn't do that. But we tried that."

Palmatier asked her two more questions. He would use them as control questions on the exam. Control questions were formulated to cause subjects to answer deceptively or at least have a doubt about the veracity of their answers. They were used as a measure against which the relevant questions can be compared.

The first control was: "Do you now remember ever telling an important lie."

"I lie all the time," Cathy said.

He posed the second: "Do you now remember doing something you don't want anyone to know."

"No," she said.

Through the interview, he had been urging her to rid herself of baggage from the past so she could pass the exam. Palmatier left the room for five minutes, saying he would return with the final questions. When he did, she wanted to confess to some past sins in light of the last two questions. She said she had stolen and peddled needles from Alpine Manor. She frequently took a friend shoplifting. She said she implied to Gwen Graham that she had continued killing in Alpine after Gwen went to Texas. Cathy said she had not.

She paused, then continued.

"And there's a letter that Tom has . . . I went through the letters and there is one. We used to write in code. This bothers me so much, but I didn't do it. I just wrote it. If you wrote something, but didn't really do it, is it still bad?"

"What is it?"

"I don't want to tell ya. But I want to pass this test . . . Well, Madeline, how she had contractions. She's dead now she was going to be the one that I would do, if I ever did anybody. So we used to write in code: ILU, I love you, stuff like that. Well, there's one letter . . . it said IGTKM. *I'm going to kill Madeline.*"

He suggested she tell Tom Freeman about that after the test.

"I want to pass this test," she said again. "It's so important. I would rather go to prison than have people think I made this up."

Before linking her to the instrument, Palmatier read her all the questions, allowing her to respond. There were five relevant questions in a total of eleven, including the two control questions. She answered each one.

"Did you make up this story just to get back at Gwen?"

"I failed that one before, and it was the truth before . . . I might have brought it up to hurt her, but I didn't make it up to hurt her."

"Did you ever suffocate even one person at the Alpine home?"

Cathy smiled.

"No. I like that question, thanks."

"Were you ever present when Gwen suffocated even one other person?"

"Work maybe, but not in the room in any other time."

"Did you lie to your husband or friends about you, Gwen and the murders?"

"No."

"Was there one other person who was suffocated and Tom not told?"

"No."

She wanted her shoes off for the exam itself.

"Only if you're more comfortable," Palmatier said.

"When I'm done will you be able to tell me how I did right away."

"Yes, but honestly, see that's the difference here . . . This time, you already know how you're going to do, and that's the difference."

He cautioned her about people who try to beat the test with muscle contractions and such.

"If I see somebody purposely messing those charts up, what would be the only reason someone wouldn't want me to see the truth?"

"Lying?"

"Kind of stupid, isn't it?"

Suddenly, she blurted out another past lie. She seemed preoccupied with the control questions. She said she and Shawn Thatcher had talked prior to Freeman's interrogation of him. She had told Thatcher to not disclose certain details.

"I don't want Tom not to trust me," she said. "He's the nicest man I've met in a long time. I think if it wasn't for him, I'd already be in jail by now."

"He's just interested in seeing things done right," Palmatier said.

"For some odd reason, I don't want to disappoint him. I don't know what it is."

"It may be that you never had anybody trust you."

She sounded earnest, almost naive.

"Yeah, he told me the truth about everything. He hasn't lied to me once. You know I try to catch people lying to me, and he hasn't."

The entire session had revealed a telling double standard: Cathy Wood expected everyone else to be truthful, and judged them harshly by that criteria, while she herself admittedly ran rampant with deception.

Palmatier put the blood pressure cuff around her arm and attached a galvanic sensor to her right fingers. As he put the respiratory band around her chest, he complimented her.

"And see, you thought you were a big girl."

"I *am* a big girl."

"I've had ladies where I've had to add straps."

"Oh, you're sweet. I think you made that up, but you're sweet."

Palmatier would ask the set of questions three times, taking a short break between each. On the first, he asked her to respond to the questions internally. She closed her eyes as the needles of the polygraph charted her responses.

The first completed, she blurted out another secret. She was still worried about those control questions.

"There's something I thought of I wouldn't want anyone to know . . . When I was living at home, I was maybe thirteen or fourteen. There was this little boy who lived down the street and we were in the bathroom and touching, things like that. That just popped into my mind." The boy was five or six years old, she said.

She had other confessions. She had a tendency to be "a child abuser." She couldn't stand kids, "even my own daughter." "There were times I had her when she was quite young that I wanted to get quite violent." She added that when she was ten she used to slap her younger brother so hard she left finger marks on his face.

Palmatier complimented her for the disclosures. Then he conducted the test a second time. She answered aloud in a steady voice. As he let the air out of the blood pressure cuff, she wanted to know her results.

"I don't know yet," he said.

He wondered if there was something that kept coming to her mind on the control question about telling an important lie.

"No," she said, her voice rising. "I can't tell you. I can't tell you that."

"I just want to be sure. I just want to get you through this thing."

She switched subjects. She was worried about the question as to whether she had smothered someone.

"Why do I get so nervous when you ask me that question? I'm afraid I'm going to fail that one, not because I did it, because that would be awful."

Then she answered his earlier question. Masturbation, she said. She had started masturbating after Gwen had left. That was her secret. Palmatier dismissed it.

"That's the most natural thing in the world."

"No you don't," she said, sternly. "You don't touch yourself. You don't have the same mom."

As he started to pump up the blood pressure cuff for the third test, she became anxious about the suffocation question again.

"Did I ever suffocate anybody? You're already taking into consideration that you already knew that I held their nose and all that."

"Sure," Palmatier said.

He asked her the questions a third time, mixing up the order.

Afterwards, he unhooked the equipment, removed her charts from the instrument. He said he would return shortly with the results. She acted embarrassed.

"God, I've told you everything about myself. That's awful."

The total session lasted nearly three hours. She had admitted to chronic lying, patient abuse, accessory and conspiracy to commit murder, criminal cover-up and physical and sexual child abuse.

Palmatier played his role right to the end.

"I hate to tell you," he said, "but you're disgustingly normal. You didn't do anything a few million other Americans haven't tried."

For fifteen minutes she fidgeted, playing with her lip and teeth with her fingernail. Everyone was fixed on the television monitor when Palmatier returned to the exam room to deliver the results. He was very businesslike, but he was no longer infallible.

"On these tests, I can make three decisions. I can say a person is telling the truth. I can say the test is inconclusive, or I don't know what is going on. I can say that they're not telling the truth. Also, Cathy, I tell everybody that there's always a chance I'm making an error."

She interrupted.

"Oh no," she whined.

"Well, there isn't anything that's one hundred percent."

"Well, did I do bad?"

"No, you passed."

"All right," she said. She cheered it, in fact.

"There were some things on those questions about the past, I was asking you about . . ."

"I don't mean to . . ."

"I know, but in each of our lives there's something there."

She started laughing with delight.

"You're so *cuuuute,"* she said. "Thank you so much!"

Seconds later she asked, "So I passed on am I making this up?"

"All of the five relevant questions."

He suggested now was the time to "really open up" to Tom Freeman.

"Oh God!" she said.

She was squealing with delight. She wanted to see Tom Freeman's face when Palmatier informed him of the results. He told her to stay put.

"I'll go find him."

As he closed the door behind him, everyone watched Cathy on the monitor.

"All right," she cheered in the first second, alone. *"All right."*

In the next second, there was a smiling sigh.

"Oh God."

Exactly at the point the sigh ended, her mouth closed and instantly opened. It opened into a pained grimace as surreal as the mask of tragedy. The transformation was seamless. She looked to the heavens and wheezed.

"Aaaaaaaaaaaaaaaaaaaah."

She began to weep, painfully and deeply.

By then, Palmatier was in the other room, watching on the monitor as well. He commented to police psychologist Gary Kaufmann and the cops from Walker.

"Look at that," he said. "This happens."

Freeman was euphoric over the polygraph results, but shocked by the instant transformation of Cathy.

"Holy shit, John, you didn't see the way she snapped when you left."

"This is a person who has told the truth," Palmatier told everyone calmly. "She's crying because someone believes her."

He said he had seen it before. It was "an emotional dumping."

"It's true catharsis," he said.

"I don't know what to think now," said Bill Brown. "I'm basically confused."

Kaufmann was exceptionally intrigued. He later said Cathy Wood reminded him of the cartoon character Baby Huey, the rotund duck in a diaper who was always running into one thing or another. Everyone wanted to take care of that duck.

Kaufmann remained surprised Palmatier had called her truthful, but now he found himself agreeing with the polygraph examiner as he watched Cathy weep. Still, he couldn't sort it all out.

"I thought, this is bizarre," he later said. "This woman is going up the river, and she's crying because someone finally believes her. It was like: What is wrong with this picture?" Palmatier formalized his results on Department of State police stationery, for not only the Walker police, but for the Kent County Prosecutor's Office. He also provided a videotape of the entire session. Cathy's breakdown would do as much to convince the doubtful as the test itself.

The snowball would soon be rumbling down the hill.

However, many months later, Palmatier would be asked again about the results. His former state police colleague John Hulsing wanted to know what would happen if his polygraph charts were submitted to blind analysis. What would they show? In other words, did the charts pass Cathy Wood, or had John Palmatier.

"It was the totality of everything," Palmatier would say. "If they were subjected to blind analysis they might come up within the inconclusive range. They really might."

No one in the room knew it—then, or for many months to come. In arguably the most important decision of the entire Alpine Manor murder case, the chopper pilot was flying by the seat of his pants.

John Palmatier had made a judgement call.

The tears were dried when Tom Freeman went to the exam room to get Cathy.

"So I heard you've been a good girl," he said.

As they left she was holding a cup in her hand.

Earlier, as Palmatier went to calculate the polygraph's results,

Cathy made what she termed "a strange request." She requested a clean, disposable coffee cup she could take home. Palmatier had returned with a cup just like the one she had sipped from during the interview. It had the State Police logo on it. Cathy Wood wanted one badly.

On the way home she showed off her souvenir.

Chapter 87

Robin quietly protested every time Gwen wanted to bring the subject up. No, she didn't want to discuss what she was going to do—where she was going to live—when the police came back.

"Gwen, the police aren't coming back."

There were never shouting matches. They rarely argued anyway. Now they talked quietly. Gwen was convinced the trailer was bugged. When Robin refused to discuss it, Gwen would sulk out the door and mount her motorcycle.

Finally, they went to a Taco Bell to hash it out.

"I want you to stay, and live in Texas if they come for me," Gwen said. "If they take me back to Michigan, I want you to stay. And you don't have to say anything to the police."

Robin nodded.

"Okay, but now I just don't want to talk about it anymore."

She couldn't fathom life without Gwen Graham. She was her lifeline. She thought, *nobody*, neither the police nor Cathy Wood, is going to take Gwen away from me.

Working at Mother Francis Hospital had become stressful. The hospital had transferred Robin to days. She lost her shift differential. She suspected it was so supervisors could scrutinize her work. She felt watched.

The job was their only income. Gwen was supposed to be job-hunting, but she was smoking a lot of pot. Mornings she told Robin she would spend the day looking for work. Robin usually came home to find her stoned. Gwen was quiet, preoccupied. She was passing hours just cruising the rural roads of east Texas on her motorcycle.

One night they dropped by to see one of Gwen's old friends in Tyler. Gwen told her all about the police visit, how Cathy was playing a head game.

"If there's anything I can do, just call me," her friend said.

"Take care of Robin for me," Gwen said.

"What kinda questions were they asking?"

"Well, Robin told her about Cathy," Gwen said.

"Yeah, and they made me write it out," Robin said.

Gwen looked at her wide-eyed.

"I can't believe you did that."

Gwen sulked for the rest of the night. She bought a case of beer on their way home, and spent the evening drinking and smoking joints.

Robin faced her own stress. She was paying the rent and $141 a month in the $760 restitution a judge had ordered Gwen to pay on the bad checks. In November, they decided to move to a cheaper, small apartment in south Tyler. One day, Gwen admitted she was not job-hunting at all.

"I went to one nursing home, but they wanted to pay me minimum wage," she said. "I can't do that after making seven dollars an hour in a hospital. I'm better off on welfare."

Gwen wanted to go to school. She applied to the nursing program at Tyler Junior College.

She's making big plans, Robin thought, but we have hardly anything to show for ourselves. In the apartment they sat on two wicker chairs and slept on foam padding. Robin used a box for a makeup stand. Gwen's sister donated a very used dresser. Robin tried to spruce it up by painting it black.

Gwen wanted to visit the library. Robin checked out books on crafts and beauty. Gwen checked out books on Spanish, prisons and the law. She was reading every night. Gwen's sister and husband had gone to Mexico to do missionary relief work.

"I've done that before," she said. "I'm not working. I could help them build houses in Mexico."

One night, as Gwen lay reading on the foam mattress, Robin asked her about the prison book in her hands.

"It's not that bad," Gwen said.

"What?"

"Says here Michigan prisons aren't that bad. There are worse ones. Yep, there sure are."

Robin wondered what Cathy's next move would be. Cathy had threatened in the parking lot to pull her into the quagmire about the murders. She had threatened her that night in the Alpine parking lot.

"You go to Texas with Gwen, you're gonna be part of it," Cathy promised.

One day at the hospital, a woman had invited Robin to attend a Catholic church in Tyler. Robin had neglected Mass for many months. By late November, she was attending every Sunday. Her prayer was simple: "Please God, help me." She prayed it often. She sent her parents religious cards, telling them how much she cared about them.

Robin sensed changes underway.

First, her mother called. She was worried. She had heard rumors that police were investigating murders involving lesbians at Alpine Manor.

"Robin, are you, and Gwen?"

She had asked the question before, and Robin had always denied it. Gwen, however, had been bugging her to tell her parents about their relationship ever since they moved to Texas. Now, she decided she had nothing to lose. How could things get any worse?

"Yes, Mom," she said.

"Are you okay?"

"Yes."

"You know you can come home any time."

"But Dad won't even talk to me."

"He's worried. We are both worried about you."

"Just don't worry, okay? Promise me you won't worry."

A few days later, Robin was at the hospital and noticed a familiar figure walking toward her down the hallway. She saw her aunt and cousin who lived in Austin. They told her they wanted to make a surprise visit. They went to dinner. Afterwards, they met Gwen. Robin figured her parents sent them to check everything out.

"Oh, she's just fine," her aunt told her mother from a pay phone.

On another day, Robin ran into Gwen's old friend Deborah

Kidder in a convenience store. She was in her Navy uniform. They
were excited to see one another. She was stationed out of state, but
had just returned to Tyler.

"What's Gwen up to?"

"Not much now. She got fired from work."

"Why? Pot?"

Robin told her about the visit from the Walker police and
Cathy's games in Grand Rapids.

"They came down acting like Gwen had murdered people and
everything."

Debbie listened in awe.

Within hours she called the apartment. Robin answered, but
Debbie didn't wait to find out who had picked up the phone.

"Gwen, I can't believe you did that," she shouted. "I can't believe you did it!"

"Debbie, this is Robin."

Debbie was hurried. She wanted Gwen.

Robin watched as they talked, then argued. Gwen turned red,
then yelled, "No Debbie, you can't do that."

She slammed the phone and turned toward Robin.

"She's gonna ruin it for me, for real."

"How can she ruin it?"

Gwen plopped down in one of the wicker chairs. She was sulking,
distant. She looked away as she talked.

"There's only two people who could ever hurt me. There's only
two people who could ever put me away. Debbie and you."

What about Lisa Lynch, Robin wondered.

"I didn't tell Lisa anything, really. And I don't think Lisa would
say anything."

Robin thought, what about me? I won't say anything. No one
would ever understand anyway. No one would ever understand
Cathy's games and the way she spoke half-truths.

Robin looked at the woman she loved. Her shoulders were drawn
together, her eyes fixed on some imaginary image. She seemed to
have disappeared inside herself. She seemed frightened.

Robin dropped to her knees in front of her.

"I won't tell, Gwen. I promise. I will never tell. You can count on
me—forever."

She reached out and embraced her legs. Gwen didn't move. She moved up and hugged her body. Gwen put her arms around her, but she felt cold and unfeeling.

Robin had never known her to be like that.

Chapter 88

By the end of November, the luxury of secrecy the Walker police had previously enjoyed was fast eroding. The Grand Rapids news media knew sketchy details of the Alpine Manor murder story.

On Monday, November 28, fifty-three days after Ken Wood had walked into Wyoming PD, an article appeared on the front page of the *Grand Rapids Press*. The headline: POLICE PROBE SUSPICIOUS DEATH AT WALKER NURSING HOME IN 1987. Walker Police Chief Walter Sprenger told the paper that police indeed were looking into "rumors" of a possible homicide. A tipster, the paper reported, had been calling both the newspaper and local TV stations.

"Hey, someone has opened their big mouth," Freeman told Cathy Wood.

Cathy said she knew the source. Needing cash for an apartment, Cathy had borrowed three hundred dollars from Katherine Brinkman, the aide who had been beaten up on K-Mart Hill. She told Brinkman about the police investigation. She didn't pay back the loan. Katherine Brinkman would later deny it, but Freeman figured the aide was probably settling some old scores.

Freeman could not complain about the results from either the press or Palmatier's polygraph five days earlier. Finally, he felt the case was getting the attention it deserved from the Kent County Prosecutor's office. The news media pressurized everything. Chief Sprenger was running interference with reporters. Alpine Manor, meanwhile, hired one of Grand Rapids' top public relation firms. They could stall reporters for a few days, but eventually a decision would have to be made on arrests.

The news media were both a curse and a blessing, Freeman decided. Reporters were time-consuming and could scare off some witnesses. Stories, however, also could produce new information and bring forward previously unknown informants.

Things would happen quickly now. When Freeman met with Dave Schieber, the assistant prosecutor agreed.

"Now the clock is ticking," Schieber said.

Cathy called Freeman in a panic. A persistent *Grand Rapids Press* reporter named Ken Kolker had dropped by the restaurant where she worked on Monday. He wanted an interview.

"Don't talk to the reporter, Cathy," Freeman said. "Come in and talk to me."

She arrived at Walker PD Tuesday morning. He wanted to talk about the acronym IGTKM on the bottom of her love letter to Gwen.

Freeman turned on the tape recorder. She asked him to turn it off. She was concerned about the acronym being misinterpreted. She was worried Freeman, the prosecutor or the courts would think the "M" represented Marguerite Chambers instead of Madeline Young.

Cathy Wood did not want anyone to think she did any hands-on killing. It was an important distinction for her. Freeman stood up, and threw a little tantrum.

"Damn it, Cathy. Don't you know who the head of this investigation is? I won't let that happen. I would never let that happen."

What he didn't say was that, under the law, it didn't really matter. If she planned the deaths with Gwen, she was as vulnerable to a first-degree murder conviction as the killer who did the dirty work.

He put the tape recorder back on. Cathy explained the acronym. As for Madeline Young, Cathy said she had recently died of natural causes in Alpine Manor.

Freeman tried to pin her down once more on Wanda Urbanski. She could have been the "U" in the elusive M-U-R-D-E-R plan, Cathy said. She remembered Gwen "holding her," but she couldn't remember if the attack had been deadly.

When they were done, Cathy asked if she had to testify against Gwen Graham. He suspected the presence of the news media in the case was making her jumpy.

"I'll check that out," he said. "It depends on the prosecutor. It depends on the attorneys."

He was on his way downtown to see Kent County Prosecutor Bill Forsyth and David Schieber, in fact. There was some paperwork. He would ask them then, he said.

She wanted to go with him. Freeman passed.

"Cathy, they'll think I'm crazy bringing you with me."

Later, she called wanting a favor. She wanted the courtesy of a phone call.

"Would you let me know in advance?" she asked.

"Let you know what?"

"When you're going to arrest me."

As Cathy Wood left, a young woman was waiting for Freeman in another room. The former Alpine aide had phoned the department earlier. She had more information about the murder story she had read about in the *Press*.

Freeman had heard the former aide's name from Cathy, but knew little about her. She said she knew Gwen Graham. She knew Robin Fielder. And she knew Cathy Wood, all right.

"Cathy ruined a lot of things in my life," she said.

The woman said Gwen once told her she had smothered a couple of patients, with Cathy serving as a lookout. Gwen had told her it was a mercy killing.

"Did they mention any patients' names?"

"Edith Cook," she said.

The former aide had dismissed the conversation in her trailer all these months as a "head game," until she read the paper.

There was more, much more.

Her name was Lisa Lynch.

Six weeks earlier, Freeman had taken the medical records to Kent County Medical Examiner Stephen Cohle. During several meetings they discussed the case and Cathy's statements in detail.

From the start, the pathologist predicted the chances were slim of finding the subtle pathological evidence of suffocation, considering the victims' ages, condition, and nearly two years of interment. The best candidate for a post mortem autopsy was Belle Burkhard.

Her arm supposedly was bruised or twisted. Alpine records listed her as Catholic.

"Damn, she won't be cremated," Freeman said.

Not only had Belle Burkhard been cremated, but so had Myrtle Luce and Mae Mason. That left Marguerite Chambers and Edith Cook. Cathy had been so unclear about Lucille Stoddard, Ruth Van Dyke and Wanda Urbanski, Freeman and others wondered if,—for purposes of prosecution—they could be considered on Gwen Graham's hit list.

After Freeman called Dave Schieber with details of the statement by Lisa Lynch, the prosecutor's office began preparing a legal petition. Evidence or no evidence, if there were to be arrests, the exhumations would have to be done.

"We are absolutely obligated," Prosecutor William Forsyth said in one meeting. "Imagine us trying to go through a trial without doing it."

The city of Walker would have to pay overtime to the gravediggers, plus replace the opened vaults. The total bill would be nearly five thousand dollars per body.

There would be many other costs, the kind that couldn't be calculated in dollars.

As she had been that night on Dover, Marguerite Chambers would be the first.

Chapter 89

Strangely enough, Ken never fielded any real criticism from Cathy for going to the authorities. She called him within two weeks after her first statements to the Walker Police.

"Ken, I want to see Jamie now," she said. "I want to pick her up and have her spend the night."

He was angry at the proposition.

"Cathy, no way. You didn't give a shit for two years, and now that you're in trouble, suddenly you want to be a mother again."

Her proposal worried him. Maybe, he thought, she just wants Jamie to get back at me. She'll kidnap our daughter and leave the state. He hoped she didn't try to pick up Jamie one day from school.

Before she hung up, she threatened to go to court to enforce their visitation agreement.

He called Tom Freeman.

"I don't want her with Jamie," he told the detective. "If the custody people get on my case, I'm sending them to you."

"I wouldn't let her go, either," Freeman advised. "But I've got to be careful. I've got an investigation underway. I've got to stay on Cathy's good side."

Then, Cathy simply dropped the request.

By late November, Ken was confused about the investigation. Cathy had been feeding him bits and pieces during regular phone calls. Sometimes he tried to advise her, telling her to make sure she received consideration for her cooperation. He didn't want her to go free, but he also didn't want to see the mother of his daughter thrown in jail and punished like a common criminal. Despite all the misery, Ken still loved her. After all, she once had been his wife.

"My goal all along was to see she got help so that she could live a normal life," he later said. "Maybe some kind of court-ordered treatment."

When he worried out loud to her that the police weren't really looking after her best interests, she chided him.

"Well, Ken, you're the one who went to the police."

He had no apologies.

"Cathy, you should have never told me this, and not gotten help. You had to know I couldn't live with this. You had to know I'd go to the police."

The phone was silent. Then her voice was very calm.

"No, Ken, I did the right thing."

One night, in the last week of November, she stopped by his apartment. She complained she couldn't get a court-appointed attorney until she was arrested. She needed one before that, she said. She had found a woman attorney, referred to her by her friend Nancy Harris.

"I don't want a man," she said. "All they want to know about is what women do with each other. All they want to talk about is sex."

She seemed convinced she was going to jail, but ultimately would be released in a couple of months.

"I'm waiting for a phone call from the police," she said. "I could be arrested any day."

Ken handed her $250 for the retainer. Next, she wanted to talk to Jamie.

"I might not see you for a while, Burger," she told her. "We won't be able to spend Christmas together. But we *will* spend a Christmas together. We'll just celebrate a couple months later—just you and me."

Ken thought, she seems so loving, so caring. When she takes the time she's so good with Jamie. Her problem is: She never takes the time.

"Hey, stay Cathy," Ken said. "Why don't you stay awhile."

In some crazy way, he missed her. She still could make him feel hope. He didn't know if the hope was cultivated by her, or his own wishful thinking.

He missed her. He missed the family they never really had.

"C'mon out to the car, there's someone I want you to meet," she told Jamie.

Ken followed.

Sitting in the passenger seat was a girlfriend.

As Cathy drove off in her Luv Truck, Ken Wood was angry all over again.

Chapter 90

Only a week earlier, Jan Hunderman had driven by Rosedale Memorial Park on an errand. She was with a girlfriend.

"Hey, this is where my mother is buried. I wanna stop. I wanna stop and see her."

Jan gazed at her grave in the section called Garden of the Gospels. She had found a certain measure of acceptance. Yet, both she and her father found something about her mother's death incomplete. Her father frequently dreamed about their life together. Jan still broke down when she talked about her mom.

"There just were no final words, no telling her that we loved her," she told a friend. "Somehow, her death just didn't feel right."

The rapping on her door came late on a Monday afternoon. On the doorstep were two Walker detectives and Ronald Westman, the owner of Alpine Manor. The three men had already talked to her father. She invited them to sit at the kitchen table.

At first, Jan's mind raced over her mother's finances, the applications to the state for help with her care. She thought, did we do something wrong? Are they here to arrest me, put me in a jail?

"We're investigating your mother's death as a possible homicide," Tom Freeman said.

Jan thought, *my* mother?

She leaned forward over the table.

"But my mother never left Alpine Manor," she said.

She looked at Ronald Westman. He was sitting only half on his seat, as close as he could get to the wall. She thought, he looks like he thinks I'm going to hit him.

Then it hit her. Murder, in Alpine Manor!

"I'm sorry," Westman said.

She collapsed back into her chair.

"How?"

Tom Freeman gave few details.

"We think she may have been suffocated with a washcloth."

They said the medical examiner might have to do an autopsy.

Jan and her father spent the next couple days together. They talked. They remembered. They tried to negotiate with their own memories.

Her father said he could no longer sleep in his own bed, the one they bought as newlyweds. It cradled a nightmare, a bad dream that repeated every night. They were there, the two women, holding their hands over Marguerite's face, he told Jan. For months to come, Ed Chambers would sleep on the couch.

On Wednesday afternoon, Jan opened her front door again to another Walker policeman. He was silhouetted by thick falling flakes of the season's first snow.

"Are you Jan Hunderman?"

"Yes."

"I have this here, to exhume your mother's body, and I need you to sign this paper."

Her mother was a Catholic, she protested inwardly. The body was sacred, reserved for the Resurrection. Jan also was afraid. She was afraid what the police said was the truth.

"What if I don't want to sign it."

"Well, they'll just get a court order."

Later she found out they already had. The paper was a courtesy, but she never expected it would happen so soon.

The next morning her husband Gary yelled to her.

"Hey, look it, you gotta watch this. Something about your mother on the TV."

She rushed into the living room and saw the morning news. There was footage of the cemetery, of the Garden of the Gospels. She saw images both pure and unclean. She saw virgin white snow and ugly dark dirt. In the middle of the picture was a high-low. Its shovel had dinosaur's teeth. The arm was mechanical, hydraulic. It lifted, jerking, then devoured more earth. Jan saw the leafless maple that sheltered her mother's grave site.

The voice on the TV said: "Kent County Medical Examiner Dr. Stephen Cohle performed an autopsy late last night on Mrs. Chambers . . ."

Last night. Jan felt herself coming apart. She had woken in the middle of her sleep *last night*. There was a white light, above her. It was long and fluorescent, but tinted that odd hospital green. It had wings, and hovered. She swiped at it with her hands, as though it were a moth. Her hands went through it. Her screaming woke Gary up.

It was the examination light of the coroner, Jan told herself. Above her. Last night. That's when they were opening my mother with their stainless steel scalpels.

She thought, I am my mother, lying on that table.

She felt like someone was cutting out her heart.

Chapter 91

The phone message to "call detective Freeman" was driving Dawn Male crazy. She kept thinking, what part of my past in Grand Rapids is catching up with me now?

She was back in Lakeview, working third shift as a cook at a truck stop. She had a new job, a new apartment and a new roommate. She had left Grand Rapids a year and a half ago, broke and jobless. After all the mind games of the summer of 1987, even the return to the little town she once loathed offered some relief. She hadn't heard from Cathy Wood in months, Gwen Graham for well over a year.

During a break before sunrise, Dawn picked up an old newspaper somebody left in the truck stop. The phone message made sense when she saw the news headline about Alpine Manor. A few hours later she arrived at the Walker PD. It was early Thursday morning, December 1. Her memory of Cathy and Gwen's little chat about murdered patients was still intact.

"They wanted me to believe them," she told Freeman. "They even went so far as to show me articles they had taken from patients that they had supposedly killed. I did not believe them. I thought it was just, I don't know, an ignorant joke."

She told the detective about the anklet Cathy had showed her. She explained Cathy's penchant for mind games.

"Cathy was the best at it, that was just her hobby . . . One day you'd be her best friend. She just couldn't confide in you more. The next day she hated your guts for something . . ."

"Of the two, who was the most likely to commit violent acts?" Freeman asked.

"Gwen. Cathy is not violent."

"Why do you say Gwen?"

"Because I know Gwen is violent."

She would give two statements, one a week later. Dawn later said police already had made up their minds as to who was the dangerous half of the Wood-Graham partnership.

"They seemed to know what the hell they were talking about," she later told a friend. "I sometimes wondered what they even needed me for. Cathy was the poor little innocent one who kind have got sucked into it all. And, at the time I probably agreed."

It was a role Dawn Male knew all too well.

The autopsy on Marguerite Chambers produced little from a pathological standpoint. The extensive news coverage of the Wednesday's exhumation, however, brought sources forward and widened the investigation into Cathy's old Alpine Manor circle. On Thursday and Friday detectives talked to more than a half dozen new people. Their statements were not consistent with Cathy Wood's self-portrait as Gwen's timid lover.

Tom Freeman interviewed former aide Ladonna Sterns. She told him she had had a brief affair with Cathy after Gwen left for Texas. She had heard Cathy was holding "something" over Gwen's head. Ladonna now was shocked by everyone's past in Alpine Manor.

"We used to all be good friends. Things got a little bit mixed-up . . . we all kind of went crazy. We all left our husbands . . . We kind of lost touch with reality at one point."

Ladonna told of rumors of sexual abuse of patients, including one that Gwen or Cathy fondled a patient's breasts to watch the nipples get hard.

"But by the time I confronted Cathy Wood, she would deny everything that was going on," she said.

She detailed the way both women would show up at work with bruises and scratches. "That's the way they got their kicks, hurting each other when they made love."

Ladonna also knew about the shelves in Cathy's bedroom. She said they were full of cute items, "like dolls, stuffed animals, stuff like that."

Violent, sadomasochistic sex. Murder. Death souvenirs next to *stuffed animals.*

Freeman thought, what kind of women am I dealing with here?

"Of the two, Cathy and Gwen, who is the most domineering one?" he asked.

"Cathy," she said.

On the other hand, Gwen Graham's persona continued to emerge as troubled and tough. Her old roommate Fran Shadden added some insight. Roger Kaliniak first interviewed Fran at her apartment. Then she came to the Walker PD. Freeman was looking for bizarre behavior by Gwen in Alpine. She remembered one example, but thought Gwen wasn't serious.

"Well, the thing on my mind is the fact that when Gwen was living with me, she had come home one day and she talked about how she had a sexual feeling from one of the older people there."

On the other hand, Fran explained, Gwen was heartbroken when she saw her first patient die. She told Freeman about Gwen's past, their fights and her self-mutilation. She detailed Gwen's stories about brawls, stealing and break-ins in Texas. She amended the stories.

"I didn't know whether to think it was just bragging, 'cause she liked to portray herself as a little tough," she added. "You know, *I'm a tough person, nothing or nobody can hurt me* sort of exterior."

She said Gwen was two people.

"A lot of times I think Gwen's got two totally separate personalities, 'cause she can be as different as night and day," she told Freeman. "She can be so gentle and kind and wanting to help people around her, and she would help anybody . . . At times she was just kind of violent."

Fran told the detective she thought Cathy Wood, Dawn Male and most of the Alpine crowd she met at softball practice were over the edge.

"Would you classify Gwen that way?"

Fran paused, then nodded her head.

"I guess deep down I always felt that Gwen was mentally ill."

There were more interviews with nursing home workers. Most produced no hard evidence, but plenty of suspicion.

Roger Kaliniak talked with Tish Prescott, the night supervisor. She now was retired from nursing, but remembered Cathy Wood and Gwen Graham quite clearly. She told them about the "uneasy feeling" she always had about the two and their inability to stay at their assigned stations.

A former aide named Brian Bruin called Walker PD after reading about the exhumation of Marguerite Chambers. He wanted to

advise Freeman that he was the aide who discovered her. He cleaned
her up after she died, he said. Gwen Graham assisted him. He
couldn't recall any suspicious behavior, adding he worked there
only six weeks.

Kaliniak talked to Paul Lopez, Robin Fielder's old boyfriend,
interviewing him on the job at another nursing home. He said that
more than a year ago Shawn Thatcher had relayed to him Cathy's
story about killing patients. He confronted her with it, but had a
hard time believing her.

"And after you asked her if it was true what did she say?"

"She said, yeah, it was true. And I asked her who was suffocated
and she wouldn't tell me. And I asked her if I could name off names
and she could tell me if they were the ones or not."

He mentioned two names. Kaliniak did a double take.

"I named off a couple of names, Marguerite Chambers and
Edith Cook. She never said yes or no. She never said anything. But
she said there were more."

The two patients were the case's leading victims. Unbeknownst
to Lopez, Cook's body was being exhumed as they talked. It was late
Friday afternoon.

"Why did you mention Marguerite Chambers?"

"I just didn't think Marguerite was ready to go."

"How about Edith Cook?"

"Edith wasn't very good, but I just didn't expect her to go so
quick."

Former Alpine aide Tony Kubiak was relaxing with his roommate Jessie in their apartment when he saw his first report that
Alpine Manor was under investigation. Police had two suspects, but
didn't name them, the newscaster said.

"It's got to be Cathy," Kubiak said.

He thought, she's evil enough to kill. But who else? They speculated on several possible partners. They considered Gwen, but only
as a possible subordinate.

"We definitely both agreed on Cathy," he later said. "It wasn't
Gwen and somebody. It was *Cathy* and somebody."

Kubiak talked to Roger Kaliniak and his tape recorder. He
showed up at Walker PD on Thursday, offering to shed light where

he could. He told them about the practical jokes and the fights between the women.

"Of the two people, which one would be more docile and which one was the more violent person?"

Kubiak, son of a Grand Rapids newspaperman, didn't take the language lightly. Docile meant "easily led." Violent meant just that. One didn't necessarily preclude the other.

"I think Gwen was more violent, I really do," he explained. "Cathy was quite dominant, was twice as big as Gwen, but I really think Gwen was more violent."

He gave a few anecdotes. He knew about Gwen's reputation as a street fighter. However, he also described in detail how Cathy had pulled Gwen into the bedroom by her hair.

They talked with the recorder off as well. He explained how Cathy masterminded paybacks and pranks at the nursing home. He was concerned she would try and drag him into the crimes. Kubiak remembered her threat that he was on her revenge list.

Cathy Wood was a threat, Tony Kubiak told Kaliniak.

"She's insane," he said.

He didn't mean the legal definition.

"Look it," he said. "Cathy Wood is sick in the head."

Chapter 92

Before it began Saturday morning, Dave Schieber's second autopsy in less than four days immediately produced one good result. Unlike the postmortem exam of Marguerite Chambers, a pathologist's exam hadn't offered the assistant prosecutor a day-old sweet roll, just before the cutting began.

Some sort of macabre pathologist's initiation, Schieber guessed. In fact, the attorney's presence was extraordinary. He *never* went to autopsies. And, this was an extraordinary case, he decided, from a legal standpoint, not to mention the basic facts. He knew any sign of foul play on Edith Cook's body would prevent a host of potential legal problems ahead.

Kent County Medical Examiner Dr. Stephen Cohle began his work at 9:30 A.M. It was December 3. A hearse had brought the coffin over from Resurrection Cemetery to Blodgett Memorial Medical Center the night before. Dr. Cohle identified Edith Cook for the record by noting her name was on her coffin. She was clad in a blue dress and brown hose. There was a gold ring on the third finger of her right hand and a copper one on the fourth finger of her left. Rosary beads were wrapped around her hands.

Attendants lifted her body onto the examination table. There would be a complete autopsy, including tests for poisoning. Dr. Cohle was concentrating on specific areas. Removing her makeup, he would examine Cook's face for lesions and bruises. He would inspect the mucous membrane that lined her eyelids for tiny hemorrhages, sometimes an indicator of suffocation. He would cut the mortician's wires that held her mouth shut, removing the cotton stuffed into her oral cavity during embalming.

Everyone was hopeful that evidence of a struggle would turn up in her mouth. Cathy Wood had said Cook had been killed with her false teeth in place, before they were removed and thrown away in the Alpine Manor trash.

Schieber and Prosecutor William Forsyth opted to avoid the sights and smells of the procedure and headed for a waiting room. They talked over the next move. The Alpine story now was getting quite detailed in the *Grand Rapids Press.* Reporters had not only identified Marguerite Chambers, they had talked to her family. They were developing nursing home sources. Saturday's paper had identified Edith Cook.

Schieber knew Walker police were frustrated by the office's reluctance to issue warrants. Tom Freeman had been asking for weeks. However, until Lisa Lynch gave her statement, prosecuting Gwen Graham was a long shot at best, if Cathy Wood also was charged. The reason was a court precedent called *Brutin versus the United States.* Unless Wood agreed to testify, *Brutin* dictated that her statements to Walker police could not be used to prosecute Graham. The concept came from the established legal principle that Graham had a right to cross-examine her accuser. If Wood was charged, and chose to evoke her right not to testify, Graham's attorney would not have that opportunity.

A plea agreement in return for her testimony would change all that. But first Wood and Graham had to be charged and bound over. Also, there had been little consideration of offering Wood a deal, at least early on.

"We were hesitant," Schieber explained later. "We were hoping Gwen would say something. We were still looking to find out if Cathy was telling us everything about her role. We had a lot of discussions about what idiots we would look like if we cut Cathy a deal and it turned out she was the one who actually did the suffocating."

Lisa Lynch's statement, however, had solved the *Brutin* problem for purposes of arrest and arraignment. Now, with all the publicity, Schieber wondered if Gwen Graham wouldn't soon bolt.

"How long can we leave a serial killer out?" he told Forsyth. "It would be awful easy for her to just flee. She's the type that can just blend in somewhere."

Whatever the autopsy's results, they suspected they had to move forward with the arrests. The Palmatier polygraph had carried a lot of weight with Schieber and his boss. William Forsyth said he was a believer.

"In my mind, I was not about to exhume anybody's body, unless I was convinced it had to have happened," William Forsyth later said. "If it was my mother, I wouldn't want somebody doing that."

Tom Freeman called Cathy Wood from the hospital during the autopsy, asking her a minor detail about Edith Cook's death. Cathy was anxious to know why and when she might be arrested.

"Why are you going to charge me if they're going to drop it?" she asked.

"Drop what, Cathy?"

"The charges. You said you would have to arrest me and then they would drop the charges against me. But that I would have to be in jail at the time so I could testify against Gwen."

Freeman thought, that doesn't even make sense.

"No, Cathy. I didn't say that."

"Oh yes, Tom, you said that."

Freeman probed his memory. Jesus, he thought, there she goes again, making me doubt what I've even said. Then he resolved the internal debate.

"No Cathy. You've got it wrong. I never said the charges would be dropped. I know damn well I never said that."

She sounded angry when she hung up.

Chapter 93

"Please don't hang up on me."

Alpine supervisor Marty Slocum recognized the Texas drawl of Gwen Graham.

Gwen sounded baffled. She told Marty about the police showing up in Tyler. Then she cracked a joke about Alpine Manor's oldest and most feisty patient.

"Marty, two things came to my mind when I saw the police. A bounced check and that I hadn't given John Gerken his coffee."

They both chuckled. Gwen became serious again.

"Cathy is becoming more weird all the time," Gwen said.

She reported Cathy's threats to Robin Fielder in the Alpine parking lot, adding that everything was a head game, an act of revenge. Cathy also called her in Texas, she said. Cathy claimed to have killed a patient named Deana Feenstra.

"She knew I liked Deana. Marty, she was laughing about it, for real."

Then she said something the supervisor thought a little odd.

"I still love Cathy, Marty. But I don't like what she's doing."

Gwen sounded more puzzled than fearful. She denied having had anything to do with any killings.

"We shared a lot of things, but we didn't share *that.*"

It was just after 1:00 P.M. Sunday afternoon, December 4.

* * *

Three hours later, Danny Alexander picked up Tom Freeman and Bill Brown at the Tyler Airport. Freeman carried with him a murder warrant for Gwen Graham's arrest. Once Graham was in custody, he or the deputy chief would call Grand Rapids. The Walker police then would execute a similar arrest warrant on Cathy Wood.

She would not get a courtesy phone call.

Freeman was pumped. Fifty nine anxious days had passed since Ken Wood had walked into the Wyoming PD. Now, as the three detectives pulled into the Five Star Mobile Home Park in an un-marked Tyler car, he was anticipating his biggest arrest as a cop.

The lights were on in the trailer. But no one was there. They went to the manager with a question.

"Say, have you seen Gwen Graham and Robin Fielder?"

He chuckled.

"Man, they're *gone*. Hell, cops were here a month or so ago. As soon as the cops wére gone, they were."

Freeman turned to Alexander.

"Damn it, Danny. You told me you were going to keep an eye on them."

They drove to Mother Francis Hospital. The personnel office was closed. They convinced a supervisor to call in an office clerk to check the employment files.

"Yes, right here's the address for Robin Fielder."

It was the old address at the mobile home park.

Freeman could feel the blood rushing to his face. As far as they knew, Gwen Graham was in Mexico. He could only hope she was still living with Robin Fielder. They could stake out the hospital and follow Robin's car. She was scheduled to work on Monday. They started out the door of the hospital, then Freeman stopped. He decided to take a precaution.

"We better go back and tell this broad not to tell anyone the police were here," he said.

A few minutes later they were at a red light on Dawson Street, waiting to turn on a five-lane highway called Beckham, just in front of the hospital. It was dusk.

"Golly Tom," Danny Alexander said. "Looks like we're fixin' to be in for a long hunt."

He turned and smiled. Freeman wasn't smiling.

Alexander turned back toward the intersection.

"Well I'll be darned. You see what I see."

"What?"

"There!"

The coincidence was astounding in a city that numbered 80,000 people. A Mustang was passing through the intersection, heading south on Beckham. Robin Fielder was in the passenger seat. Gwen Graham was at the wheel.

"Danny Alexander," Freeman said calmly, "you're the luckiest sonovabitch in the world."

Alexander pulled behind the Mustang. They followed the car for twelve miles, radioing coordinates to a dispatcher. They were waiting for a marked unit to intercept and make the stop.

When the squad car pulled over the Mustang, Freeman told Alexander to alert the other car.

"You tell them I'm going to approach the car."

The Walker detective walked up to the driver's side and looked in the window. Gwen was wearing sweats. Her hair was a mess, her hands covered with grime. Later, she said she had been working on the car.

Tom Freeman had wanted to say the words for weeks. It was almost 8:00 P.M., his time.

"Gwen Graham, you're under arrest for murder."

In seconds, they had her out of the car and in handcuffs. They kept Robin Fielder in the Mustang. They had already planned their strategy. They wanted to minimize the chance of another screaming fit.

Robin was calm, compared to her last performance.

"Tom, they've talked about it," Bill Brown later told Freeman.

The assistant chief studied Gwen Graham. The statements, the polygraphs and the autopsies hadn't convinced him. The look in Gwen Graham's eyes now did.

"She was completely different than the last visit," he later recalled. "I saw fear. Terror, in her eyes. She knew her number was up. She was struggling to control herself, somewhere deep down inside."

It was nearly an hour before midnight when Roger Kaliniak rang the buzzer for the upper apartment at 108 Lexington. The large figure descended the steps, wearing only a flimsy nightgown.

"Who is it?"

"It's Rog, Cathy."

She opened the door. It was not only Rog, but Chief Walter Sprenger and two Walker patrolman. Cathy was irritated she was being bothered so late at night.

"Cathy, we have a warrant for your arrest on the charge of murder."

She wanted to change her clothes. They followed her up the steps. Kaliniak found her words at the top of the steps ironic, considering the charges she faced and the fallout yet to come when the families learned of the arrest.

"You're not going to be mean to me, are you?" she said.

Chapter 94

The confusion had begun with the police cars. Maybe it began a long time before that.

Robin Fielder remembered all the flashing lights, the way the color seemed to blemish her skin. She remembered looking out the car window, seeing someone, a woman, her family, pulling open her living room curtains. They were watching the arrest scene on the street. They were watching her and Gwen.

Robin had asked the detectives after they took Gwen away.

"What are you going to do to me? What do I do?"

"You can bring her some clothes to the jail," someone said.

"Where do I go?"

"You can go back with us," said Bill Brown.

"Where?"

"To Michigan."

"I'm not going anywhere with you."

She asked again.

"Where do I go?"

"Why don't you go home?" one policeman said.

"Where is my home?" she said, loudly.

Robin Fielder only knew where she lived.

Now she was there, in the apartment, mixing lemonade, a quart of lemonade. She was drinking it right from the pitcher. She was chain-smoking.

Before she had gone to church that night she had talked to her mother.

"Are you all right?" her mother had asked again.

They had been reading all about Alpine Manor. A couple of days earlier her dad had called. It was the first time they had talked in more than a year. He was crying.

"You gotta get out of there, honey," he said. "You gotta get out of there."

Robin picked up the phone, not to call her parents, but Gwen's uncle, the attorney. There was no answer. She called the number, over and over. Finally he answered. He told her to take Gwen's clothes and essentials to the jail.

She became lost on the way. She didn't know the city. She didn't know much of anything about Tyler, Texas. She had always left everything to Gwen.

When she finally arrived, there was a deputy at the desk. He looked into the brown bag of clothes and toilet items she held.

"No, she can't use that," he said.

Her heart sank. She began to cry.

"They told me to bring it. What do I do with it?"

"I don't care what you do with it."

"I wanna see Danny Alexander. I wanna see Freeman and Brown."

"They're not here right now."

She stood around, in front of the desk. The desk officer said something into a microphone. A pay phone rang in the waiting area.

"Are you Robin?" said somebody who answered it.

She nodded.

It was Gwen.

"I'm okay," she said. "Robin, you go home."

She walked to her Mustang. The engine wouldn't turn over. She put up the hood. The same thing had happened in the church parking lot earlier. Gwen had bummed a ride to the church to rescue her and the car. The arrest came on their way back.

Robin was crying again.

"Can I help you, m'am?"

He was a uniformed officer. He did something to the battery cable. She started the car.

Back at the apartment, midnight approached. She was drinking more lemonade, smoking more cigarettes, sitting alone in the chair. She had a Bible open in front of her. The phone rang. It was Angie Brozak and Ladonna Stearns.

"Are you okay?" one of them said.

"No. They just picked up Gwen."

Five minutes later the phone rang again.

It was her dad. Later, she found out Ladonna and Angie had called her folks.

"Honey, are you okay?"

"No, Dad."

She began to cry again, but these were different tears.

"Dad, I wanna come home," Robin Fielder said.

Chapter 95

Attorney John Engman wanted a professional courtesy. He wanted to see exactly what the police and prosecutors had that led them to believe his mother-in-law Mae Mason was a murder victim.

When he called William Forsyth with the request Monday, the Kent County prosecutor was reluctant. Engman knew about the politics of the office. He had worked there as an assistant for ten years. He offered Forsyth a choice.

"Look, do you want me to throw a fit in the *Grand Rapids Press*, or do you want to show me what you got?"

The weekend had been a very long one. Early Saturday morning they had just returned from breakfast when Alpine Manor owner Ronald Westman called to warn Linda of a pending news conference and ongoing investigation.

"Your mother is one of eight people supposedly murdered at the nursing home," he told Linda.

Within the three hours of the call they were closing doors and hanging up on one reporter after another.

"Don't talk to anyone," John said.

They didn't want to talk to reporters. They wanted to talk to the police.

"Why isn't somebody from the police department calling?" Linda said. "Anybody. Somebody."

By Sunday, John and Linda had talked themselves out of the possibility Maisy had been killed. By Sunday night, they had come full circle. Linda gazed out their big windows, the ones that faced the Thornapple River.

"John, I just can't handle this anymore. You've got to go to the prosecutor's office."

By Monday afternoon he had read the documentation of the prosecutor's case. John Engman called his wife.

"I think it's true, honey."

"John, what about Stephie?"

Their eldest daughter was the worry now. For three months after her grandmother died, Stephanie had worn the color black.

Al Van Dyke could tell the woman on the other end of the phone was reading a prepared statement. She said she was calling for Alpine Manor. It was about the investigation. She named several potential victims' names.

"Your mother is also mentioned," she said.

The former detective considered the possibility far fetched. Hell, he thought, I was with her up until a couple of hours before she died. When the names of the suspects and the eight possible victims were published in the newspaper, Van Dyke found himself becoming more defensive. Never even had a divorce in the family, he thought, let alone a murder.

"Being in homicide as many years as I was," he said later, "I didn't like the idea of somebody killing one of mine."

He refused to entertain the notion his mother might have been killed, even after he talked to the Walker police chief and later Tom Freeman. However, the M-U-R-D-E-R he saw in the newspaper gnawed at him. Was she the last letter? Was Ruth Van Dyke the R? Had he left her alone, to killers?

That was sad, he thought. That was damn sad.

Tom Freeman told him there were five much stronger cases than his mother's death. Let them do their job, Van Dyke decided. He would have expected the same. On one matter, however, he drew the line. Freeman asked him about the possibility of exhuming her body. Van Dyke knew the detective didn't need permission, just a court order.

"Look it, she couldn't have been murdered, understand?" he told Freeman. "As far as you're concerned, I was with her at her death bed."

Donald Urbanski, the seventy-year-old nephew of Wanda, received two calls, one from police and one from Alpine Manor. The retired UAW local president had been his aunt's legal guardian for five years. He read her name in the newspaper list of eight.

The aunt Urbanski remembered worked as a bookkeeper until she was seventy-five. The one he visited at Alpine Manor for five years was ninety, diabetic and all but comatose. She never moved or talked. He had been told she died of pneumonia.

"After I was called about the murders it hit me like a bolt of lightning," he later said.

In the year before Wanda Urbanski died he had received a half dozen calls from Alpine Manor. The staff reported his aunt had been discovered in her bed with bruises, and in one instance, a laceration. The nursing home attributed it to her hitting her head on the bed rail and other accidents.

"How can she get bruises?" Donald Urbanski always asked. "The woman never moves."

Nancy Hahn received her second call from the *Grand Rapids Press* reporter Ken Kolker late Monday. He first called Saturday, but was evasive.

"I don't even know what this call is about," she told the staff writer. "I'm not going to answer your questions."

In Buchanan, Nancy was one hundred miles away from the first news coverage of Alpine Manor. By Monday, she still knew nothing. The reporter broke the news to her on the second call.

"I can't believe no one has told you. But your mother is on the list, and she's got to be one of them."

Nancy asked, what list?

When he explained she felt her breath leave her. After she hung up, she called the Walker police. The detectives were out. Early the next day she called Ronald Westman at Alpine Manor. He apologized for not calling.

"I'm sorry, it was an oversight," he said. "Besides, I'm not even sure the murders happened."

As the news was carried throughout the state, and the country, the details hit Nancy Hahn hard. Everything in her life seemed to be going haywire at once. Her teenage son was in the hospital for jaw surgery. She and her husband were not getting along. Now there was guilt, again. Everything had to be rethought, refelt.

My mother had *not* died in peace, she thought. There had been no dignity in her death.

"I felt like I was a rotten wife, a rotten mother and a rotten daughter," she later recalled. "I felt I couldn't do anything right."

The crying became incessant. She seemed to stop only so her body could recuperate for an hour or two. Then it would resume again.

She picked up the phone and called a referral service. Nancy Hahn had decided she'd better get some help.

The first call Ted and Maxine Luce received from the nursing home kindled their imaginations.

"When I think of her in that position and someone *deliberately* . . . ah . . . cutting off her breath," Maxine later said. "That's the horror of the thing. When they're so helpless—like children."

The second call, from the police, dashed their hopes. Ted and Maxine Luce had been hoping the news wasn't true.

The cursory involvement by police with the families was by design. The small department's limited manpower already was taxed. Walker Police Chief Walter Sprenger had made an arrangement with Alpine Manor. The nursing home agreed to inform some families of the suspicious deaths.

The fact of the matter was that the Walker police still weren't exactly sure who would be on the final murder list. They arrested Gwen Graham on an open charge of murder for the death of Edith Cook. They arrested Cathy Wood on open murder charges for Cook and Marguerite Chambers.

By Tuesday, December 6, two days after the arrest of Gwen Graham and Cathy Wood, the *Grand Rapids Press* had published a list of eight possible victims: Marguerite Chambers, Myrtle Luce, Mae Mason, Ruth Van Dyke, Belle Burkhard, Wanda Urbanski, Edith Cook and Lucille Stoddard. The list was gleaned from a formerly suppressed search warrant and interviews with families.

As the week unfolded, families learned more from news sources than anywhere. Some would have nothing to do with the news media. A surviving nephew of Edith Cook and his wife refused all requests from those wanting to know more about Alpine's oldest possible murder victim. They appeared to consider the possibility of discussing the matter untidy.

"We're proud to say we have talked to no one," the nephew later said.

As police and prosecutor feared, they lost control of the story. National and statewide media carried reports. Ken Wood was giving interviews to reporters. He was widely quoted as saying his wife and Gwen Graham had murdered the patients because "it was fun." The M-U-R-D-E-R plan was widely reported. Graham killed for "emotional release" stories indicated.

Motive, however, largely was elusive.

"Motive is something we don't have to prove," Dave Schieber told one reporter flat out.

By midweek, the "L word" was in play. Chief Sprenger told reporters that the murders were not a matter of "thrill-seeking." He said that "a lesbian relationship was the motive of the case."

Television cameras and reporters converged on gay bars looking for background and footage. The Alpine group's old haunt, the Carousel, had closed. News media invaded Club 67 on South Division. Arthur Laham, a manager there, tossed a cameraman out who tried to shoot customers at the bar. Other customers complained they were getting needled by reporters.

Laham remembered Cathy Wood. She often hung out by the pool table. She was always snitching on pool players who gambled at the table, a violation of the bar's rules.

"Watch out for that one over there," she would always tell him, pointing out a patron who had wagered a small bet.

The focus on homosexuality shocked both conservative western Michiganians and many gays as well, but for entirely different reasons. Gay spokesmen protested the media was unfairly spotlighting homosexuals.

"Pathological behavior like that crosses many different socioeconomic levels," one gay leader told reporters. "It doesn't have a damn thing to do with what your sexual orientation is."

The publicity, talks with Walker detectives and reports from friends who worked at Alpine Manor pushed Jan Hunderman's imagination into the unthinkable.

"You wouldn't believe some of the things that went on down there," one officer had told her. There were pranks, jokes, fights and slashed tires, said a friend. There was a group of lesbians who drove pickup trucks and necked in the parking lot. Jan knew nothing about lesbians. She agonized over all the talk.

"Why not do it to patients when the urge strikes them?" she later asked. "Were they touching her, abusing her, sexually molesting her, when she couldn't do anything back?"

The news coverage, like the case, centered around Cathy Wood. Reporters gleaned first details of the murder from the affidavit attached to the search warrant for Gwen Graham's trailer. It was sworn before Cathy Wood implicated herself in the crimes. She was a passive witness. In interviews, Ken Wood emphasized her subordinate role. She was a troubled, overweight young woman who came forward to clear her conscience, he maintained. She wanted "professional help," he said. He quoted her during a tearful phone call from Kent County Jail.

"This is an awful scary place," she reportedly said.

Wood's mother Pat also pled her case. She told reporters her daughter was "innocent," adding Ken had "exaggerated" her confession. He was telling police "half-truths."

Alpine Manor had nothing but praise for Cathy Wood. Staff was ordered not to talk to reporters. Ginny Seyferth, a leading Grand

Rapids public relations executive, appeared at joint news conferences with Chief Walter Sprenger. Seyferth said both suspects were caring, sensitive workers, especially Cathy Wood. Reporters were not told about the pair's disciplinary reports, drinking and physical and psychological wars, on or off the job. There was nothing about Wood's frequent altercations with the patients.

"Her reviews were great," Seyferth said earnestly. "You couldn't ask for anyone more professional. Cathy was very popular. She was a favorite."

Both Sprenger and Seyferth portrayed the nursing home as an unknowing victim. Seyferth said a psychologist had been retained to counsel troubled staff and patients. The nursing home later claimed to have lost only one resident because of the murder story.

While Seyferth practiced damage control in a large briefing room in the Walker Community Building, detectives listened to quite a different story unfold in the small interview room at Walker PD. Cathy Wood was intoxicated with power and struck fear into other aides, one former worker said in a statement two days after Wood's arrest. She withheld food and water from patients unless they bent to her will.

"Cathy appeared to have a split personality," a former aide named Jean Marie Grep told Roger Kaliniak. "She could be very kind and generous to the families, to the residents, when she knew she had to be. But on the other side, she could be very cruel . . ."

Gwen Graham, meanwhile, remained an enigma. The public would learn little more about Gwen Graham than the violent, domineering persona that had been fashioned largely by Cathy Wood. Most of those who could have added some balance to the coverage had no plans to brave the press. Graham was a transient, an outsider in a Texas jail. She planned to stay in Texas as long as possible. She was fighting extradition to Michigan.

One of the sources reporters did find in Tyler was a sixty-three-year-old newspaper dispatcher named Ruth Weaver. Her quotes were buried at the bottom of stories. Gwen Graham delivered the *Dallas Morning News* for her from 1983 to 1985. She said Graham was likeable, her situation "sad."

"Her life was always difficult," she told a newspaper reporter. "I would say she was definitely an abused child. Her parents were divorced. They were a poor family. They never had much of anything. I think they moved around a lot."

She remembered the series of cigarette burns up her arms. She remembered Gwen's traffic accidents. That was one thing about Gwen Graham, she said.

Bad luck just seemed to follow her around.

Chapter 96

Tish Prescott left nursing and Alpine Manor, but was finding little comfort in retirement at the age of sixty-five. She was receiving threatening phone calls. They began shortly after the arrests.

"They have friends out there," the caller always said. "Don't think you're off the hook."

The calls usually came after dark. Sometimes the caller was a man, sometimes a woman. She found them terrifying, dangerous in fact. Tish's own health was not good. She had diabetes and congestive heart failure. The calls frequently left her out of breath.

Repeatedly, she called Walker police. She knew they thought she was being a nuisance.

"Tish, I don't understand these threats," Tom Freeman told her. "People who have given far more damaging information, are not getting threats. You, who have told us nothing incriminating, are getting them all the time. It just doesn't make sense."

The phone kept ringing. Soon, she was able to predict it. The calls always came after a splash of publicity on the case.

"Don't think you're off the hook!"

She contacted Grand Rapids attorney, Nancy Gage, an old family friend. The lawyer voiced concern to the prosecutor's office. Tish's name was on the list of possible witnesses on the arrest warrants. Cathy Wood had told police she thought Tish suspected something odd when she blurted out that Marguerite Chambers had died.

Tish couldn't even remember that incident. However, she

thought, God knows how many times I walked in on them alone in a patient's room. Maybe they think I saw something.

In late December, Tish received a subpoena. She was being called as a witness in Cathy Wood's preliminary exam, set for early January.

She received another call.

"Don't think you're off the hook."

She was afraid to pick up the telephone anymore.

Two days before Christmas, she was driving on Hall Street in East Grand Rapids. It was midafternoon. The intersections were lined with school children waiting with crossing guards at the lights. As she came to the intersection at Breton Avenue she saw a driver roar up behind her in her mirror. The vehicle swerved around her, then cut her off. She screeched to a stop, rather than swerve toward the school children.

Shaken, she watched the motorist speed off. She couldn't see if the driver was man or a woman. She could only see the back of the vehicle.

It was a pickup truck.

Tish moved in with Nancy Gage until the preliminary exam. On January 4, the court heard testimony from, among others, Dawn Male, Ken Wood and pathologist Stephen Cohle. Tish Prescott was not called. District Judge Sherwin J. Venema decided there was sufficient evidence to bind Cathy Wood over for trial for the murder of Marguerite Chambers and Edith Cook.

Back at her apartment in Grand Rapids' Heritage Hill district, Tish's fears were fueled again. She found her storm door shattered and footprints in the snow. The Grand Rapids police installed a special alarm.

"Don't think you're off the hook," the caller said again.

Nancy Gage complained to both the prosecutor's office, and later to Cathy Wood's attorney, Christine Yared.

"Would you have your client call her friends off," she told Wood's attorney.

After the preliminary exam the phone calls eased up. Then they came to a stop.

Chapter 97

The letters from Gwen came daily. Some days, two or three letters were waiting in the Notre Dame mailbox in front of her parents' home in Walker.

Most were amply illustrated. Gwen traced the images on stationery and envelopes in jail. Robin saw unicorns and rabbits and mushrooms and raccoons and clowns and birds. There were full-page drawings: A yellow bird poking out of a bird house, its wing holding a letter addressed "For Robin Fielder." A robin in a tree. A rabbit with a cane and top hat, saying "You sing, I'll dance." A sleeping baby in a cradle, hanging from a bow.

The correspondences upset her father. Robin suspected he might even have snatched some on Saturdays when he got the mail. He was reading the newspapers.

Robin thought, can these letters be from somebody who killed people? Gwen wrote words of love, in letter after letter.

"If there's any way I can make this easier on you, let me know," she wrote.

For Christmas, Robin sent her an outfit: a sweater, plaid shirt and some slacks. Robin received a jail-made Christmas card. Gwen drew a heavily decorated tree with a scroll that read:

Hope is not pretending that troubles don't exist . . . It is the
trust that they will not last forever, that hurts will be healed and
difficulties overcome . . . It is faith that a source of strength and
renewal lies within to lead us through the dark to the sunshine
. . .

"Merry Christmas pretty girl. I love you," she added.

These are not the words of a killer, Robin thought. She was reading the newspapers, too. She kept waiting to read that it was all over. She kept waiting for Cathy to tell everyone it was all a big joke.

She opened another package, a Christmas present sent via Gwen's sister. Inside was a sweatshirt. Her name was on it in big letters, along with a big Tyler rose.

She was bawling when her mother got home from work.

"What is it honey?"

She showed her mother the sweatshirt. Then Robin threw the box. She was mad at Cathy. She was mad at the cops. She was mad at the whole world.

She just wanted to be left alone.

She was, every day. Her routine began the same way every morning, and ended when her mother came home at midafternoon. Robin perched on a stool at the breakfast counter, drinking pot after pot of coffee, chain-smoking her Virginia Slims. She sat under two bright lights with metal shades that hung by long chords from the ceiling. They looked like interrogation lamps, and she felt interrogated by the voices of her own mind. She passed hours looking out the window toward the street. She was sure one day the police cars would arrive.

She hardly ate. In December, she had lost nearly twenty pounds. Her father was talking about hospitalizing her. She told him she was troubled because she hadn't been entirely honest with police. He suggested she clear her conscience.

"Just tell the truth, honey. That's all you have to do."

Her family sought the help and counsel of an old family friend, a Kent County Sheriff's deputy named Bob Hiner. Robin and Hiner paid a visit to the Walker police in mid-December. She gave another statement to Tom Freeman. She had told him in Texas that she saw Gwen and Cathy kidding with one another about some big secret. She cleared that up, but left with many more secrets of her own.

"It's not true," she told Freeman, of the kidding.

"Okay, then why did you bring it up?"

"Because I was mentally confused. I didn't know what was going on."

Back then, she was hysterical. Now, Robin didn't know who, or what information, she could trust.

"Did you ask her if she did kill anyone at Alpine Manor?" Freeman asked.

"Yes I did."

"What did she say?"

"She said, no, she didn't."

"Did you believe her?"

She paused a few seconds.

"Yes."

"Why are you hesitant?"

"Because you have evidence, that's the thing that's going in my mind. I don't know, she said she didn't do it, but if you have evidence, I don't know what to think."

Robin was doing all her thinking on the kitchen stool, under the lights. She thought, the police would never understand what Gwen told me. They won't believe it's probably a joke, a mind game. They certainly don't understand Cathy. She could see from the newspapers no one really knew how truly evil she was.

They will crucify Gwen, she thought. Robin remembered the marks on Gwen's body. She has suffered all her life already. She saw her as a kind of suffering Christ, victimized by the sins of others. She thought, if I tell I will be Judas. I will be a pawn in Cathy's plot.

She thought, I promised on my knees.

By January, Robin still was losing weight. She was finding it difficult to write Gwen anymore. She had only sent a half dozen letters. Writing only upset her more.

One day she stopped in at Alpine Manor to say hello to Marty Slocum and others. They all complimented her about her figure. This is not the way to lose weight, she thought.

"There's no murders," she told Slocum. "Why won't Walker police believe it? Cathy's playing head games again."

The internal turmoil only became worse, under the lights. She decided to spend more time out of the house. She would pick up Gwen's letters, then head to the Grand Rapids Zoo.

Robin had a favorite spot, there in the January cold. She always sat on the same bench, next to the duck pond. She shivered and smoked cigarettes and cried. The water was frozen, but the mallards stayed near their haunt. One duck always was quacking and toddling around alone, apart from the flock.

She began thinking, that's me. That small brown one. She's trying to join the rest, and they're running away. I'm alone. I have no more friends. Everyone thinks they know what I've become.

She thought, nobody can understand this. Nobody can understand the way I feel for Gwen. I can't tell my parents. I can't tell anyone—about what I feel for her, let alone what she may have said.

By mid-January, Robin had lost thirty pounds. She was down to

135. Once in a while, Gwen called. She had to get to the telephone before her father, before he told Gwen that she was not home.

One Monday night in mid-January Robin picked up the phone.

"If I ever get out of this, Robin, will you come back to Tyler to live with me?"

Robin had recently received an anniversary card from Gwen, for two years from January 8. She had been thinking of everything Gwen had told her about Cathy, about the murders. What she once wrote off as a joke and a mind game now posed far too many questions.

Maybe, Robin thought, I should just be like the duck. Maybe I should just stay away from everyone.

"Robin, will you come back?" Gwen asked again.

She answered quietly.

"Gwen, I don't think so. I don't think so, not now."

The next day, January 17, the female inmate being held for murder on a one-million-dollar bond in Smith County Jail made a ruckus.

"Get me back to Michigan," Gwen Graham shouted. "I want to go back to Michigan."

There were two dozen pictures of Robin Fielder taped all over her cell. She also had a laminated photo she always took with her into the prison shower.

"Robin and I are showering together," she sometimes said.

A half hour later, Gwen Graham stood before District Judge Bill Coats. She declined a court-appointed attorney.

"She didn't want anything," the judge later commented. "She wanted to get it over with. She wanted to waive everything and go back."

She seemed elated by the prospect of the trip back to Grand Rapids. In the courtroom, Gwen Graham was talking and joking with guards.

Chapter 98

Ken Wood was not content to sit back and read the newspapers. He talked periodically with Assistant Prosecutor David Schieber about the legal process his ex-wife faced. In early February, Ken brought up the subject of a plea bargain for Cathy.

The prosecutor's office already was dealing. Gwen Graham was back from Texas, arraigned and jailed in the Kent County Jail without bond, waiting for her preliminary exam later in the month. The prosecutor wanted Cathy's testimony against Gwen. With it, she could be bound over easily for trial.

Ken knew Cathy was considering an offer. She gave him the details in one of her weekly phone calls from jail. She could plead guilty to one count of second degree murder and conspiracy to murder. It would mean a prison term, but, unlike first degree, a chance for parole.

"Has she said anything to you about it?" Schieber asked. "Is she going to take it?"

Ken offered an opinion.

"Second degree murder is no bargain. Why don't you give her a real deal?"

"We can't afford to have a jury think we bought her testimony. That will not help our case."

"Look, Dave, I don't give a shit about your case. All I care about is Cathy. All I care about is getting Cathy some help."

The assistant prosecutor didn't budge.

"Ken, it's the best we can do."

Later, Ken received a collect call from Cathy. She had been transferred to the jail in Montcalm County, forty miles away in Stanton. Her attorney had requested she not be housed in the same lockup as Gwen.

Ken mentioned that he had talked with Dave Schieber about the plea bargain. Cathy was livid.

"How do you know that?" she snapped.

Ken didn't understand why she was making such a fuss. He reminded her that she had told him all the details.

"But he talked to *you*," she fumed. "He's not supposed to do that."

Christine Yared was a year short of thirty, and only in her fourth year of lawyering. However, the Grand Rapids attorney didn't need much tenure to spot a good offer when she saw one.

Yared was in her first year of private practice, but had learned plea bargaining on the fast track. When she was an assistant city attorney, she prosecuted misdemeanors for the city of Grand Rapids. Mornings were spent facing a line of defense lawyers in sixty-first District Court. Few wanted a costly trial, most wanted to negotiate.

Yared wanted her client Cathy Wood to think about a trial and its potentially grave consequences. She had studied Cathy's statements, particularly the videotape of the session with John Palmatier. Ultimately, Yared would be the only one in the court case who would make a written transcript of the tape. Cathy's admissions about planning Marguerite Chambers' death, Yared decided, made her exceedingly vulnerable.

"They could have easily tried her on first degree murder," she would later recall. "And, they could have convicted her."

Under Michigan law, that meant life in prison—mandatory or "natural life," as convicts called it. It was Michigan's harshest sentence, a living death penalty. The law dictated there was no opportunity for parole.

Yared knew the prosecutor wanted the maximum penalty for Gwen Graham. However, trying to convict her without Cathy's testimony would present a host of evidentiary problems as well as leave a great gap in the story for a jury. The second degree murder offer was a good option for the client who had thrust the young attorney into one of the most publicized murder cases in Grand Rapids history.

In late February, the offer became public, but not in the way Yared originally intended. Cathy Wood had called to complain that the prosecutor's office had been talking to her ex-husband. Ken knew all about the details of the plea offer, she said.

On February 20, Yared filed a motion, arguing that the prosecutor's office had violated Cathy's attorney-client privilege. She argued the "prosecutorial misconduct" hampered her client's defense. The motion asked that Ken Wood be prohibited from testifying. First, it asked that all charges be dismissed.

Maybe Cathy Wood could do better than a plea to second degree murder. Maybe she wouldn't need to make a deal at all.

Chapter 99

Dave Schieber watched the ember on Robin Fielder's cigarette speed down the length of her Virginia Slim in short, hot bursts. Soon, a long ash hung from the tip.

It was their first meeting. She had agreed to come downtown with her father, Tom Freeman, and Sheriff's Deputy Bob Hiner. Schieber was preparing for Gwen Graham's preliminary exam in February. They were sitting at the big conference table in Bill Forsyth's office.

The assistant prosecutor wasn't expecting a statement. He was hoping to establish some kind of rapport. He could tell from the case details and the speed of that cigarette ember that the girl had been through a lot.

"Robin, I know all this has been traumatic, and I know you have to go at your own pace. I won't push, okay? You just tell me the truth. But you only have to tell as much truth as you think you can."

She talked, but said little of substance. That was better than lying, the attorney figured. He would rather not have her say something for the record that a defense attorney could later use to impeach her on the stand.

Before she left, he asked her for a favor.

"If you remember something important," he said. "Just take a piece of paper and write it down."

Robin saw Gwen only once—on TV, as she was led through Kent County Airport by detectives in late January. Gwen was wearing the outfit she sent her for Christmas. She was thirty pounds thinner. Robin wasn't the only one who was losing weight.

Robin spent the rest of that night in tears.

There were more letters, now postmarked from Grand Rapids. Gwen was sending jubilant predictions she would be freed at her preliminary exam. She sent a prayer card, St. Francis of Assisi's prayer, "Lord, make me an instrument of thy peace." She sent a lock of her reddish hair.

Robin wrote back, but did not visit. When she did not show up at the jail Gwen wrote a four-line letter:

"No visit today. I was surprised. Shrug shoulders and say 'oh well.' I still love you Robin. Guess I'll go."

Later, she wrote:

"Have I lost you? I don't know. Only you know that answer. I'll never let go, Robin . . . I cry a lot more now."

Robin hadn't been able to bring herself to visit. She hadn't been able to bring herself to do *anything*, but sit on the kitchen stool, under those two bright lights.

"You will be called to testify and you will have to tell the truth." She kept hearing those words. They were Dave Schieber's. She no longer feared police cars coming for her. She feared the secrets she was keeping deep inside.

Then, she received the subpoena for Gwen's preliminary exam. She thought, I'll have to go there, in front of everyone, in open court. Everyone will hear my name. Everyone will hear me lie. Or, everyone will hear the truth.

Robin didn't know what the truth was. She knew only words, conversations. She thought, should I tell them conversations? Are they the truth? And, what was more important, telling them conversations, or my word? She had promised Gwen. She promised she wouldn't say a thing.

On a cold afternoon in February she found herself driving to Meijer's. She parked her Mustang in its massive lot. She walked among the hundreds of shoppers in the sprawling discount department store. She walked past the clothes and the toys and the hardware and the food. She saw many faces, but she felt entirely alone.

She walked back from the pharmacy department to the long line of cash registers. The cashier thanked her for the purchase, but Robin didn't smile back. She picked up the bag of Sleepinol. It was just an over-the-counter sleeping medicine, but maybe it still would work quick.

As she drove, she had one hand on the wheel, the other cupped at her side. She thought, you're gonna take them, or you're going to throw them out the window.

She put her hand to her mouth. She took a big gulp of Diet Pepsi, washing down fifteen.

She thought, go home now. Lay down. Lay down and forget about Cathy and Gwen and Alpine and the court.

She was driving down Richmond Street, maybe ten minutes from home. She looked at herself in the mirror. She looked at her tired, red eyes. In her black pupils there was a hint of reflection, a tiny little window of light.

Then she began to shake.

You *asshole,* she thought.

"I don't want to die."

She said it aloud.

"I don't want to die."

She thought, I've done nothing wrong. I have no reason to be ashamed. I've told no jokes, talked of killing no one. I'm innocent. Why should I be the one to die?

Her Mustang was already aimed in the direction of West Catholic, her old high school. She sped down Richmond then up Bristol. There was no time now to call her father or her mother. They were at work. But there was West Catholic, where she was safe, before her whole life came apart.

Her brother was there, at wrestling practice.

She ran inside to find him.

"I don't want to die."

Her father met them both at Butterworth Hospital, in the emergency room.

"I don't want to die."

"I know, honey."

She meant it. She really meant it.

"I don't want to die, Dad. I just want to get some help."

Later, on one of February's coldest days, Robin returned to the Grand Rapids Zoo. She sat at her favorite bench at the duck pond, but she wasn't there to watch the lone mallard. She had paper and a pencil.

This time, Robin Fielder was making a list.

Chapter 100

By mid-March, Cathy Wood still hadn't made a plea agreement and appeared headed to trial. Her attorney's motion to dismiss the case because of Ken Wood's knowledge of the offer had been denied. Now, she was making an effort to beat the murder charges.

Earlier, she told Ken police had double-crossed her.

"Ken, I won't give them anything," she said in another jailhouse phone call. "I'll serve time for the two murders, and let Gwen go. And Ken, you know I'll do it."

Cathy's complaints were formalized during two days of testimony in an evidentiary hearing before Kent Circuit Judge Robert A. Benson. Judge Benson would determine if her statements to the Walker police could be used in her pending trial. Graham's preliminary exam, meanwhile, had been delayed.

Christine Yared was arguing that the police had violated Cathy Wood's rights with promises and threats. Her statements should be disallowed, she said. If Yared prevailed, such a ruling would gut the prosecutor's case.

Prosecutor William Forsyth argued for the state. He put Roger Kaliniak, David Schieber, John Palmatier and Bill Brown on the

stand to recount their dealings with Wood. He introduced a half
dozen cards she had signed during the investigation, cards that
acknowledged she understood her constitutional rights.

Yared tried to show that behavior by police and the prosecutor's
office had lulled Wood into thinking she really wasn't a suspect, that
she mindlessly had signed the Miranda cards as a formality. Yared
culled some embarrassing testimony. There was the trip to Burger
King; Cathy changing her clothes in the basement; the sex jokes that
first Saturday at Walker PD; Tom Freeman pretending to be Cathy's
boyfriend.

The attorney who ultimately would argue the Alpine Manor
murder case for the people found himself on the defensive. Yared
asked Dave Schieber about his discussions with Cathy at Walker PD
about lesbian sex positions.

"Do you recall what those statements were?"

"Yes. It was fairly lurid. I asked her a variety of questions in terms
of some sexual practices, what her role was in the sexual relationship with Gwen."

He explained that he was trying to determine who was the dominant partner in the relationship.

"I recall asking her—I was looking to see who was dominant so
I recall asking her who was dominant in sexual play . . ."

Yared introduced the video of John Palmatier's polygraph. She
contended that he had come on as a friend and confidant. She
argued that he had hinted she might avoid a jail term.

Forsyth brought Freeman back to the stand to explain Wood's
demeanor after the Palmatier polygraph.

"She was the happiest person on earth," Freeman said.

"Did she tell you . . . why she was so happy?"

"Because now someone finally believed her."

Cathy Wood took the stand. It was her first court appearance in
two months. The only hint of her wilder days was the remaining
bleached strands of her hair. The platinum now appeared like frost-
ing on a head full of dark roots. Her long waves were shorn into a
conservative bob. She wore a pink, V-necked, knit sweater and appeared to have lost some weight.

Wood testified that Freeman had promised that "coming to the
window first" about the murders would help her. Yared asked her
how that made her feel.

"I believed it," she said quietly. "Because I was taught police don't lie to you. So I believed it."

She also believed Dave Schieber, she said. She contended he told her that she didn't need an attorney, as long as she was "telling the truth." She also said she wanted to pass the polygraph because Freeman made her feel she would be arrested for providing false information if she didn't.

"I decided if I'm going to be arrested, I'm going to be arrested for something that happened then something that no one believes me about. That's why I was so happy I passed it. I wanted to go to jail for the right thing and not for something not true."

She also said she told people—friends and police—about the murders as a matter of personal conscience and civic duty.

"I told so many people along the line about what had happened, and it was eating me inside. And if no one believed me, what I was telling them, it could have gone on and on in Texas. It could have gone on for a long time. I didn't have any control on it, and I had to stop it somehow."

Ultimately, she testified, Freeman had promised her that charges against her would be dropped, and now police had reneged.

Those were the promises, Yared argued. The threats were she would be jailed for false information.

"She was told these things over and over in different forms and different ways," Yared told the court.

Benson ruled on March 15. First, the judge indicated there was nothing improper about police providing camaraderie to a suspect. "I'm thinking when we have robocops or we get computers to do the interrogating, then we'll get a really natural affectation."

Second, Judge Benson disagreed with the contention that Wood had been threatened or coerced. He based that determination on Cathy Wood's own statements in his court. He also watched the Palmatier video. By her own admission, Benson said, she had given police statements because she wanted to be believed.

Apparently, she had made Judge Benson a believer as well.

"The police were actively trying to conduct an investigation of the case which is hard to investigate because of the helplessness of the victims and the lack of physical evidence . . ." the judge told Christine Yared. "The only key they had to this was your client, who,

I think, had a conscience and was willing to participate the best she could."

Wood had lost the evidentiary hearing, but gained a conscience. It would serve her quite well in the days to come.

Chapter 101

A month later, on April 19, families, attorneys and the curious gathered in the Walker courtroom of District Judge Sherwin J. Venema for the preliminary examination of Gwendolyn Gail Graham. The people had a new star witness. Her name was Catherine May Wood.

In exchange for her testimony, the prosecutor agreed to take her guilty plea to second degree murder and conspiracy. They were the same terms of the original offer, before all the maneuvering.

Wood's participation spurred additional murder charges against Graham. She now stood accused of six counts: Conspiracy to murder and the killing of five patients—Marguerite Chambers, Myrtle Luce, Mae Mason, Belle Burkhard and Edith Cook.

Wood's presence on the side of the prosecution also scuttled an ongoing legal argument by Graham's lawyer, James Piazza. The thirty-eight-year-old attorney was a senior staffer with the Defender's Office, a group of nine lawyers which handled most of Grand Rapids' court-appointed defenses. Piazza was the veteran of 2,500 cases and 140 jury trials not only in western Michigan, but also in the demanding criminal courts of Detroit.

Piazza had begun the legal infighting early. He believed Graham's case stood a good chance of never reaching a jury. His approach was favored by a concept in the law called *corpus delicti*. The term meant the fundamental fact necessary to prove there was the commission of a crime. In a homicide, that meant the prosecution first had to establish there was a death, and that death had been by criminal means.

The hitch was that corpus delicti usually had to be established before any statements by defendants could be considered. In the Alpine Manor murders, wrongful death had been established by medical examiner Stephen Cohle. The pathologist, however, had based his wrongful death determination not on signs of foul play on the bodies, but on conversations with Tom Freeman. Freeman had based his belief on statements by Cathy Wood. These statements were hearsay and should be excluded until the corpus delicti was established, Piazza argued.

"They couldn't establish anything," Piazza later said. "They were trying to bootstrap the case."

Graham's preliminary exam had been delayed by weeks as Piazza launched his assault based on the corpus delicti rule. He had unsuccessfully sought to have Judge Venema disqualified because he had presided over the preliminary exam of Cathy Wood. Piazza's formidable ability to argue the corpus delicti issue was one of the main reasons a deal was offered to Cathy Wood, Dave Schieber later said.

Now, the argument was all but moot.

"With Cathy Wood testifying," Schieber pointed out, "the whole corpus delicti problem simply would go away."

After medical examiner Stephen Cohle testified as to the reasons he had ruled the deaths of the five victims homicides, Cathy Wood was sworn.

Watching from the prosecutor's table was Tom Freeman. Still anxious over her game of hide-and-seek during their sessions, and her about-face during the evidentiary hearing, the detective had no idea what to expect. He had fallen in her disfavor. She no longer talked to him. She had aligned herself with Dave Schieber in the preparation of the case against her former lover.

"When she walked into the courtroom I sat there and thought, Jesus Christ, this is going to be a nightmare," he later told a friend. "I thought, what in the hell is she going to say next about this case."

Wood crossed her hands in front of her. She wore a pink turtleneck. Her platinum strands now covered only the hair below her ears. With her lower body concealed behind the stand, and her voice low, she appeared almost frail.

Gwen Graham, without expression, studied Wood. It was the first time they had been face-to-face in nearly two years. Graham wore a red-and-white short sleeved sport shirt. Cathy avoided her stare.

The idea of murdering anyone, Wood testified, had started with a joke by Graham as far back as October, 1986. The first possible victim: Robin Fielder.

"We started talking about killing people, and she said she wanted to kill Robin. And it was just a conversation. It was just like a joke, something to joke about. It wasn't anything I took seriously."

The joke escalated into a real plan by Gwen to suffocate a patient in Alpine Manor, Cathy said. Throughout most of her testimony she distanced herself from the planning. There was no mention of her choice of Marguerite Chambers. It was Gwen's idea to hold Marguerite's breath longer.

For the first time on the record, she gave her version of the hours after the first murder. They had gone home to her house on Effie. Gwen tied her into the bed with restraints, she said.

"She went to the dresser and she got a pair of tube socks and she put them on her hand. She came over to the bed and she put one knee on either side of me and—she had to hold me different than Marguerite—but she started to suffocate me."

"Well was this all sport, or what was it?" Dave Schieber asked.

The tears began to flow. Throughout her testimony, Cathy frequently would make use of a box of tissue.

"No, I—I couldn't move. I—I couldn't open my—she had to hold my lips. I couldn't open my lips. I—all I could do was cry. And I sort of cried and she untied me real fast and she kept saying she was sorry."

Afterwards Schieber wanted to know why she didn't go to the police.

"I always did what she told me to do . . . I never—never turned her down. I always did what she told me."

One by one, Cathy elaborated on each murder, fixing their locations in the nursing home for each one. The stories were like previous statements—the rolled washcloths meant to scare Cathy into submission, the two of them pinching the noses of potential victims, Gwen's killing to "relieve her tension."

"She was always happy after one of them died," Cathy said.

Up to twenty patients were considered for death, she testified. Schieber wanted to know about any trends among the victims.

"They progressively got better. They went from Marguerite to Belle . . . Belle fought big-time. It just kind of progressively got so they were healthier."

Cathy said she had picked one victim, Edith Cook, as a matter of mercy.

"Edith was so sick. And, I thought that if someone had to die, at least it could be someone . . . that wasn't healthy, that was real sick."

Then, the news media and ultimately Grand Rapids finally learned the nature of the series of methodical killings, as Cathy saw it.

"After—after Myrtle, Gwen and I were at home and I was real—I was real insecure with our relationship. And, I said now you can never leave me. She said she wouldn't but she wanted some assurance that I would never leave her. So, we were supposed to take turns."

She explained her inability to kill Madeline Young.

"What was your motivation for being involved in this at all?" Schieber asked.

"I thought that Gwen was the first person to ever love me and I didn't want her to go away. I didn't want her to go away no matter what. I put myself before those patients. If she—she told me that she had to and I didn't stop her."

"How would (taking turns) prevent you from leaving her?"

"Because then she could have something over my head just like I did for her."

Several hours later Graham was bound over for trial on all charges. That, however, wasn't the lead news of the day. Cathy Wood herself had provided the final ornament on a case already adorned with the sensational. Grand Rapids finally had been given a reason for the serial killings. Local news media improvised a widely-used catch phrase.

The pair killed as part of a "lesbian love bond." From now on, that's how the reports usually went.

Mae Mason's granddaughter Stephanie Engman sat among the spectators, her eyes captivated at first by the rows of scars on Gwen Graham's arms.

She thought, you're sick. You're very, very sick.

Stephanie had insisted to her mother that she be allowed to attend. She had to do *something*, some act to avenge her Nanna's death. She put on her best suit and sat very proper on the bench. The drama student would act the role of the perfect court watcher. Inside, she endured wave after wave of rage.

She had tried to drown everything after she heard the news of the murder by secretly drinking for eighteen days straight. She screamed at reporters who kept calling the house. Now her grades were plummeting. She couldn't concentrate, let alone study. One day she just stood up and walked right out of class.

As she watched Cathy Wood, she only became more infuriated every time the witness dabbed her eyes.

"I thought, how dare you cry," she later told a friend. "If anybody should be crying, it should be me."

As she watched, the eighteen-year-old high school senior was struck by two inconsistencies. The size difference between Graham and Wood was overwhelming.

"It just astounded me that a three-hundred-pound woman could feel so afraid of Gwen Graham," she later recalled.

And, she thought, all this remorse. Yet, all the coldblooded planning. The two didn't fit.

"She was too sorry," she later said. "She was *too* sorry for what she had done."

Later her wrath turned to Graham. Dawn Male took the stand, talking about fistfights she used to have with the defendant. Graham had her hands at her mouth. Then Stephanie noticed. She was giggling.

My God, Stephanie thought, you're facing murder charges and you're giggling. Something in this woman was way off.

Jan Hunderman and Ed Chambers wanted to know exactly what had happened. They had come to the exam hoping to find out how Marguerite Chambers had spent the last moments of her life.

"Marguerite was making noise and she—she was jerking," Wood testified.

Jan closed her eyes, but had to open them quickly. When she turned to study Graham she saw something flash near her ear lobe. She had an earring, a little crucifix hanging from a chain.

"How could anyone who wears a cross believe in killing people, just to relieve her tension?" she later said. "I looked at her earring and just wanted to yank it out."

Chapter 102

> *"I don't care what those people say. I went into it
> knowing what I was going to do, knowing what it
> was going to make me look like, and knowing what
> it was going to do to the nursing home, but I had to
> do what I had to do. As long as Gwen can't hurt
> anybody else, I'm good with anything else that
> happens."*
>
> —Cathy Wood, October 24, 1990.

A twenty-year-old Grand Rapids woman named Raquel Payne sat in
her upper flat on the city's southeast side, telling a visitor about the
time she was jailed with Cathy Wood. In 1989, she spent ninety days
in the Kent County Jail for probation violation on an old unarmed
robbery case.

"We were in the same cell for a month and a half. We were
friends. We used to talk all the time. She used to always tell me, 'I
don't know nothing. I don't know nothing.' Then when it started
getting close that I was leaving I said, 'Cathy I just want to know one
thing, did you guys really do that?'

"She said, 'No, I made it up.'

"I said, 'Damn Cathy, you're gonna spend a lot of time in prison.
You're gonna spend the rest of your life in prison and nobody did
anything. Nobody was killed . . . Why did you do that?' "

"She said, 'Because I loved her. I love her and I want to be with
her.'

"And she figured that was the only way . . . She knew they would
end up in the same prison and said Gwen would have no one to turn
to. And when they got in that other prison, she said she would be the
only one Gwen could turn to—and all her problems would be
solved. She said the only thing she would miss was her truck.

"I believed her. Listen, Cathy ain't the sweet person she makes herself out to be. I thought she was real sweet, until she told this big black woman, 'Look, if you're having a problem getting out of here, I'll push your big black ass right through those bars!' That lady never said nothin' else.

"Cathy's crazy. She's mentally disturbed. She wants what she wants when she wants it. And how she gets it, she doesn't care."

A nineteen-year-old Grand Rapids woman doing six months for soliciting heard a somewhat different version. Margaret Mann was sitting in the day room in cell block number six, listening to Cathy Wood talk about the murder charges she faced.

"Yeah, I did it," she said. "Gwen was the lookout. Gwen watched my back."

For weeks, former polygraph operator John Hulsing eyed the news coverage in disbelief. He couldn't believe the profile of Cathy Wood that was developing.

When one article reported that Wood had passed a second polygraph with another examiner, Hulsing acted. He placed a call to James Piazza at the Defender's Office. He knew the contact would make some of his friends in law enforcement unhappy, and the decision also carried a certain personal risk. Hulsing had a new career as a clinical psychologist in a state prison east of Grand Rapids. If he became involved in Graham's case, and testified, news coverage could expose his police background to inmates. Many of his patients were murderers; some were cop killers. His rapport would be destroyed. He would have to leave the job.

He called anyway, but Piazza was difficult to reach. Hulsing left several messages. Finally, he caught the attorney in the office.

"I don't know why they are going forward with this case," he told the attorney. "Cathy Wood simply isn't telling the truth."

Hulsing explained Wood's failed polygraph and her manipulative behavior with Tom Freeman. The cop turned psychologist did not consider it odd that Wood had become the center of attention in the story. With her narcissistic orientation, he thought, she probably found it exhilarating.

"Jim," he told Piazza. "Cathy Wood isn't this angel that everyone seems to think."

*　*　*

The more administrators at Alpine Manor read about the murders the more they disbelieved. Stories about Cathy Wood's pathological lying and revengeful vendettas filtered up from the stations to people like Jackie Cromwell and Margaret Widmaier. Later, they read her statements to police. These didn't square with basic facts.

For example, Wood told police she had listened in the room intercom and heard Gwen Graham struggling with Belle Burkhard. She even said she heard the rustling of sheets. Any staffer at Alpine Manor knew that the system was of such a quality that it was difficult to detect a distant voice in a patient's room, let alone the soft sounds of bedding.

"The police never took the time to come out here and check basic facts like that out," Jackie Cromwell later complained. "Nobody did their homework, neither the prosecution nor the defense."

There was more. Marty Slocum couldn't remember being occupied by Cathy with gossip the night Mae Mason died. The administration was never concerned about the position of Belle Burkhard's arm, as Cathy told police. There was preliminary exam testimony of a red heart from a patient's mobile being a murder souvenir. Many recognized the item as belonging to another patient who was unconnected with the list.

If Cathy and the police couldn't get the smaller details right, they reasoned, how could anyone be expected to believe the major issues—like murder?

The first list of eight murder victims was suspect as well. A charge tech had reported that she was with Wanda Urbanski for ninety minutes, right up until the moment of her death. Cathy Wood was not on duty for Lucille Stoddard. Two staffers were with the patient when she died.

As for complaints about Cathy and Gwen roaming the halls by former supervisor Tish Prescott, Widmaier and Cromwell considered Tish too strict, a chronic complainer. Marty Slocum never reported such problems.

"This is our Sherlock Holmes," Jackie Cromwell later said, pointing to Slocum. "She's a real detective. She knows what's going on. If anything was going suspicious, I'm sure Marty would have come forth."

As for Cathy's frequent injuries from patients, they reasoned that she was often called up to handle the more difficult residents because of her size. She was bound to get injured, and she reported injuries more than other aides.

In early January, the Michigan Department of Health sent the nursing home the results of its investigation into the deaths. Someone had complained to the state about the murder reports, resulting in the probe. The investigation determined that management simply had no reason to suspect foul play, or even patient abuse.

It wouldn't stop the court case and all the publicity. However, those who ran the nursing home would consider it some vindication. That was something they would take anywhere they could.

With one news report, hairdresser Maureen Haverhill's conversation with her former customer took on a disturbing new meaning. My word, she thought, maybe Lucy Vanderveen was telling the truth. Someone *was* trying to kill her.

The newspapers were full of dates and months, but Maureen was unsure of her own. There was no way for her to know that Lucy Vanderveen was admitted to Alpine long after Gwen Graham had left the facility.

She felt horrible for ever doubting her old customer. She felt like she had done Lucy Vanderveen an injustice. She only wished she could apologize.

She couldn't. Lucy Vanderveen died at Alpine Manor in early 1988.

Chapter 103

Adjournments repeatedly postponed into summer what promised to be one of the most sensational murder trials in Grand Rapids history. The legal infighter James Piazza kept looking for ways to gain an advantage, while Dave Schieber familiarized himself with his star witness.

Piazza, who also had an ongoing Defender's Office caseload exceeding one hundred clients, was calling on every resource he could. He sent extensive medical records of the victims for independent analysis. He cross-checked and referenced the more than three dozen statements taken by police. He sent out his investigator to interview nurses and aides. He drew up an organizational chart of the many sexual liaisons among the staff of Alpine Manor.

Piazza believed Gwen Graham was innocent, and it wasn't simply a public posture. His research in the nursing home and meetings with Graham did not reveal the remorseless monster portrayed by Cathy Wood. Like the rest of Grand Rapids, he also kept seeing the often-repeated TV footage of the high-low excavating Marguerite Chambers' grave. He believed publicity rather than substance pushed the prosecution.

"I think the prosecutors backed themselves into a corner and *had* to go ahead with this case," Piazza later said. "By the time they had exhumed the bodies, they had made their own beds."

Piazza was encouraged. Neither fibers, hair nor prints linked Graham to the bodies. Not one of the widely reported souvenirs had turned up. The prosecution didn't even have bodies for three of the charges. They were ashes. The only eyewitness, Cathy Wood, arguably had a lengthy hidden agenda. Wood, in fact, wasn't even a true eyewitness. She had claimed to see Graham suffocate one patient, but had not remained until the moment of death. Graham's role in the rest was hearsay.

In June, Piazza filed a motion for an independent psychological evaluation of Wood that he could use in Graham's trial. He argued that Wood appeared to be a pathological liar and had a split personality. Kent County Judge Roman Snow denied the motion. Piazza tried to secure files from Wood's former psychologist. Judge Snow examined the records privately in his chambers, then told Piazza there was nothing there he could use to impeach the witness. With all due respect, that was the court's opinion, Piazza pointed out. Again, he was denied.

David Schieber told reporters there wasn't a "shred of evidence" to support Piazza's claims about Wood. "I've talked to her and she's fine," he said.

In fact, Schieber was doing more than talking. What reporters didn't know was that the assistant prosecutor was taking her out to dinner as he prepared his own case. Schieber dispatched Tom Freeman at least four times to Montcalm County Jail to pick up the witness for preparatory interviews before the trial. The idea of eating in public with the codefendant in a spectacular serial murder case made Freeman nervous.

"I thought, Jesus Christ, how can we be doing this?" he later recalled.

They went to a downtown bar called Beason's and a popular restaurant chain called Schelde's that featured food and drinks. She wore no handcuffs. Schieber later acknowledged that he considered the possibility he was being manipulated by Cathy Wood.

"But there's a human element that comes into play here. I came to know Cathy. On a lot of levels I like Cathy. She is intelligent. She does have a sense of humor. She's vulnerable. She's a *very* human being. When she describes this period with Gwen, she describes it almost as another lifetime."

Another time Schieber put it this way: "You ought to get to know her. Actually, she's a real nice person, for a killer, I guess."

Once the Alpine Manor case's greatest detractor, Dave Schieber now was sold on Cathy Wood's story as well. He later said he was astounded by her recall of events nearly three years ago.

"When I interviewed her and we had the employment records there, she was simply amazing. She would say: Mae Mason was killed, this person was on duty, and we did it during break, and we had worked a double shift. And you looked at the records, and that was it. It was impressive—her memory, her faculty."

Meanwhile, back at Montcalm County Jail, Wood often bragged to other inmates about the assistant prosecutor. One was Dawn Male. She was an inmate in the same lockup, serving a sentence for her second drunk driving charge. Cathy boasted to Dawn that Schieber would come to the jail when she called.

"Basically she felt she had him under control," Dawn later recalled. "She would ask him for special little favors. Little things. We weren't allowed to have legal paper. We weren't allowed to have ink pens at all. He would bring her special ink pens, legal paper, little books to read. She asked, he brought."

In his thirty years on the bench, Kent County Judge Roman Snow had developed a reputation as a fair jurist known for staying current with the ever-evolving law. His rulings, however, were generally safe ones. Grand Rapids attorneys knew he rarely broke new legal ground. He didn't like being reversed by the Court of Appeals.

By late August, finally it appeared Gwen Graham would finally face a jury in Judge Snow's court. Her trial date was set for September 11.

Ten days before trial Jim Piazza surprised both the judge and the prosecution with a new motion. Previously, he had asked Dave Schieber to run Gwen Graham with a State Police polygraph examiner. He wanted the same courtesy the authorities had extended to Cathy Wood. The assistant prosecutor declined.

"Our experts tell us she's a psychopath," Schieber said. "And they don't test on polygraphs because they don't have any conscience."

Piazza then had Graham tested by a private polygraph examiner on August 29. She passed a test with five questions about the killings. On September 1 the attorney filed a motion asking for dismissal of the murder charges, based on the test. Though polygraph results couldn't be used before a jury, Piazza cited cases where they had been used in pretrial motions and in certain federal cases.

While Judge Snow ultimately denied the motion, the fallout quickened the wits of the opposing attorneys. When Piazza informed reporters of the polygraph motion, the prosecution lambasted the move in the judge's chambers. Schieber and William Forsyth complained that Piazza's chats with the news media were unethical. He was tainting potential jurors with the polygraph results. Piazza argued that when it came to pretrial publicity, the prosecution already had that area cornered.

"Every time you see this case on the television you see that exhumation, that coffin coming out of the ground," Piazza complained. "Who alerted the media to that? It was not my intention to influence a jury."

Both sides would be hard pressed to find someone in western Michigan who didn't know about the story. The two lesbians were both the fodder of jokes and the objects of disgust. News reports constantly referred to Graham and Wood as "lesbian lovers," a redundancy. Sexual preference was reported in the semantics of witchcraft. One newspaper report would describe the gays in Alpine Manor as a "covey of lesbians." Ken Wood appeared on the Larry King Show. In the Defender's Office jokes were flying. Piazza would brilliantly argue the case, one went, then write a book. The title: "The Dikes of Death."

While gay leaders called the Alpine Manor news coverage "exploitative" and "hateful" to gays in general, they kept a certain distance from Gwen Graham. Piazza was surprised there was no public outcry from gays for a fair trial. Basically, gay leaders considered the pair's behavior too far out, and Graham didn't ask for help.

"Some of the reason we didn't get involved in the situation was connected to the lack of [mental] health," Gwen DeJong, head of the Gay Community Network of Western Michigan, later recalled. "I think the kinds of folks who participate in gay organizations have their shit together a little better. These were not those kinds of folks."

In the courtroom, Graham would face her accusers virtually alone. Neither parent planned to come to the trial. Her father Mack Graham was trucking. Her mother would remain in Texas. Her old friends from Alpine Manor would be sequestered as witnesses. Only Fran Shadden, her old roommate, planned to have a courtroom seat.

Piazza's final pretrial skirmish was a motion to move the proceeding to another county because of the publicity. Judge Snow delayed any decision about a change of venue. A pool of two hundred jurors was available in Kent County.

"Let's wait and see if we can seat a jury here," he said.

* * *

On September 7, Cathy Wood entered her guilty plea before Kent Circuit Judge Robert A. Benson, formalizing her agreement with the prosecution. The judge would sentence her after Graham's trial. As Judge Benson asked her questions to determine if she was pleading voluntarily, Wood was shedding tears.

Wood reached for tissues over the bench. The hands passing them to her belonged to the circuit judge.

Chapter 104

The steps at 333 Monroe ascend to a dignified facade of massive panels of stone composite. However, the interior of the Hall of Justice suffered. Dissatisfied clientele littered and left other mementos, like the defiant "Fuck you" scratched into the stainless steel panel of one courthouse elevator, or its companion etching, "Fuck me too."

As jury selection for Gwen Graham's trial began on Monday, September 11, Grand Rapids still was talking about the day the Hall of Justice was stained with blood. Graham's trial was the second sensational murder story in a year. In late 1988, a Grand Rapids cop walked into the courthouse at high noon and discharged a single slug from his nine millimeter semiautomatic into the base of his wife's neck as she sat in her chambers. She was a popular district judge. A manslaughter verdict inspired petitions, thousands of letters of protest and "justice" rallies on the front lawn before her killer was sentenced in June.

There was no surplus of benevolence in the All-American city in the late summer of 1989. Now came Gwendolyn Gail Graham. She was charged with five killings. The entire city of Grand Rapids had only six homicides that year.

When Tom Freeman helped retrieve the city's most notorious defendant from her holding cell behind the courtroom for her first day in court, the detective found the little Texan plastered against the cell door, her eyes full of terror. The lockup had an imposing commercial commode.

"Get me the fuck away from this toilet," she pleaded. "Please, get me out!"

The plumbing in the Hall of Justice, Gwen feared, was about to suck her down.

Nearly all of the people in the first pool of sixty prospective jurors admitted to reading or hearing about the case. Thirty-seven were dismissed by the judge or challenged by the two attorneys before twelve jurors and two alternates were seated. There were eleven men and three women. The voir dire took a day and a half.

Sitting with David Schieber at the prosecution's table was Tom Freeman. At the right table was Piazza and Graham. She wore a horizontal striped shirt and gray pants. Her hair was pulled back, but cascaded in thick reddish blond waves nearly to the middle of her back. With her turned-up nose and short stature, she might have appeared cute, had it not been for her furrowed brow. Throughout the trial, her face wore a permanent pout.

With opening statements Wednesday, September 13, everyone was offered a preview of two young trial lawyers quite experienced in the practice of their trade. They looked scripted for the contest. The prosecutor was blond and blue-eyed, a local lawyer for the people. Piazza was tall and bespectacled, but his black hair and penetrating dark eyes betrayed his Italian origin. He was a former Detroit defense attorney representing a tough lesbian from the South.

Piazza was both studious and streetwise. He liked trying to make new law, as evidenced by his pretrial motions. He also played a biting blues guitar in local jam sessions in off-hours, avocation that took him into an array of subcultures. He understood the kind of petty power struggles that were often played out on society's lowest rungs.

With Graham's case, Piazza was continuing a recent run of bizarre defenses. Earlier, he represented a client who had killed a drug dealer in an effort to earn a place on a sixty-seven-year-old transvestite's will. He had argued self-defense for another man who had stabbed someone in front of the Carousel Bar after being attacked by a posse of gay bashers. For Graham's trial, he had just come back from a much-needed vacation.

A competitive long-distance runner in his off-hours, Dave Schieber simply hated to lose. His professional sights were set on lofty establishment heights. He said he became a prosecutor because "I'm real good at it, and I like it." He hoped a judgeship was in his future. Schieber didn't know the Kent County Prosecutor's Office success rate in trials, but he certainly tracked his own. Going back to his first year in 1981 he could rattle them off like sports seasons: "Let's see, 5-5, 6-4, 8-2-1, 12-1, 3-1-1, 8-2, 8-2 and 9-1."

Schieber still had his wind from a previous contest. He had successfully prosecuted the O'Brien golf course murder case. The trial was filmed from gavel to gavel by a tabloid TV show. Under new state rules, cameras now were allowed in Michigan courtrooms. Schieber decided the O'Brien coverage gave him an edge.

"I thought I had an enormous advantage," he later explained. "I thought I could block it out. I thought, Piazza is going to be more nervous . . ."

Schieber also had not forgotten the time Jim Piazza beat him on an armed robbery case early in his career. The case had looked open and shut. A woman had been robbed downtown by a man. But under Piazza's careful cross-examination the victim admitted her work habits. She was a hooker, and that was the end of David Schieber's case.

Now experience had imparted to the assistant prosecutor a proven trial strategy. A case had to unfold like a climactic story, he believed, but it also had an ebb and flow. The story had to be told with the strongest characters of the moment. Also, he counted on two surprises in every trial: One good, one bad. Take the former as a gift, and expect the latter. However, don't let it rewrite your tale.

In his opening, Schieber told the jury to expect a narrative like none they had ever heard before.

"This is a bizarre case, and it was committed by bizarre people," he said. "And you can't hope to understand this case unless you understand those people."

Specifically, they had to understand Cathy Wood. Schieber planned to lay out a tragic account of the overweight, submissive Wood, willing to do anything for love, including cover for her homicidal lover. Not only were patients killed, the two of them had also conspired to murder fellow workers.

Piazza told the jury they should look for a different story. Cathy Wood was a liar, a manipulator, a ruthless accuser bent on revenge. Either no murders occurred, he argued, or they were committed alone by Cathy Wood. Gwen Graham was now a victim of what she thought was one of Cathy's jokes. He downplayed the homosexuality.

"We're asking you not to judge these people's morals or lifestyles, but just listen to the testimony, listen to the content of it. Because you're going to hear about love. You are going to hear about jealousy. You are going to hear about hatred. You will hear, through the testimony, about revenge. All [can be found] in heterosexual relationships. The same emotions are going to play here before you in the next week . . ."

With his very first witness, Dave Schieber gambled. He didn't like the hostility he had sensed when he talked to Alpine administrator Jackie Cromwell earlier in the day. He had planned to use Cromwell to introduce documentation from work records that Gwen Graham and Cathy Wood were working on the appropriate shifts at the time of the deaths.

When she was called, he decided not to risk putting her on the stand that long, though he was leaving a giant hole in the proofs. He elicited from Cromwell a verbal picture of the nursing home, its shifts, its employees, their duties. He had her describe "total care" patients, which all the victims were.

"Total care patient is one that has to have all their needs met by the nursing personnel . . ."

She was so tense she needed a glass of water.

Schieber brought up the subject of sexual preference in the halls of Abbey Lane, Buckingham, Camelot and Dover.

"Were you personally aware that a pretty high percentage of your nurse's aides were gay at the time?"

"No, I was not."

The next witness's appearance was also brief. Gary Hunderman was called, the son-in-law of Marguerite Chambers. He testified to receiving the hurried phone call from Alpine Manor about her death.

"Do you recall specifically who you talked to . . . would it be a nurse, nurse's aide, doctor, administration?" Piazza asked on cross.

"No, she did not say her name."

Throughout the morning, Jim Piazza seemed alternately preoccupied and distracted. Before everyone broke from lunch he put his complaint on the record.

"Your honor . . . during the opening statements, I personally found it very distracting of the one particular still camera in here . . . the click has been distracting . . . I ask that something be done about the still camera, or the still camera be removed from this courtroom."

The judge wanted to know if the photographer from the *Grand Rapids Press* could use a quieter camera. Before she could answer, another attorney jumped to his feet, one representing the newspaper. It was his understanding, he said, that the prosecutor had asked some witnesses not be photographed. Schieber joined the fray.

"I have a large number of witnesses who are homosexual, who are living their lives out as normally as they can, as obscurely as they can. And I have other witnesses, because this involves death and murder and emotions, who wish to testify without the intrusion of cameras, and I think in both instances, it is a reasonable request . . ."

The mood in the courtroom was combative. Spectators were murmuring. The trial was off to a tense start.

Judge Snow settled the dispute by giving each party something. The noisy camera would stay, but the photographer had to go to the back row. If there was good reason, certain witnesses would be spared the camera's lens.

Now, the ground rules for the rest of the trial were set. After lunch the prosecution planned to produce its star witness.

"We are in recess," Judge Snow said.

Chapter 105

Heads sleepy from two-hour lunches quickly cleared when the prosecution summoned the first witness of the afternoon. "Your honor, I would call Catherine May Wood . . ."

Wood was the image of contrite restraint. She had perfect, brown bangs. Her helmet cut was shaped neatly around a turtleneck of pure white, complemented by a smart, patterned shirt of largely white as well. Only a few strands of bleached hair remained, just visible at the back of her head. Cathy Wood looked like a nun in an order that had just ditched its habit.

First, Schieber asked her to detail her plea agreement for the jury.

"And what do you now face potentially as a sentence?"

Her voice was hardly audible.

"Life."

"Is there another part of the plea agreement?"

"That Gwen and I are kept separate at all times."

"And at whose request was that included in the plea agreement."

"Mine."

Then the whole sad story began. Schieber began with David/ Debbie, Wood's cross-dressing girlfriend. She was a pubescent victim of her own naïveté, the questioning went.

"How would you describe yourself, that is, a mature fourteen, or what?"

"No I didn't leave—I didn't leave the house much. I stayed in my room and read a lot."

Piazza stood up. The last thing he wanted the jury to hear was a sympathetic story.

"Well, Your Honor, I hate to interrupt at this time, but, personally, I don't see the relevancy of a relationship this lady had when she

386   *Lowell Cauffiel*

was fourteen years old, as it pertains to the issues that are here before this court regarding my client."

Judge Snow looked at Schieber.

"How does this become material in the matter before the court?"

". . . In order for us all to understand this case, we have to understand Catherine Wood, and that there were certain key things about her life that, no matter how painful, are going to have to be made known. And I think both these events of her past, and certain parts of her relationship with Miss Graham, are relevant to help explain the dynamics of this relationship, and how and why things took place."

Snow overruled.

"I will permit the questioning," he said.

Despite Piazza's frequent objections, Schieber drew the whole story out, including David/Debbie's seduction of Wood with a strap-on dildo. People in the courtroom were transfixed. Sexual devices. Lesbianism. Deception.

All this figured into her dating Ken, Cathy said.

"This first time we had a date, he took me to his apartment and—I started to take off his pants, just—just so I could see if he was a boy or a girl. And then when I saw that, I just quit, and he was surprised, but that's—I had to do *that.*"

She drew out the word.

Cathy told the jury about their marriage, her pregnancy, her weight gain of two hundred pounds. She testified about isolating herself in her apartment, being afraid to do laundry in public, being told to go to the grocery store to weigh herself on the bulk scale. She told about being hired at Alpine and her separations from Ken. Dawn Male moved in with her. Dawn Male cheated on her, deceived her, like everyone else.

She met Gwen Graham, who moved in and became her lover.

"Is that person here in court now?"

"Yes."

"Could you point to her for us please."

Wood gingerly lifted her index finger. The defendant glared back.

Wood described her discovery of the Carousel and new friends: Ladonna Sterns. Angie Brozak. Robin Fielder. Paul Lopez.

"At some point did Gwen ever express an unusual desire to you?"

"Yes."

"What was that?"

"She wanted to kill somebody."

She claimed the conversation took place in October of 1986.

"What was your reaction to that?"

"I thought she was teasing, and she says, 'Well, let's kill Robin.' And I said, 'Oh, no, she's too nice.' "

There were other potential victims, she said, including Catherine Brinkman. Wood said she thought Gwen was joking.

By the New Year, Gwen wanted to kill a patient, she said.

"We were at home in the bedroom and she said she wanted to kill somebody at the Manor, and I just—that was about it, I didn't pay much attention."

She was speaking very softly. The jurors were leaning forward in their seats.

Later, she said, they had another murder conversation in bed, she said. They might even have been playing backgammon at the time, she added.

"I asked her how, and she said she wanted to do it—was going to suffocate them, and I said something about, with a pillow, and she said no, she—that they would turn their heads, so that she would use washcloths to hold their nose and then their mouth. And I had asked her why, and she says to keep—because she would have to apply so much pressure that they would have indentations or bruises from pushing."

"Did you ask her at the time who?"

"I don't think so."

". . . did you ask her why?"

Schieber had to be careful. He was digging himself into a hole with a question that had yet to be fully answered in the hundreds of pages of statements and testimony already taken in the Alpine Manor murder case: *What precipitated the first killing?*

"No, I don't think at that time I'd asked her why, either, because I—no, I don't think so."

"Can you give us any reason why you wouldn't ask that question?"

"No."

Schieber changed the subject.

"How would you describe your relationship with Gwen at that point?"

"I loved her. I thought she loved me."

"As between you two, in your judgement, who was more dominant?"

"She was."

It was an important point in the prosecution's case. Wood *had* to be submissive. She, after all, had been given a break by the prosecution. There also had to be some reason why she didn't immediately go to the police.

For the next hour Wood gave her final version of the killings themselves. They were terse, confident descriptions. She located her and Gwen on shifts and stations in the nursing home. Gone were the "I don't know's" of the past.

Marguerite Chambers was tried twice, she said. Gwen came up with the idea to hold her longer after she stopped breathing. There was no hint that Wood had picked her out, as she had previously told John Palmatier.

"She had come over and she had told that she was going to do Marguerite, and that she needed more time, so I was going to stand outside the door."

Cathy Wood began crying, quietly, as she sat there, clad in white.

"She was on the far side of the bed and she had a washcloth on Marguerite's nose and one under her mouth and she was suffocating her, and Marguerite was making noises—and I don't know."

"Did you see Marguerite make any movement?"

"Yes, she was—she was jerking."

Gwen helped clean up the victim for the funeral home, she told the jury. She and Gwen helped lift her body to a stretcher. Cathy told the kind of anecdote someone might attribute to a merciless psychopath.

"I held her head when we pulled her over, and it kind of dropped, and I thought she was going to open her eyes, and I looked at Gwen and she was laughing, smiling at me."

After they went home, Cathy began drinking Jack Daniel's, she testified. She was afraid to take a shower, to go in the basement, she said.

"I thought Marguerite would be down there and that she would get me."

She told the jury the story of Gwen putting her in restraints, trying to smother her with her hands clad in socks. She said Gwen had straddled her with her knees. She demonstrated to the jury how Gwen held her nose and lips.

"That night, when she tried to suffocate me, then . . . I knew what Marguerite had felt . . . I had to stop it or say something. I knew I had to do something."

Before moving on to more murders, Schieber would try to establish that Wood's fear and submission to Graham was based on her brute force. Gwen restrained her on three occasions, Cathy said. The second time she bit her. The third, much later, Gwen pulled out a gun. Now, Wood reported for the first time publicly the act that Graham had told to at least two others about the hours after it happened. However, the roles in Cathy's version were reversed. Cathy was the victim.

"What happened that time?"

"That's when she pointed her gun at me."

"Where did she point the gun at you?"

"At—at—at the vagina."

"Were you naked?"

"Yes."

Spectators looked at one another. Some commented on a break that they were more sickened by what was going on in the bedroom in the little house on Effie than the murderous activity in Alpine Manor.

Cathy testified about Graham's burn marks, how she told her she used to "play chicken" with lit cigarettes. She described fights with Dawn Male and her living room wrestling match with her husband Ken.

After Marguerite Chambers was killed, Cathy said, Gwen made a promise. ". . . I wanted to tell, and she told me she—it wouldn't happen anymore, and I believed her."

But when the patient Maurice Spanogle died after struggling with Graham in the bathroom, Gwen took it as a sign "she was supposed to continue," Cathy testified.

Next was Myrtle Luce. Cathy offered a macabre anecdote, steeped in infidelity and sex.

"We were sitting at . . . Abbey Lane, and it was break time and we were left alone in the station, and we were talking about how many people we had slept with, and we would just—we were making slashes, and I had finished."

"You're making slashes, what do you mean?"

"Like when you make four and cross it off, that would be five. We were doing that."

"How many did you write down?"

"Three. And she was doing hers, and then she stood up and said, 'I'm going to do Myrtle.' "

"What did you do?"

Briefly, Cathy fell into her old "I don't know" habit.

"I don't know if I started rounds, or I don't know if I stayed at the desk, I can't recall that . . ."

But the next thing she knew, she said, she heard that Myrtle Luce was dead. When she went into Luce's room she saw what she called Gwen's calling card: A rolled washcloth.

"She would put them over the shower, she would leave them on my cart at work. She left them everywhere, because she knew it scared me."

"Did you have any conversation with Miss Graham after Myrtle was killed?"

"Mm-hmm. Yes, that's when I asked her why?"

"What was Miss Graham's response?"

"Because, that it relieved tension. She was always real happy afterwards."

"How did you feel?"

"Awful."

Cathy sniffled, pushing her right hand into her hairline and staring down at the stand.

She didn't stop the killings, however.

"I wanted her to be happy."

Each murder had its own particular character, its own unique set of facts. Next was Mae Mason.

"Gwen was on Abbey and I was on Camelot, and Gwen came and told me that she was going to do Mae, and I said, "No, you can't, you're over there with two other aides and a nurse and I'm nowhere around . . . and what if they walk in on you?"

She explained how she detained supervisor Marty Slocum with gossip. Afterwards Gwen, she said, handed her the little house—a souvenir. She detailed the others: The balloon with MOTHER written on it from Marguerite Chambers and a sock from Myrtle Luce. (Later, she said there was an earring and a handkerchief, but she didn't know which one belonged to Belle Burkhard and which to Edith Cook.)

She detailed Belle Burkhard's violent struggle, as she heard it on the intercom. Then she saw Gwen walk out of the room with a washcloth flapping out of her back pocket, she said. Gwen told her she had mangled Belle's arm as she struggled, Cathy testified.

Cathy talked about Edith Cook. Cathy said she had picked that victim. She felt sorry for her as she suffered from gangrene, she said. She admitted throwing away her teeth.

Schieber wondered how she was feeling about all the later deaths as they occurred.

"In a way, I tried to pretend it didn't happen. I tried to pretend it wasn't happening, but there was so much going on . . . there was just so much, Ken, work, the neighbors, and then this, and I just tried to pretend it just all wasn't happening."

The prosecutor and his witness covered the testing of potential victims, the unsuccessful plan to spell M-U-R-D-E-R (Schieber: "Whose idea was that?" Cathy: "I don't know"); their pledge to take turns, her inability to kill Madeline Young. He introduced Proposed Exhibit Number One, the letter to Graham with I-G-T-K-M, "I'm going to kill Madeline."

". . . We were supposed to take turns so we could never leave each, so that we could say something about each other."

Cathy was crying again. Her nose was red.

"Oh, I was so insecure, every—everybody was having affairs with everybody. Alpine Manor was like—everybody was sleeping with everybody, and I thought, I thought that this was going to happen. And I didn't want her to ever go away, and so that's why I said that."

At one point, Schieber asked her about love.

"Did you consider your love for Gwen to be genuine and true?"

"Yes."

"Legitimate and strong?"

"Yes."

He asked her if she could compare her relationship with Dawn and Ken to that with Gwen Graham.

"No, I never loved anybody the way I loved her, no."

At another juncture in the questioning Schieber wanted to know why the killings stopped after Edith Cook.

". . . Soon after Edith, Gwen, she quit Alpine and she went to other nursing homes."

Actually, "soon" was nearly three months. But rather than dates, they discussed more homicidal plans.

"Did you and Gwen make plans to kill anybody else?" Schieber soon asked.

"In the home?"

"Anywhere."

"Dawn and Angie."

Cathy explained the plot. Gwen had had an affair with Angie, she said. Gwen could get Angie to say "real outrageous things" on the telephone, while Cathy listened on the extension.

Piazza objected. Relevancy.

"[Graham's] ability to control other individuals is important in this case," Schieber argued.

Overruled.

Schieber asked again, "Did you and Gwen make plans to kill Angie?"

"Gwen and I? I listened to what she told me . . . I knew what I was supposed to do."

Cathy explained she was supposed to hide at the fish ladder, while Gwen lured Angie Brozak to the riverside park. Gwen picked out knives from the kitchen drawer. Everyone would think Angie's husband or Ladonna Sterns had killed her because of their love triangle, Cathy explained.

"I was supposed to help . . . and I was supposed to stab her."

As for Dawn Male, Cathy later testified that Gwen considered her disposable. That's why she was told about the killings and shown the souvenirs.

"Because she was going to die, so it didn't matter if she knew."

Schieber eventually got back to the subject of the patients.

"Did you ever reduce to writing what you and Gwen had involved yourself in?"

"Yes."

The attorney reached for a single piece of paper. He and Piazza had argued about its admission earlier outside the presence of the jury. Like the I-G-T-K-M letter, it was obtained in the search of Graham's trailer in Texas. Now it would serve as a climax in the testimony of the woman everybody figured was the people's star witness.

Proposed Exhibit Number Two was a poem on "nurse's notes" stationery:

I love you Gwen
I think you're great
For this afternoon
I can not wait

That's when we'll wake up and
That's when I'll kiss you.
That's when I'll hold you
Oh Gwen I miss you.

Bunny hop
Over here
And let me lick you
On the ear.

I want to get married.
Right now right away.
Don't make me wait
Till the day.

When you're mine
Oh please say
You'll be mine
Forever and five days.

". . . Do you recognize this writing here?" he asked Wood.

"It's mine."

"This is a poem written to whom?"

"To Gwen."

"Is there a stanza or a line there which has any significance to what we're talking about here?"

"Forever and five days."

"Explain to us how that stanza means anything."

"When we first got together we were supposed to be together forever. And then after a patient was killed—but it wasn't the first one—but after a few patients were killed, it was supposed to be forever, and however many days went with however many patients were killed. So this was after the fifth one, but I don't know if that includes Maurice or not."

Earlier, the courtroom had heard a tighter explanation. Judge Roman Snow had asked to see the poem outside the presence of a jury. The revelation had all the compelling impact of a twisted romance title.

Wood had just handed the poem up to the bench.

"What does this 'forever and five days' mean?" the judge asked.

"That meant five patients had died . . . every time a patient would die, it would be forever and a day, forever and two days, forever and three days, so I know that was (written) after the fifth one . . ."

At 4:12 P.M. Cathy Wood stepped down from the stand. She had testified for nearly three and a half hours. The jury would sleep on her testimony. Many were exhausted already.

With Wood's testimony laced with uncomfortable sexual detail and punctuated by crying jags, more than one juror was glad the day was done.

Chapter 106

As he began his cross-examination Thursday morning, Jim Piazza tried to demonstrate that Cathy Wood's teary conscience was situational at best.

"Miss Wood, when you first . . . saw or knew about the death of Marguerite Chambers, you immediately, of course, went to one of the nurses or supervisors . . . to explain what happened, is that correct?"

"No."

"You did not? You told the police, obviously?"

"No."

Victim by victim, he asked the same question.

"You didn't say anything about any foul play at the time?"

"No."

They covered the friends she told.

"Yet the police came to you some fourteen months afterwards, or so, and when they confronted you with this, you told the police that none of this was true, on your first statement is that correct?"

"Well, I made a statement that it was a joke . . ."

The defense attorney was relentless. He had been anticipating cross-examining her for months. He asked Wood to read her taped statements, then pointed out contradictions. He probed her pact with the prosecution. She admitted she formerly thought charges against her would be dropped. He pointed out she could be out of prison in just ten years. She admitted that during the investigation she worried about being locked up in a mental hospital.

When Piazza brought up the fact that Wood had seen psychologists, Dave Schieber looked for help from Judge Roman Snow, who had ruled previously that Wood's psychological history was off-limits. Piazza argued that the prosecution had already introduced the issue into the trial, allowing him to pursue it in his cross-examination.

"The fact that she had sex with a female at the age of fourteen, I didn't see the relevancy, but the prosecutor wanted the jury to understand her," Piazza explained. "I believe the jury should understand the fact that she's seen a psychologist while she was in jail, and prior . . ."

Piazza maintained the prosecutor "opened up the door" to the subject.

Judge Snow, however, slammed it shut.

Piazza went back to basics. Questioning Wood, he demonstrated she had seen not one victim die, that the victims' initials hardly resembled M-U-R-D-E-R. He covered Wood's threats to Robin Fielder to imprison Graham. Then he went to the issue of dominance. He asked Wood her weight and height.

"Stand up, Gwen."

Graham stood up behind the defense table, her head slightly down, her arms hanging at her sides.

"She is about five-foot-three, is that correct?"

"I don't know."

". . . And you were afraid of this person?"

"Yes."

Piazza brought up the gun.

"Isn't it true, Miss Wood, that it was you who tied up Gwen Graham. It was you who took a gun, put it up her vagina, and threatened to kill her if she left you?"

She denied it.

Piazza brought up the plot to kill Angie Brozak. He asked if she had ever told her ex-husband: "I wonder what it would be like to stab somebody, to push a knife through them."

She denied it.

The attorney attacked I-G-T-K-M.

"Couldn't that be: I'm Going to Kill Myself?"

No.

If there were souvenirs, did she have any to show the jury?

No.

Piazza put the washcloths in context. Yes, Wood admitted, rolled washcloths were often used for routine care in Alpine Manor.

Piazza tried to get the jury thinking about another motive.

"Miss Wood, isn't it true that you were going around telling people that Gwen Graham was involved in . . . killing people . . . not because Gwen Graham did it, but because you didn't want people to take Gwen Graham away from you, isn't that true?"

"No," she said.

"No further questions of this witness," Piazza said.

On redirect, Dave Schieber questioned her again about who she told about the murders. One of her answers caught the assistant prosecutor by surprise.

Yes, she admitted, she was afraid at first of going to jail, but when she began talking to police she wanted the truth known.

"Why?"

She spoke very matter-of-factly.

"When she was killing the people and I didn't stop it, I felt bad enough, but then when she was in Texas and she would call me on the phone and say she wanted to smash a baby up against—"

Piazza cut the witness off with his objection. Her testimony was inflammatory.

The jury was sent out of the courtroom. Judge Snow wanted to hear what she had to say. She told him Gwen, while working in a Texas hospital, told her she "liked going past the nursery, because she wanted to take one and smash it against the window."

"She wanted to what?" the judge asked.

"Smash it up against the window."

"Smash *what* up against the window."

She sounded almost flippant.

"One of the babies. I had—I had to do something, I didn't care about myself anymore."

Her explanation dominated television newscasts that evening. The jury, however, never heard it. The judge considered it too prejudicial. Among those who knew the chronology of the case, however, Wood's reasoning still didn't make sense. Graham would have made the baby statement a year before Wood was involved with the police.

After the jury was seated again, Wood explained the reason she first told police the murder story was a "joke."

". . . If anybody heard us talking about it, that's what we were supposed to say."

Before she stepped off the stand twenty minutes before noon, Schieber tried to resolve an underlying contradiction in Wood's story.

"You've expressed that you wanted Gwen back once you had lost her?"

"Yes."

"And that you also feared her?"

"Yes."

"Explain what you mean, that you would both want her and fear her."

Wood's voice was analytical.

"Well, violent relationships were normal for me. I almost thought that's the way they were supposed to be, because that's all I had. So I wanted her back."

When she stepped down, everyone broke for lunch.

Gwen Graham later told several people what happened during the noon break after Cathy Wood's testimony:

"They took us back to the county jail for lunch. She was downstairs and I was upstairs. I didn't know she was in the building. When I came back down to go to the trial, you go out past two holding cells. And there, out of the corner of my eye, Cathy was sitting there. Our eyes met, and then she turned, looking down, and started giggling . . . She started laughing. Yep. If I didn't think that door was locked, I would have been in there. That would have looked real good at my trial. But I wouldn't have cared by then."

* * *

As everyone's lunches settled, medical examiner Dr. Stephen Cohle took the stand. He adjusted his glasses and led the courtroom in detail through the autopsies of Marguerite Chambers and Edith Cook. He described the condition of Chambers' body, working from his notes.

"Well, first of all, the eyes were shrunken. This was due to having been buried and dead for a number of months. I could not determine eye color . . . there was some mold, particularly on the face, the back of the neck, and the arms and legs."

He explained what he looked for in suffocation victims. There might be injuries around the inside of the mouth, a fracture of the nose.

". . . There may be small hemorrhages, around the eyes most prominently, they may be elsewhere on the face. And these hemorrhages result when blood vessels break because of the efforts of the victim to breathe."

There may not be anything.

"All these findings I am talking about are in the best-case scenario, in the situation in which the individual is able to struggle . . . Absolutely nothing may be found in someone, particularly someone in either extreme of life, extreme old age, with the person who's helpless, or in infancy. There may be absolutely no findings in autopsy, and the entire diagnosis of suffocation would be made by both a positive history of suffocation and a lack of other findings to explain death."

And, simply, that was the case for both Marguerite Chambers and Edith Cook. He could not establish the cause of death based on his examination alone. There was no pathological evidence of suffocation. Cook, he noted did have one tooth, but there were no signs of a struggle. There were no abrasions in her mouth. Neither patient had hemorrhages around the eyes.

However, Dr. Cohle pointed out, there also was no overwhelming pathological evidence that natural conditions had caused their deaths. Marguerite Chambers did not have a heart attack, as was indicated on her death certificate. Chambers certainly had Alzheimer's Disease, but "she could have lived perhaps several months, or possibly years longer," he said. Edith Cook had narrowing in her coronary arteries, but the condition was not life-threatening.

"It's not that she couldn't have died of it, but it isn't very likely," the pathologist said.

On cross-examination, Piazza pointed out that the bodies of three victims were not available for autopsy. Only two of the five death certificates introduced by the prosecution had been amended by Dr. Cohle to "homicide." Cohle acknowledged that he could not amend the other death certificates because he had not examined the bodies. His conversations with Tom Freeman, he testified, had provided the impetus for changing those of Chambers and Cook.

"Okay," Piazza said. "So, Doctor, the bottom line is, in your autopsy of only those two individuals . . . you found no physical evidence to substantiate the cause of death being asphyxiation by suffocation, is that correct?"

"That's correct."

And, Dr. Cohle acknowledged, without the conversations with Freeman about the case, his determination of cause of death would be natural causes. There also was the possibility his determination was tainted, the pathologist admitted.

Piazza asked, ". . . If the information you received from Detective Freeman was incorrect, then your opinion might be incorrect? Might be?"

"That's correct," Dr. Cohle said.

If the jury was looking for reasonable doubt, Jim Piazza decided that with his cross-examination of both Cathy Wood and Dr. Cohle he had already served up a multiple choice.

On Thursday afternoon and again on Monday, the prosecution produced eleven more witnesses. Many did little to offset the lack of physical evidence.

Aide Pat Ritter told the jury how she discovered that Belle Burkhard had expired. This was the victim with the supposedly twisted arm. On both direct and cross Ritter said she couldn't remember anything unusual about her arm.

"You didn't notice anything out of ordinary with this?" Piazza asked on cross, making the point again for the jury.

"No I didn't."

Ritter did notice that Cathy Wood appeared nervous as she cleaned up Burkhard's body.

Another aide described finding Myrtle Luce. There was "nothing unusual" about the body, she said under cross. A mortician told the jury Edith Cook arrived for embalming with no teeth, but said under cross-examination he saw no signs of foul play.

Angie Brozak testified, followed by Ladonna Sterns. Brozak was terrified. She had talked with Schieber beforehand.

"Why am I being subpoenaed?" she asked him. "I know nothing about these murders. And I can't say one good word about Cathy Wood."

Schieber told her she was his basis for his conspiracy to murder charge. He needed to establish certain facts. On the stand, the assistant attorney had her testify that she had left her husband, lived with Sterns and knew Graham.

"Here's a fun question," Schieber asked. "Did you ever sleep with either one of them?"

She looked out at the TV cameras and the packed courtroom, stammering with her answers. Earlier, Judge Snow had granted her request that she not be photographed. She had children in school. Still, she felt the only purpose to the assistant prosecutor's questions was to put her sexuality on display.

When Piazza was offered a chance to cross-examine her, Brozak was eager. She wanted to tell the jury all about Cathy Wood, her mind games, her vindictiveness. She wanted to tell the jury she was a pathological liar. She was shocked when Graham's attorney didn't stand up.

"No questions, thank you," he said.

Ladonna Sterns also had been ready to cooperate with Graham's defense as well. Both Brozak and Sterns felt the Walker police had discounted their input about Cathy Wood's personality. Sterns had called Piazza's office several times, leaving messages. She never got a call back.

Sterns, however, was no help to Graham as a prosecution witness. She testified about a car ride with Graham before she moved to Texas.

"And I had asked her, why would Cathy call the cops on her. And then she said, 'Well, Cathy couldn't really call the cops because, if she did, they would both go down the drain.' "

During cross-examination, she admitted both of them were drinking during the car ride. Then, the defense attorney sat down.

"Thank you, nothing further."

One prosecution witness, Tony Kubiak, sought Piazza out in the courthouse before the day of testimony began.

"Look, I think they got it all wrong here," he told Piazza.

Later, he complained that the transcript of his statement to the police did not accurately reflect what he said. Certain words had not been transcribed, making him look like he supported the prosecution's case.

The Cathy Wood he knew was a psychopath, Kubiak said.

Schieber wanted to wave Kubiak as a witness, but Piazza declined. Under a court rule, Schieber called Kubiak, but had no questions. Piazza had questions, though he would have preferred to dress up the surprise witness first. Kubiak took the stand wearing a jean jacket, his sunglasses propped on top of his head.

"Would it be a fair statement to say that Cathy Wood was the dominant person in that relationship between Cathy Wood and Gwen Graham?"

"Yes."

Kubiak testified about Wood's manhandling of Graham in the little house on Effie.

"What I remember seeing is Cathy grabbing Gwen by the hair and pulling her back into the bedroom . . ."

He described mind games.

"Well, they got involved in other people's lives, and basically would tell one person one thing, tell another person the other thing, and just basically try to destroy the bond between them people."

"You say 'they.' Who would be an instigator of these mind games?"

"Well, it usually pointed back to Cathy."

When Piazza finished, Schieber avoided a redirect. He wanted to get Kubiak off the stand. Schieber told himself, there's the bad surprise. "He just laid Cathy out," the attorney later said.

The assistant prosecutor remained on course. He produced people who heard about the murders directly. Ken Wood told his story. Lisa Lynch testified about Graham's admissions about suffocating Edith Cook. Dawn Male told about the souvenirs, but could hardly place the conversation in a meaningful time frame. Schieber brought forth a witness from out of town.

"Your honor, I would call Deborah Kidder, please."

Kidder described herself as an ensign in the United States Navy, stationed at the Naval Hospital in Orlando, Florida. She told the jury about Graham's story about murdering patients after their barbecue in Tyler.

"Did she say how many patients?"

"It was about a half dozen. She named names, but I can't recall the names, it's been a long time ago."

"Did she say who did the suffocating?"

"She did."

"Gwen did?"

Kidder nodded.

On cross, Piazza tried to soften the impact.

"You thought . . . she was pulling your leg?"

"Yes, sir."

A few minutes later, Schieber asked, "When Miss Graham told you this, was it in a joking fashion?"

"Not really, no."

"Was anybody laughing?"

"No."

"Nothing further, Your Honor."

As the prosecution came to its final witnesses, Jim Piazza still felt his client's defense was in fine shape. All those who had heard murder conversations still fit his defense theory that the whole matter was a joke. Whether they took it seriously or not didn't really matter. In cross-examination, he had clearly established for the jury that both Wood and Graham liked to mess with people's minds.

Dave Schieber's confidence, however, also was growing. After Piazza had made an issue about the fact that Cathy Wood couldn't produce souvenirs, he was approached on a Thursday break by Gary Hunderman.

"Look," he said. "My daughter remembers that balloon. The kids gave it to my mother-in-law as a present."

"Get your daughter here," Schieber said.

However, by Monday, the assistant prosecutor changed his mind.

"Don't worry about getting your daughter out of school," he said. "I think we have enough."

By late Monday, Schieber was extremely pleased. He had endured his bad surprise, and counted his good one as well. He hadn't expected Deborah Kidder to be such a powerful witness.

Schieber also was encouraged that the defense had become so fixated on Cathy Wood. Now, he had one more witness. He was about to offer up a surprise of his own.

He didn't think Jim Piazza would describe it as very good.

Chapter 107

Robin Fielder woke up the morning of September 18 knowing that the day had finally come. The fact that it was her twenty-third birthday was secondary. Today she was scheduled to testify. Some birthday present, she thought. If she made it through the day, that alone would be a very special gift.

She had come a long way since her suicide attempt eight months earlier. There were several sessions with a psychotherapist. She shared some facts about Alpine Manor, Gwen, and Cathy, but nothing incriminating. She didn't want her new confidant drawn into the case. Instead, they talked about family and loyalty and friendship and the kind of guilt that carried internal punishments.

The therapist helped her with what she felt was like a tightly wound spring, twisting inside her since she went to Texas, maybe longer.

"No, I'm not hypnotizing you," the therapist said. "It's called relaxation therapy."

Robin lay back, listening to her soft voice. She asked her to take several deep breaths. The therapist had her conjure up images of Gwen and Cathy. She could see them in her mind's eye. She took another deep breath.

"Now, Robin," the therapist said. "Throw it all away."

They walked down an imaginary staircase, letting all her troubles go. When they walked back up she was to feel positive, stronger. At the top of the stairs was courage. When it was over with she felt wonderful, for the first time in many months.

Robin made her own decisions. She chose to make two more statements to police. She went back to work, as a secretary in her father's office. Her weight stabilized at the level she had always wanted it, before Alpine Manor, before all the madness began. She chose to stop writing to Gwen.

"Do what you want to do," she remembered one of Gwen's last letters saying. "If you want to tell the truth, it won't hurt me. Go ahead."

On her birthday she wanted to put on blue jeans and a T-shirt. Instead, she chose her most colorful skirt. Its sheer fabric was printed with peacocks, sporting colors of magenta, purple, green and royal blue. She complimented it with a magenta top, the one with a big black button, sewn right over the top of her heart.

Everyone who loved her was trying to help. Her father gave her a pep talk. Her mother stayed home from work to see her off. Robin had renewed her friendship with Lisa Lynch. Lisa would pick her up for court. She would be met there by family friend Bob Hiner. Her parents said they would be in the courtroom for support.

"You can do it, Robin," Lisa kept saying as she primped in her bathroom. "You can do it."

Before leaving, she had a real good cry. She still didn't know if Gwen was guilty or innocent. She still didn't know what the truth was. She fixed her makeup and pulled herself together. I may not know the truth, she thought, but I certainly know what has been said.

There was a conference in Dave Schieber's office.

"You'll have to look at her and point at her," he said.

"I won't."

"You'll have to."

"I'll look at her, but I won't point at her. Can I just describe what she has on?"

She would follow Lisa Lynch. She was the last prosecution witness.

Robin was waiting in an office, away from the reporters and the crowd, when suddenly Dave Schieber stuck his head in the doorway.

"C'mon let's go."

She felt like she was inside one of those jostling, fast-moving camera shots in a cheap cop show. A TV cameraman, in fact, was waiting in the hallway. The assistant prosecutor began barking orders. Dave Schieber was hollering, in fact.

"My witness has a *right* not to be on TV! Do you understand?"

The cameraman backed away. In the courtroom, there would be no pictures, no footage. The judge had exempted her.

Yes, the courtroom. Schieber and Bon Hiner were leading her there. The main doors swung opened. For a second, Robin Fielder thought she was going to pass out. People, their heads turning, filled the limits of her peripheral vision. She dared not look at the face she could sense staring at her in the corner of her eye. She dared not look at Gwen.

She put her head down and followed Dave Schieber's heels. She sat and was sworn. She looked up at her hand. It was shaking. She looked out at the courtroom. She was looking for her mom and dad. She thought, where are you? *Where are you?*

"Robin, how old are you please?"

She looked at the attorney.

"Twenty-three."

"As of when."

"Today."

Schieber looked at the jury. She looked at the jury. They were all smiling. She could have sworn the assistant prosecutor said "Happy Birthday." The court transcript later showed no such thing. But it made her smile. It made her relax.

He asked her about working at Alpine Manor. Did she know Cathy Wood and Gwen Graham? Yes.

"Are either of them in court here now?"

"Gwen."

"Point to her for me, please."

Robin turned. She looked above her. She couldn't look her in the eyes. She thought, what does she think of me, betraying her? She felt her right arm come up, her finger extended.

"She's over there," she said, her voice quaking.

There, she thought. I've done it.

She looked out in the courtroom. She saw her father. He gave her a thumbs up sign. He was smiling at her. She saw Tom Freeman. He was smiling.

As she told the jury how she met Gwen and began their relationship, she felt herself smile. It wasn't the memory.

She thought, *I've done it.* I'm going to make it through this. I'm getting this over with. She felt euphoric.

For a second, it worried her questioner.

"Excuse me, your honor . . . Robin, you keep smiling. Why are you smiling?"

"Just smiling," she told him.

She straightened her back. She was ready, for any and all questions. Soon, the smile left. There were quiet tears, painful recollections.

"Was there a time when Gwen Graham told you about some unusual activity?"

"At Family Foods."

She explained their conversation in her car.

"We were just sitting there talking, and she told me she had killed six people, and she started crying, and then I started crying."

"Do you remember any of the names she told you at the time?"

She took her time. She thought real hard. She felt like everybody in the courtroom was hanging on everything she said.

"Yes. Marguerite Chambers, Edith Cook, Mae Mason."

They covered two years in less than an hour. Robin told about Cathy's threats in the Alpine parking lot, Gwen leaving with her that night, the conversation at Lisa Lynch's trailer, fleeing to Texas, Gwen's incessant joking, and the barbecue with Deborah Kidder. She detailed that talk.

". . . And she had mentioned names, she had said she kept—they kept souvenirs. She said that she would be the one who killed them and Cathy would stand outside and watch."

"Did she make any other statements about it?"

"She had said that—she mentioned Belle Burkhard, and that it was hard for her to do this, because Belle was fighting back and it bruised her arm."

"Did she say anything about Edith?"

"She had thrown her teeth in the trash, and that the only way they could probably prove it was—"

Piazza objected. Robin still didn't look toward Gwen.

Overruled.

Robin continued.

"She had said the only way they could prove that this had been done is because Edith had a tooth in her mouth, and it could probably scrape her mouth or bruise it."

Robin told the jury about the first visit by police, her frame of mind then.

"Were you in love with Gwen at that point?"

"Yes."

There were other tears in the courtroom besides Robin's. At the defense table, Gwen Graham was wiping them from her cheeks with her fingertips.

"How did Gwen treat you?"

"Like a queen."

Schieber eased into the next question.

"Did Gwen ever tie you up?"

"No . . . I wouldn't let her."

". . . Who was the dominant one?"

"Gwen."

The attorney wanted to know what happened after the police left.

"Did you confront Gwen?"

"No, she confronted me."

Yes, she confronted me, Robin thought. Under the bright metal lights in her kitchen, Robin had gone back to that day many times. It was the day after the Walker police had left Tyler. In her own mind, she could see Gwen and the trailer and their bedroom. They were there, getting ready for work. Gwen was really disturbed. It all seemed so different now.

"Did you do it?" Robin asked her then.

Tears were rolling down Gwen's cheeks that day as well.

"Yes," Gwen said.

That day, she did not want to hear that. She did not want to believe the words.

"No, you didn't do it," Robin told her.

Gwen grabbed her by the shoulders and shook her.

"I did it, Robin. I *really* did it. I know you can't believe it. I know you don't want to believe it. But I did it."

Gwen fell onto the bed, bawling. Robin lay down beside her, holding her. She turned to Robin.

"The police, they will be back," Gwen said.

In the courtroom, Robin heard the voice of David Schieber.

"What do you mean?" he asked.

Now, she had to tell him, tell them, the jury. She spared the detail.

"I kept telling her that I didn't believe it, and she said she did it."

"She said she did what?"

"She had killed these people."

Her questioner made sure the jury heard it again.

"After the police were there, she admitted she did the killing?"

"Yes."

Yes, she *did,* Robin thought, and I couldn't believe her.

There were only a few more questions, about moving from the trailer, about the library books Gwen checked out.

"What did she say?"

"She didn't really say a lot about it, she just was trying to find a way out?"

"What do you mean?"

"So she wouldn't get the total blame for it."

Schieber wondered if she mentioned any other killings.

"Yes, she did say she—her and Cathy wanted to kill Angie."

All the old conversations were clicking again in her mind, but in a new way. Schieber asked about the Alpine victims.

"When she would say . . . 'I killed six people,' would she mention the names."

"Yes."

"And were they always the same names?"

"Yes."

"Did she ever say that Cathy Wood was the one who did the killing?"

"No."

"Did she always say that Gwen was the one who did the killing?"

"Yes."

Robin didn't expect the defense attorney's cross-examination to be so short—not even ten minutes at the most.

"You did not believe these statements, otherwise you would have gone to the police, is that a fair statement?" Piazza asked at one point.

"Yes."

Then, finally she heard those words.

"Nothing further, Your Honor."

Robin Fielder looked at the jury, then the courtroom. All these people, she thought. This is reality. This is the truth: Gwen killed those people. She's a killer, and so is Cathy Wood.

At that moment she decided that for good, beyond a reasonable doubt. All the jokes, all the macabre details she thought were attempts to scare or irritate her, now made perfect sense. All the conversations fit. She saw motives. There was a reason to kill Angie Brozak, she decided. There was a reason to kill me. We had Gwen's eye, her attention. We were threats to Cathy.

"We were supposed to kill you too, Robin," Gwen once told her. "But I wouldn't let her. I said you were too nice."

Yes, and when that couldn't be done, Robin decided, Cathy chose someone Gwen could kill—the old, the sick, the defenseless. She remembered what Gwen had said: Cathy proposed the idea to kill patients as they worked on crossword puzzles. Then, the first was Marguerite Chambers. She was dead on January 18, ten days after she caught us together.

It was me, she thought. It started because of *me*. The realization would send new rushes of guilt through Robin for months to come.

She thought, it *was* a game, a game of deadly secrets, one that no one but Cathy could possibly win. That's why Gwen kept writing Cathy from Texas, to placate her. She remembered what Cathy said in the Alpine Manor parking lot: "What if I took Gwen away from you and put her away."

Robin thought, and now I'm helping her do it. I've become part of her plot, here in the courtroom, simply by telling the truth.

A few minutes later, Bob Hiner led Robin into the private corridor off the courtroom. Through the door she could hear the court adjourning. Then she watched the men and women of the panel file past her. She felt their eyes examining her. She thought, what do they think of me?

After the jury passed, the court officers came by escorting Gwen. Robin felt herself being guided into a doorway, but she could see Gwen straining to see her, lifting her head up with yearning eyes. Gwen yelled: "I still love you Robin!"

Down the hall she could hear Gwen yelling.

"Let me go. Let me go."

There was a guttural scream. Gwen was being wrestled away by the bailiffs.

Dave Schieber closed the door of the office behind him as Robin lit a cigarette in the silence. She was in tears, but she wasn't hysterical. There would be no more hysterics, not in this twenty-third year of her life, at least.

"You all right, Robin? You were a terrific witness, maybe my best witness ever."

She took a long drag off her cigarette and exhaled a stream of smoke halfway across the room.

She looked at the attorney. Then she nodded her head.

Gwen Graham battled her jailers all the way back to the elevator. When the doors closed she began screaming at the top of her lungs. At the jail, a psychiatrist would be summoned to calm her.

As the elevator descended, downward into the bowels of the Hall of Justice, she seemed entirely oblivious to the damaging nature of Robin Fielder's testimony. Consciously, at least, that was not the source of Gwen's hysterics.

"It just dawned on me that I would never see her again," she later said.

Chapter 108

Jim Piazza spent Tuesday morning trying to overcome a defense attorney's nightmare: A prosecution witness who appears to have all the reason in the world to help a defendant, but rises to a higher standard. Piazza could only hope that in Robin Fielder's case, the jury didn't think the higher calling was the truth.

His cross-examination on Monday was brief by design. He wanted to get her off the stand, where she could do no further damage. However, the entire defense effort also appeared brief, especially in light of Piazza's extensive preparation. He began at 9:50 A.M. and ended seven minutes past noon.

Piazza offered four witnesses, the last the trial's grand finale. She had been silent since her arrest. Now, in her own defense, Gwen Graham planned to take the stand.

Piazza called Dr. John N. Campbell, the medical director of Alpine Manor. He was also Edith Cook's personal physician.

"After your knowledge of Edith Cook and reviewing Dr. Cohle's autopsy, would you have changed the death certificate or would you have had it remain the same?"

The doctor said he would have stayed with coronary arrest.

The attorney asked if Cook's death was suspicious, or if any of the other deaths were, would the nursing staff tell him?

"If it were suspicious, it would certainly be made—I would be made aware of it, yes."

Piazza wondered if there seemed to be an increase of deaths in the time period.

"I'm not aware of any increase. I just recall the usual number of deaths in the nursing home."

On his cross, Dave Schieber asked about the common practice among physicians at nursing homes like Alpine Manor.

"In fact, you never viewed Edith Cook's body after she was dead, did you?"

"That's right."

Schieber wondered, was it inconvenient?

"Well, it's not a matter of convenience, it's just—generally, when a patient dies in a nursing home, the nurse calls the doctor, and we release the body to the funeral home, but it is not the normal practice to go and view the body unless there is some special reason."

Piazza called former Alpine aide Shawn Marie Dougherty. She told the jury how she had found Mae Mason dead, but in the same position where she had left her. She praised Graham's work habits and detailed Wood's pettiness. She told the jury she quit because of Wood.

"Did you know her sexual preferences?"

"Yes I did."

"Was that one of the reasons or just her attitude?"

"Her attitude. Her sexual preference meant nothing to me."

"Was Cathy Wood a type of domineering person, or was she a passive person."

"I found her to be domineering."

Piazza called John Hulsing, the polygraph examiner. Judge Snow would not allow him to mention his polygraph or his former trade as an examiner, but he could quote from his interview with

Wood. He gave his occupation as a former state police officer of twenty-five years, a "specialist lieutenant," who had interviewed Cathy Wood.

"What did Cathy Wood say in reference to her observations on Marguerite Chambers?"

"She told me that she had observed Gwen Graham smother Marguerite Chambers."

"Did at some point in time she change that?"

"Yes . . . She told me that she had not seen Gwen Graham smother Marguerite Chambers, but she had been told by Gwen Graham."

"So she changed her story with you."

"Yes."

Piazza asked about their talk about spelling M-U-R-D-E-R.

"What context was that, what was said about that?" Piazza asked.

"It was during that conversation, during the interview, when I asked if that was something they had discussed. I said, 'I understand that you have discussed the term, 'murder,' M-U-R-D-E-R, and you were going to kill someone whose last name corresponded to those letters,' and her response was 'Yes, I said that, but that's not true.' "

As with Shawn Dougherty, Dave Schieber decided to pass on cross-examining Hulsing.

At exactly 11:00 A.M., Gwen Graham rose from the defense table and walked to the witness stand to be sworn. Her shoulders hunched, she had a slight toddle to her walk. She wore her gray slacks and a faint powder blue blouse with a print. With a modest application of makeup, she looked distinctly feminine.

By the eleventh question, Piazza headed for the subject of his client's arms. He wanted the jury to see a victim, not a thrill-seeking sadomasochist.

"Growing up did you have some problems with your father?"

"Yes I did."

"And what were those problems?"

"Will you repeat that question?"

She was speaking very quietly. She looked like she was quietly pouting.

"What was the problem you had with your father when you were growing up? I know it's difficult."

"Sexual—sexual misconduct. Can't think of the word."

"Did your father sexually abuse you when you were little?"

"Yes, sir."

They talked about her burn marks.

"What are the reasons for those? And when did you do that?"

"When I was sixteen, to get even with him."

"Even with who?"

"With my father."

"For what?"

"For what he did to me. That's the only thing that hurt him as he had hurt me."

They covered her background in Tyler, her decision to move to Grand Rapids, getting work at Alpine Manor. Most of her answers were one word, yes or no. She often spoke in fragments, hardly exceeding two or three words. Earlier, in preparing her for the testimony, Piazza had told Graham to tell her questioner that she "didn't understand the question" if she was confused. She took his advice quite literally, and followed it frequently.

"Did there come a point in time when you and Cathy Wood became lovers?"

"Yes."

"Okay, can you describe to the jury that circumstance?"

"I don't understand your question."

They covered their relationship and those in their social circle.

"While you were living with Cathy Wood, did you have any affairs with any other women?"

"Yes, I did."

"Who were they?"

"Angie Brozak, Dawn Male, Robin Fielder."

"Did Cathy Wood ever find out about these?"

"Yes she did."

"What was her reaction?"

"Very angry."

They talked about Cathy playing mind games, setting up people with false information.

"Would you start them, go along with them, or what?"

"Go along. I'd go along with them, yes I would."

The conversation with Dawn Male about murders was a game, an attempt to "scare her," she said.

They told a number of people about killing patients, she would say. It was a running, "sick" joke.

It was the heart of her defense.

"Have you killed anybody at Alpine Manor?"

"No, I have not."

Graham's brow furrowed. Sometimes it was hard to tell whether she was angry, pouting or overwhelmed.

She talked about leaving Cathy.

"And what was the reason for moving out?"

"Something to do with Robin, but mostly tired of playing games, tired, tired of her."

"Of whose games?"

"Cathy's. Hurting people. Their feelings. It just got out of hand."

Cathy tried to prevent her from leaving Michigan, she said. She told the jury how she went home with Cathy that night of the threats in the Alpine parking lot. She said she told her all about her long affair with Robin. Cathy wanted to sleep with her one last time.

"And it was not abnormal for us to tie each other up, and so I agreed to that."

"Who tied who up?"

"Cathy tied me up."

"Okay."

"And my—I had the gun in the house, and she stuck it, she stuck it up my vagina."

"Cathy did?"

It was one of her very few long answers on the stand.

"Yes, she did . . . While I was tied up, yes, and told me that she was going to kill me, and then she said, 'No, maybe it would be better if I let you watch me kill myself.' And then she just started crying and she pulled it out and she left the house, and she left me tied up there. And I thought she was going to go find Robin, but she came back, about three hours later, and untied me . . .."

Graham talked about her admissions to Lisa Lynch and Deborah Kidder. Yes, she talked about murders, but the witnesses had left out an important attribution, she said. *Cathy* had said there were killings. Gwen testified she told Lynch and Kidder *Cathy* said she had killed six people.

". . . Cathy had said that at one time, that I went along with it."

As for Robin Fielder, she admitted talking about murder in Texas.

"What did you say at that time, if you remember?"

"That I was scared, that Cathy was really going to do it. That she was going to get even, just like she said she was."

"Did you deny killing anyone to Robin Fielder?"

"Yes I did."

He asked her to explain why she had checked out the Tyler library books on the justice systems and prisons.

"Because I was scared?"

"Scared of what?"

"What if this—I was scared that what if this really, this was—I didn't believe that this was happening, but what if it does."

A couple of questions later, "Is there any truth to the mind game you were playing, that you killed anybody at the Alpine Manor?"

"No."

"Do you know whether or not Cathy Wood had killed anybody?"

"I don't think she did, but I can't say for sure. I don't think so."

Piazza retrieved People's Exhibit Number One and Number Two, the letter and poem on nurse's notepaper. He asked her about the acronyms, specifically I-G-T-K-M.

". . . do you know what they mean?"

"I do not know. I do not know what they mean, it's been so long."

He asked her about "forever and five days."

"What does that mean to you?"

"Forever and the amount, the amount of months we've been together . . ."

"So one day would be one month?"

She nodded.

"Mm-hmm. Yes."

Gwen Graham would not concede at the start of Dave Schieber's cross-examination that she was the controlling personality.

"Cathy was."

"And you say that because of what?"

"Because that's the way it was."

However, there was nothing simple about her answers when he began to probe their love affair. She answered her prosecutor's questions politely, punctuated by "sir" in the Southern tradition of respect. Her logic, however, made little sense. The jury would get brief glimpses of the kind of split viewpoints Gwen Graham could hold simultaneously, without being aware of any contradiction at all.

"During the course of your relationship with Cathy, you were attracted to her?"

"Yes, sir."

"And it was a satisfying relationship to you?"

"No, sir."

"No? When did it cease to be satisfying for you?"

"Never was."

"Why did you continue it?"

"Because I loved her."

She answered as though that should be obvious to everyone.

"In what fashion wasn't it satisfying for you?"

"She was an unhappy girl."

". . . and that's my question, was it satisfying for you?"

"No sir."

"Why not?"

"Because I was not happy because she was not happy."

"So why did you continue it?"

"Because I loved Cathy."

She seemed perplexed by Schieber's train of thought. There were long pauses before many of her answers.

He asked her about infidelity. She admitted telling Cathy about sleeping with Dawn and Angie.

"How did she need to know, what benefit did she accrue?"

"My honesty with her."

Except, he pointed out, she didn't tell her about Robin.

"What makes Robin so special?"

"She's a very special girl."

As she testified, one former witness had decided to remain in the courtroom to study the testimony of Gwen Graham. Within fifteen minutes, John Hulsing had already decided that Gwen Graham was up against something beyond her intellectual and psychological resources.

The state cop turned psychologist didn't know if Graham had

committed murder or not. But he did know she wasn't prepared to defend herself. She looked bemused, depressed.

"She didn't have a chance," he later said. "It was downright pathetic, in fact."

Schieber's grilling continued.

"What on earth would prompt you to attempt to prove to Dawn Male that in fact the allegations [of murder] were true?"

"Going along with Cathy's game, just going along with the game."

"Was it funny?"

"To me and Cathy."

Schieber was incredulous.

"The thought of killing old women at a nursing home was funny to you and Cathy?"

"No, the thought of messing with Dawn Male."

". . . How would killing old patients scare Dawn Male?"

"Well, if you were alone with two people that had said that they had killed people at a nursing home, you'd be scared."

Schieber condescended.

"I'd have a lot of reactions, but fear probably wouldn't be one of them."

Piazza was on his feet, asking the prosecutor's wisecrack to be stricken.

Later, Schieber peaked his cross with classic prosecutorial trial technique. He massed Gwen Graham's accusers, figuratively making her a lone voice in a crowd.

"So Lisa Lynch's testimony is wrong, at least as you recall it?"

"Yes, sir."

"Is Deborah Kidder right when she says that you said that you did the suffocating?"

"I did not say that."

"So Deborah Kidder's testimony is wrong?"

"That part of it is wrong."

He moved to Robin Fielder. When he went to employ the same strategy, Schieber found the going difficult. Graham simply could not remember major portions of Robin's testimony from the previous day. She had been too captivated by the sight of Robin, she later explained privately.

"And do you recall that she said that you admitted that it wasn't a joke, that it was all true, that you had done the killing?" Schieber said, trying again.

"Do I recall her saying that?"

"Do you recall her saying that?"

"Yes, sir."

"Is that true?"

"No, sir."

"Can you give us some reason Robin would say that?"

"I don't understand."

"You don't understand?"

"No, I can't give you a reason."

Finally, Schieber left the jury a hint of motive. The attorney had read Fran Shadden's statement about Graham's previous conflicts with her parents.

"In fact, did you tell Fran that you despise your mother?"

"No, sir."

"Let me do it this way. Have you confided to Fran that you have a love-hate relationship for your mother?"

"No, sir."

"What is accurate then?"

"That my mother and I had had some problems when I was growing up, and that we have a good relationship now."

Schieber paused, glancing at the jury.

"I am assuming nobody would do what you have done unless they had received a great deal of personal pain?"

Gwen knitted her eyebrows.

"I don't understand what you are talking about."

"In your mind, when you killed these people, who were you really killing?"

Jim Piazza jumped to his feet.

"Objection, Your Honor, that's argumentative. He's not asking a question."

Schieber didn't need to at that point.

In his closing argument and rebuttal, David Schieber covered the whole story again, right off establishing a lofty point of view.

"I guess the first thing I want to talk about is . . . that this isn't some sort of referendum on homosexuality or lesbian relationships, or anything of the kind. Surely, this can't be representative of your average gay relationship. It isn't meant to be. The dynamics of this relationship were destructive, almost cancerous, sort of feeding on each other and destroying things around them. And that could happen in a heterosexual relationship as easily."

He struck the themes he had been developing through the whole trial. Graham masterminded the murders. Wood went along because she feared that was the only way to keep Graham. However, he acknowledged, Wood herself was not without guilt.

"There's never been an argument on our part that she's pristine, that she isn't involved in this, that she didn't contribute to this. This is a destructive relationship, with each of them contributing to the destruction."

However, "You have to give Gwen some credit," he argued. "She masterminded a manner of death that would leave nothing—no prints, no bruising, not a fiber of forensic evidence. There were no witnesses, and in three, no bodies.

". . . It is the perfect crime. It's totally senseless. It's murder for murder's sake. There's no money to be gained here. There's no revenge involved here. The motive is just intensely personal. Cathy says that after these killings, that Gwen would be happy; that Gwen would say it relieved her tension.

"And we don't know enough about Gwen to know why. Surely we know enough about her to know that she's two people. One person . . . is caring and a good nurse's aide, and this other person, the person that's violent, and we heard it described, in these terrible fights; a person that would tie Cathy up, and suffocated her just to show the power that she had over her, or place a barrel of a gun to her vagina. Not to kill her, but just to show the power. Her motivations are known perhaps not even to her. But it's clear from what you have heard that she has every opportunity to be a disturbed person."

He concluded his final argument by evoking his two most important witnesses. He knew Jim Piazza would soon carry on about the lack of physical evidence.

"You heard this testimony, this testimony from a person who says that Gwen treated her like a queen. That even Gwen can't think of a reason for her to lie. And you want physical evidence? Well, consider that.

"And consider this. Consider Cathy Wood's mailing address for at least the next ten years . . . And she testified, you recall, she said, 'I know what my sentence guidelines are, I know I'm not eligible for parole'—*eligible*—'for ten years.' "

Schieber eyed the entire panel.

"What greater physical evidence can there be than that?"

In his closing, Jim Piazza spent a half hour poking holes in the prosecutor's claim that Graham was "dominant" and bashing Wood's credibility.

"I would wonder if anyone here in this courtroom would go up in an airplane, grab a parachute that Cathy Wood said, 'I packed this parachute and it will work.' Wonder how many people in this courtroom would jump out of that airplane."

Where were the souvenirs? Where were the suspicious fellow employees? Where was the increase in the death rate? He drove his argument through the hole Schieber had left for him.

"In fact, when you look at the physical evidence, the prosecutor did not even bring anybody to show that Gwen Graham worked on the shift, at the time and days when these supposed murders occurred . . . Did you hear that from the prosecutor. No."

At, another point: "We have supposedly five perfect murders, supposedly, and we have not one person, not one independent eyewitness to say anything, except for Cathy Wood."

At another: "Ladies and gentlemen, this lady has lied to you, constantly lied to you . . . who's she trying to kid? She's trying to pull this mind game that she's been working with all these years—on you! Don't let Cathy Wood get away with it."

Cathy Wood. Her name kept coming up, over and over. Piazza tried to speculate on Robin Fielder's motivation, what she might have really heard after police arrived in Texas. "The confusion there, the excitement. Maybe Robin misunderstood."

Then again, Piazza hammered away at Wood.

"Cathy Wood, she pleads guilty. Did she plead guilty to a nonexistent crime? Well, the prosecutor says we want to get inside these people; I'm not sure we did. I'm not sure we ever will. People do things, strange things . . . Maybe she pled guilty because Cathy Wood is guilty."

Like Ken Wood, Dawn Male and a cast of others that sat around her table in Alpine Manor . . . like the police, the prosecutor and the news media . . . like the city of Grand Rapids itself, attorney Jim Piazza was intensely focussed. He wasn't the first to be captivated by the twenty-seven-year-old former nurse's aide who hardly made a minimum wage.

She wasn't even in the courtroom most of the time. But even the trial of Gwendolyn Cail Graham seemed to revolve around none other than Cathy Wood.

Chapter 109

The nine women and three men met for forty-five minutes on Tuesday. On Wednesday, enough families and spectators to fill Judge Roman Snow's courtroom returned to the Hall of Justice, simply to wait, as the jury continued deliberating the fate of Gwen Graham throughout the morning.

The panel was made up of ordinary Grand Rapids folks. They included a machine operator, a cashier, a manager of a fast-food restaurant, a cook, an engineer, a factory worker and a service representative for the local phone company.

Afterwards, some of the female jurors would flee the Hall of Justice, fearful of media exposure and recrimination. One of the male jurors found his lunch breaks unsettling. He always walked up the Michigan Street hill to Blodgett Memorial Hospital where he worked. Several times Gwen Graham passed as she was transported to the Kent County Jail. She looked at him as she rode in the back of the cruiser.

"Maybe she'll figure out where I work," he later said.

Other jurors spent their breaks trying to guess who Graham's parents were. One day they pegged what they thought was a "Southern-looking couple" in the courtroom. Then they realized she had no eye contact with anyone in the courtroom.

At first the task before them appeared overwhelming, some later recalled. Late Tuesday they asked Judge Snow if they could have transcripts of the trial to study. He told them that would be quite difficult, if not impossible, and they should "talk" about the testimony among themselves.

They come up with a system that was not unlike a self-help group meeting. They moved clockwise around the table, each juror taking his turn talking about the testimony, about his or her impressions of the case. There were mixed feelings about Cathy Wood. Some saw her as a victim, others suspected a hidden agenda.

"I felt sorry for her," a thirty-four-year-old electrical engineer named Scott Russell later said. "She seemed to be looking for direction in life and never got it. I think she was a person who was in the wrong place at the wrong time, hanging around with the wrong person. I think she was a good person, somewhere down inside."

Vicki Karczewski, the thirty-one-year-old phone company rep, was not so empathetic. "I basically thought this all could be Cathy's idea, because she seemed like the person who would need that kind of hold. Overall, it took two of them to come up with this, but Gwen had played the far greater role."

A thirty-four-year-old furniture factory worker named Mary Schild found Wood unbelievable.

"I had a hard time believing the David/Debbie syndrome. How could you *not* know something like that. I was convinced murder had occurred, but was not convinced based on what Cathy had said."

Cathy Wood was not on trial, however. Many jurors agreed that they would have never reached a decision based on her testimony. Robin Fielder had stunned many of them.

"I couldn't figure out, what in the world is she doing here, with these people," said Russell.

Karczewski later explained, "When she came in you saw this sweet little girl, once normal, who fell in with the wrong person. There was nothing for her to gain. She wouldn't look in the direction of Graham. She was still hurt. You could see that. You could see it was hard for her to get up there and testify against her. She seemed to be fighting for her own self-respect. She seemed to be fighting to find a normal life for herself again."

Early on, two jurors kept the panel from a unanimous decision. On Wednesday, the panel asked the judge if the court reporter could read the testimony of Catherine Wood, but then opted to try and talk it out once more when they found out the task would take three hours. They went around the table again.

Many felt Graham had hurt her own case by taking the stand. She was too pensive, too studied in her responses to Dave Schieber. They saw her answers as contradictory. Sometimes, she simply just didn't make any sense. Her credibility was so poor, some doubted she even had scars under her long sleeves.

"If she had them, why didn't she just show them to us?" one juror later said.

When the vote became unanimous, there was a consensus: It was all, or nothing.

"There wasn't any smoking gun in this trial," recalled Russell, who later was elected foreman. "There wasn't anything concrete. It was basically looking at all the testimony, and your gut feeling. But there was a consistency to the testimony. The same names kept coming up. It seemed to us if she did one, then she did them all."

The deliberations lasted nearly six hours total.

People were standing two-deep inside the courtroom doors. Gwen Graham waited, wearing a bulky gray sweater with a design of black just below her breasts. She was chewing gum, as the jury filed back in midafternoon. Her jaw stilled as the foreman was asked to read the verdicts.

The word "guilty" sounded six times: Guilty of first degree murder on all five victims, guilty of conspiracy to murder.

Graham looked forward, hardly even blinking.

As she was led out of the courtroom in handcuffs, Jim Piazza patted her on the back. She walked with head down, her shoulders hunched.

It was as though she were there on automatic pilot.

As the courtroom doors opened, people poured out into the hallway, silent and overwhelmed, like an audience leaving a disturbing film. Reporters and TV cameras were waiting.

One of the first out was Jan Hunderman. She had attended every proceeding with her father Ed Chambers. Jan had grown increasingly frustrated with news coverage of the case. There had been too much emphasis on Wood, Graham and lesbians, she thought, and not enough on the real victims of the case. Some reports seemed to suggest the victims were little more than vegetables.

One account would report victims were smothered "as they slept," as if such a thing were possible.

"My mother," Jan later told a friend, "was *not* smothered in her sleep."

Wood's testimony of her mother's struggle had disproved that, for those in the courtroom, at least. Now there was justice.

"My mother can finally rest in peace," she said.

Ed Chambers still was not sleeping in his own bed.

"Shoot the sonsabitches," he mumbled to a reporter. Then he turned away. He didn't want the cameras to catch a grown man crying.

Linda Engman was surrounded by reporters. She was a picture of sophistication in a smart red suit, the ensemble complemented by black teardrop earrings. Her comment had primitive origins.

"As far as justice in Michigan goes," she said, "I wish we had the death penalty."

Linda wasn't sure any punishment could help her daughter Stephanie. She was in Hope College now, but in the wake of the trial publicity she would leave the school with under a C average. Before, she had never received a poor grade in her life.

Some families avoided the trial altogether. Edith Cook's family kept its code of silence. Ted and Maxine Luce watched the coverage of the verdict on TV. Myrtle's daughter, Hazel Dredge, who had cared for her at Alpine so religiously, was not at the proceedings. Now she was suffering from Alzheimer's disease. She was a resident in Alpine Manor.

My mother had a good life, better than most, Ted Luce reasoned, and the way it was ended wasn't going to take that away.

"It does make me feel bad," he said later. "But I feel bad for the girls who did it too. Their lives are ruined."

Alpine Manor had an official reaction to the verdict via a spokesman from the public relations firm, Seyferth & Associates, Inc. Account executive Craig Piersma read the statement on the steps of the Hall of Justice.

"Even though we find it difficult to believe that any of this actually happened, now that a verdict has been reached we will continue to place our trust in our system of justice, as the process moves forward. As always our primary goal is to help the well-being of our patients and their families. We will continue to provide quality care in a supportive environment in our nursing home."

Cathy Wood had her own spokesman as well, in the form of her attorney Christine Yared who talked to reporters in the halls. She spoke as though Cathy had been vindicated.

"We're happy with the verdict," she said. "I'm happy for Cathy and for the families of the victims."

As the crowd of newspeople milled around for interviews in the hallway, only one spoke up in Gwen Graham's behalf. Fran Shadden emerged from a courthouse phone booth where she had just given Graham's mother the news of the verdict.

"Oh no," Gwen's mother had simply said.

Fran believed her old roommate had problems, but didn't believe she was a killer. The testimony had failed to convince her. She was so angry her voice shook.

"I'm shocked," she told a TV reporter. "I don't understand how somebody can be convicted on no physical evidence, and just hearsay. Especially the hearsay of a bunch of gay people who do nothing but play games anyway. It's sick that somebody can play a sick game and get away with it."

Nancy Hahn had planned to go to the trial, but was talked out of it by her son.

"Mom, don't put yourself through that," he said.

David Schieber had told her, "Your mother Belle was the only one who put up a struggle."

Nancy wasn't sure she could handle all the descriptions of something like that.

Later, she repeatedly questioned the decision, but it was only one of a host of regrets. One summer day she got a call from a total stranger who had read her name out of the paper. She said she, too, had a mother at Alpine Manor. She explained her mom kept begging her to call the police. The nurse's aides were killing patients, she said. The woman thought her mother was making up stories.

Like Nancy, the woman was riddled with guilt. She seemed to be trying to apologize. She was looking for atonement, and so was Nancy.

She told herself, so many times, over and over, I should have gone and visited her. I should have been closer to her.

And, the questions. Many had asked the same ones: Was she aware enough to understand what was happening to her? Were there many attempts to kill her? How many horrifying nights did my mother spend there waiting? Waiting for *them*, waiting for them to come back . . . to finish the job.

Nancy Hahn felt smothered by her own shortcomings. I should have been alert, she thought, alert to what was going on.

She had a comment for the reporter who called her right after the verdict. She was in Buchanan, two and a half hours from Grand Rapids, from Alpine Manor, from the Hall of Justice. But she had always been too far away. She told the reporter:

"I'm glad she has been convicted, but I can't say I feel much better. I carry this very bad guilt complex because I left her in the home. I wish I had her here."

Later, a veteran Grand Rapids reporter who covered the trial called an author who was considering writing a book on the Alpine murder case.

"You're gonna have real trouble writing a book on this," she said. "There's some question as to whether it really even happened. And the victims just aren't very sympathetic. They were in bad shape. They were going to die anyway."

The reporter was wrong, murder or not.

The victims were among the living.

Chapter 110

As Cathy's sentencing approached, Ken Wood was all but certain she wouldn't be getting the kind of help he wanted for her long before she ever went to work at Alpine Manor. He figured, they will lock her up in prison somewhere, and that will be it.

Ken was struggling to bring some semblance of order and security to his own life. His severance settlement from GM was gone. He had plummeted from a $40,000-a-year income to finding spot work in convenience stores. Cathy told him her mother Pat was going to try to get custody of the child. With custody came support money from the Department of Social Services.

"Whatever you do, Ken," Cathy told him. "Don't let my mother have Jamie. My mom just wants her for the money."

Ken also suspected his ex-mother-in-law was just trying to get even with him for testifying. For months at a time, the woman made no effort to see her granddaughter.

On the other hand, Ken also periodically found himself on the defensive with his ex-wife.

"Cathy would bring it up: 'You never let my parents see Jamie,' " he later recalled. "I would say, 'Hey, your mom can call Jamie or see Jamie any time she wants. She doesn't call. She makes no effort to see Jamie at all.' "

It was a familiar territory. Pat versus Ken, with Cathy in the middle, a conduit for the conflict. One night he sat down and had a good talk with Jamie.

"Some day this will all work out," he told her. "Some day we will be able to turn this around and some good will come out of it."

As for the bigger picture, Ken knew people were suspicious of his motives in the high profile he had taken in the case. Graham's defense attorney had jabbed him on the stand for appearing on the Larry King show, and hinted in his closing argument he was looking to make a fortune on a book. He would not, though he wished he could. He wished he could somehow get paid for all the misery the case had brought.

Later, Ken appeared on a string of talk shows, making appearance with a forensic psychologist who had studied serial murder. He met families of victims of notorious medical killer Donald Harvey. He saw a video of Harvey interviewed in prison. When he saw a dark, vacant look in the former orderly's eyes, it chilled him. It was the same countenance he had seen come over Cathy.

Yet, often, Ken still defended her, trying to figure out publicly the nature of her metamorphosis.

"All these people who supposedly know Cathy are gonna have bad things to say," he later said. "I've seen the good Cathy, the nice Cathy, the humorous Cathy, the mother, and sometimes the wife.

Something snapped in her. And people, they have no right to judge her, because they don't know her well enough to judge her."

He sometimes wondered if he really did.

"At times I don't know what to think," he would say, nearly a year and a half after the trial. "Sometimes I hate her guts. Other times I feel sorry for her. Sometimes I think I'm the only one in the world who defends her."

Ken became her advocate once more before her sentencing. He wrote a letter to Kent County Judge Robert A. Benson, the jurist who had taken her guilty plea. In fact, he wrote two.

He began the first letter: "This is the most important letter I will ever write. I pray it's the best for so much may be riding on it . . .

> I know there will be pressure to give Cathy a major sentence, especially with the nature of the crime and number of victims.
>
> Several months ago, when I turned Cathy in, I was seeking one thing, help for Cathy. It's something I've been trying to do for the past ten years. Ten years ago I took it upon myself to help a 17-year-old girl who I felt I loved enough to make up for all the bad things she hadn't told me. That was the mistake of a 20-year-old boy who dearly wanted to be loved and who wanted to be an important part of someone's life. I was no match for the problems Cathy was having inside . . . though there were times when I felt it was just a matter of time before Cathy forgot about the past and learned to enjoy the life she had with our daughter and myself.

He told Judge Benson that Cathy had "a cold mother" and a "violent father" and lived in a home where "love wasn't shown." "She couldn't even recognize that my daughter and I were trying to give her our love."

He wrote he knew Cathy "better than anyone."

> And I know that Cathy cracked under pressure of married life, of not being able to deal with her past, feeling unloved by people she trusted and depended on. And that Gwen's influence and the influence of excessive drinking . . . fueled by depression, blocked her better judgement. Cathy needs our help, not our wrath or outrage.

What he wrote next was a view not uncommon in Grand Rapids, in Michigan, in America, among those who became familiar with the coverage of the Alpine Manor murder case.

Cathy is guilty of taking lives or at least not preventing Gwen from taking them. But how much life did she really take? All of the victims weren't even living. They enjoyed nothing, experienced nothing and were going to die. The families at the times of death were relieved at the end of the suffering . . . I know they had no right to play God . . . but when you decide how much of her life should be taken or lost in prison, shouldn't it be equal to what was taken from their victims?

His daughter could be the final victim, he wrote, as well as himself, if Cathy didn't get "help." For three years, he pointed out, his daughter had been without a mother.

He didn't go into detail as to why.

Chapter III

Hey Mr. Prosecutor! . . . I want to thank you for helping me. Is that strange? Do you get hundreds of thank-you letters daily? I know you must! You helped me more than I think you'll ever know.

—Cathy Wood, November 15, 1989.

Ken Wood wasn't the only one to write Judge Robert A. Benson before he sentenced Cathy Wood. He received pleas for mercy from, among others, two jail ministers, a friend of Cathy's mother and a former coworker at Alpine Manor.

Gwen Graham made Cathy do it, some wrote. Her supporters in

jail wrote about a transformation. Originally "withdrawn," she now was friendly and a "kind, caring person" ready to "serve both God and other people," one minister wrote.

There was a critical letter, from Citizen's for Better Care, a nursing home patient advocacy group. Its ombudsman blasted a comment by Ken Wood in the newspaper that the victims "were waiting to die." He urged the circuit judge to disregard Wood's reasoning: "A lenient sentence based on this reason sanctions abuse and even murder of chronically ill older persons."

Benson also received letters from Cathy Wood's family, supportive testimonies from her sister and her mother among them. A pre-sentence report prepared for the judge included an interview with Cathy, who detailed her stock disparaging portrait of her parents—the abusive father, the working mother who had little time for her.

At the request of Cathy's attorney, an aunt named Judith Terpstra, the sister of Cathy's father, wrote Judge Benson a letter. She provided a poignant anecdote about Cathy's father, John:

> My earliest memory of Cathy was when she was approximately
> three or four years old. I had invited Cathy and her family over
> to my home in Grand Rapids for dinner. When dinner was
> almost over Cathy had asked for an extra portion of fruit salad.
> Her father proceeded to scoop up large spoonfuls of everything
> on the table and heaped it over her plate. He then called her a
> ('fat little pig') and told her to eat it all. She cried and he
> slapped her for crying. I told them that it was my home and she
> didn't have to eat it, but my brother said she did. She tried to
> please him and attempted to choke it down.

She described Cathy's father as "hot and cold" most of his life. "He could be one of the warmest, kindest persons and without warning turn on you, and the sad part is, I don't know why . . . Our father, Cathy's grandfather, was a distant person, and he treated John about the same way as John treated Cathy . . ."

She also wrote "Cathy was simply not given much attention" and her childhood "was not a pleasant one."

> I remember being in their home several times in the morning
> for coffee. The children would rise, dress themselves, feed

themselves breakfast, be given instructions on what chores they
were to do and then be told to leave the room.

She remembered an adolescent Cathy Wood who wanted "to be
a doctor and help take care of people."

"She was kind and intelligent but emotionally starved," she
wrote.

After Cathy married Ken, she didn't see much of her niece,
Terpstra wrote. The aunt moved away to the east side of the state.
They met "only at rare family gatherings."

"And her weight had ballooned. She seemed pleasant enough,
but quiet and withdrawn, with occasional outbursts of extreme
laughter."

On October 11, Catherine May Wood walked contritely into
Judge Benson's courtroom, her third appearance before the jurist.
Cathy did not speak before her sentencing. Her attorney Christine
Yared read Cathy's written words. It was a quintessential statement
of contrition.

> I have been kept in maximum security and totally alone for
> most of my ten months . . . reliving the past. All of the time
> alone has given me the opportunity to take a long, hard look at
> myself and my problems. I've learned a lot from this, the most
> important one being that saying I'm sorry is not enough. Mere
> words cannot express the remorse and guilt I'll have to live with
> all the rest of my life. That, along with the fact that because of
> this I'll not be able to watch my baby grow up is a horrible
> torment. I was caught in a mess, but I do not excuse my actions
> or try to blame anyone for my part in this. I don't seek
> sympathy, I have to take full responsibility for my actions, and
> I'm prepared to face the consequences.

Under the statute, Judge Benson could sentence Cathy Wood to
life in prison. Under that sentence, she could be eligible for parole
in ten years, but the state parole board was no longer granting such
releases. A public hearing also would be required before parole.

Judge Benson turned to Assistant Prosecutor David Schieber for
some input.

"Anything you want to say about sentencing?"

"Only this, Your Honor. Ms. Wood has in all ways fulfilled our plea agreement. She has cooperated fully. She has testified to what we sincerely believe to be the truth."

Schieber explained that he was making arrangements with the Department of Corrections, so Cathy could serve her time in a federal prison, away from Gwen Graham.

Judge Benson acknowledged all the letters he had received. Then he continued.

"Several Factors that enter into my sentence in this case. I'm convinced that you truly show remorse, which I think is important ... I'm also convinced from what I know of your story, and the rather lengthy evidentiary hearing that we had, and what I read about the case in the paper, you are in fact a follower and not a leader, and this, again, doesn't excuse your actions. It doesn't justify your actions. But I think it does in the eyes of the sentencing court put you in a little different situation."

Judge Benson credited Cathy for breaking open the case.

"I'm most impressed by the fact that except for you, I'm sure this matter never would have been cleared up."

He indicated she had come clean in more ways than one.

"This is a sentence which is going to be primarily for punishment, because I don't think you need any particular rehabilitation, because if I turned you loose today, I'm convinced that you wouldn't do anything like this again."

Judge Benson sentenced Cathy Wood to prison terms of twenty to forty years on the second-degree murder and conspiracy charges. They would run concurrently.

She would be eligible for parole in sixteen years, in the year 2005.

There were no supportive letters, little fanfare and no surprises when Gwendolyn Gail Graham was sentenced twenty-one days later.

A pre-sentence report prepared by a Department of Corrections examiner for Judge Roman Snow was little more than a formality. The law demanded certain punishment for first degree murder. The report included statements from families of most of the victims. Most wanted Graham in prison and society protected. However, the relatives of Edith Cook, as they had with the news media, declined to provide any input to the court.

The examiner probed Graham's criminal background, but came up with only the bad check charges in Tyler. He noted her self-mutilation, alcohol and drug use and reports of sexual abuse. Contacting her mother, he reported: "Gwendolyn's mother reports that she was unaware of any abuse that Gwendolyn may have suffered at the hands of her father."

Graham maintained her innocence in the report. The examiner described her as "subdued, cooperative" but also "despondent."

She told him: "I'm mad as hell. I'm so angry that I can't believe it. I can't believe these people would come back and convict me of these crimes. I am not guilty of killing anybody. This was just a joke that got carried too far. I'm not going to give up though. I think that eventually I will be found not guilty, and the day will come that I will walk out of prison."

The examiner acknowledged her mandatory life sentence, but suggested the Department of Corrections treat her with "intense psychotherapy."

"She has never been analyzed or treated by members of the mental health community, and she has obvious deep-seated psychological problems that need to be properly addressed before she can learn to function in either a closed or open environment."

Gwen Graham declined to say a word before Judge Roman Snow on November 1. He sentenced her to serve a mandatory life prison term for each of the five murder counts and a life term for the conspiracy conviction.

There was no chance of parole. Only a successful appeal to a higher court or a rare gubernatorial pardon would ever free Gwendolyn Gail Graham.

PART
FOUR

1990

Chapter 112

I don't want to explain my actions so that people might like me. I don't even care if people don't like me.

—Cathy Wood, October 24, 1990.

Pam Durfee, a twenty-year-old inmate doing three-to-ten years for bad checks, explained to a visitor what Cathy Wood was like during the two months she stayed at the Huron Valley Women's Facility, Michigan's maximum security prison for females.

"Me and a mutual friend of ours, well, we got to be like the Three Musketeers, you know. We did a lot together. Then, I begin to hear some of the stories Cathy started spreading . . . and I didn't know what to think. I heard them everywhere. Deputies, officers. There were mind games, using one against the other.

"She used to lie to get things from other people, you know. She didn't have no money, or so she said. She turned around and had taken ten dollars from a girl. Cathy never paid her back. Then, all of a sudden, Cathy came up with her catalog orders and her TV and her foot locker and it's like—what's going on? How do you come up with one hundred dollars to get the TV. It don't make no sense. All of us were sitting here giving her stuff, personal items like food, cigarettes, shampoo, soap. We're helping her out and she's just using us.

"Then, Cathy went to a friend of mine, Patty. Patty is a very, very attractive woman. And Cathy started using her, first for her money . . . then she started playing with Patty's mind, playing with her emotions, you know. 'I love you.' Then, 'I need this.' Um, Patty never felt for a woman until, you know, Cathy, basically did what we call 'turned a person out.'

"The mind games she played on Patty were tremendous. She used her—abused her sexually, physically. Used her for her money, her body. She kept saying, 'I love you. I love you.' And Patty needed to hear 'I love you,' and it just started playing with her mind. And then one day, Cathy said, 'Bitch, get out of my face.' And basically, Patty was crushed.

". . . She would also show articles about her case and stuff. Pretty much bragging about it. I never knew nothing about this case, still don't basically.

"But every once in a while—this is the prison system—you will tend to get high. It's just something we do. It's not like you bring out pipes. We're talking about weed maybe once or twice a year.

"We were outside. This was 2:30 to 4:30 yard. And we were going to get high, and we were going to play a joke on Cathy, 'cause Cathy don't like to get high. So we told her it was a rolled up cigarette, and it was a joint. And she got really high and we just let her smoke it all by herself. And she just started talking. It was like somebody pulled out the cork, and it didn't stop.

"And she said something that really blew our minds away. And to this day, I can't figure out why she would do something to hurt somebody that bad.

"She said, 'I did the murders. I really got that bitch back.'

"And we started questioning her, asking her what the hell she was talking about, 'cause outta the blue she started talking about this. And one of my friends asked her, 'What did Gwen do that was so bad?'

"And she said, 'Gwen broke up with me . . . that's what she gets for breaking up with me.' And she got real serious. She says, 'I'm gonna pay Gwen back. I'm gonna take that woman's life.'

"I'm going, all this because somebody broke up with you? You know, this is *life*. After that me and my friends pulled completely away from Cathy."

Not long after Christmas, Cathy Wood was picking up some mail near the prison control center when she bolted into the prison staff lounge, strictly off-limits for prisoners. She was screaming. She had passed Gwen Graham in the hall.

Kent County jailers had sent Graham to Huron Valley before arrangements were complete for Wood's transfer to a federal prison. Guards in the prison couldn't understand what the fuss was about. There was such a vast difference in their sizes.

The next day, Wood sought protective custody in an interview with a deputy warden, a Ph.D. who used the doctorate title before his name. She gave an analytical rendition of her life misfortunes. She began with stories about systematic abuse by her ex-husband and ended by explaining the psychological motivations of her affair with Graham.

"She was exceptionally convincing," the deputy later recalled. "She was downright erudite, wanting to discuss it on a clinical basis, as though she was responding to my title."

He granted her request.

Back in Wood's hometown of Grand Rapids, the local news media was alerted to the fact that the two women were together in the same facility. The *Grand Rapids Press* featured an editorial blasting Dave Schieber for failing to live up to the plea agreement.

On February 1, 1990, Wood was transferred from the Huron Valley Women's Facility to a federal correctional facility in Lexington, Kentucky.

Chapter 113

The modern complex of one-story buildings could pass for a community college, if it were not for the fencing and tumbleweed razor wire. Inside, Gwen Graham found trouble in the prison inmates call "The Valley."

Unlike some celebrated prisoners, Gwen did not attract a following. Often, she lost privileges and was placed under "top lock" for breaking simple prison rules. She became deeply involved in a succession of relationships. She spent two months in solitary for a brawl with an inmate.

Gwen's visitors were very few. Her parents were hundreds of miles away in Texas and Oklahoma. Early on, only Fran Shadden and one of her friends sometimes made the two-hour trip from Grand Rapids. Gwen never once reached her limit of four visits a month in the first year.

During one visit by Fran, Gwen reluctantly agreed to be introduced to an interviewer. She was painfully shy in the first meeting, sometimes giggling like a bashful child. They agreed to begin talking on a regular basis. Soon, she became more relaxed, more open. She joked often. Sometimes, she sulked and pouted. Always, she was exceptionally polite. A meek "thank you" always served as her good-bye.

More often than not, Gwen gave her old partner Cathy Wood the benefit of the doubt. She avoided disparaging remarks and characterizations, always calling her "a very unhappy girl." In fact, she frequently defended her. She sided with Cathy in conflicts with Ken Wood and her mother Pat. Her feelings were clearly split about the woman who had put her away.

"Some days I would like to strangle her, if I could get my hands on her," she said one day. "Then, there's certain days that I wonder if she was here if we would be together. I still have feelings for her—not all good, not all bad."

On one point Gwen was consistent. She was innocent. She had murdered no one.

In the year the interviewer researched the Alpine murders, he rarely caught Gwen in a lie. In fact, she further incriminated herself circumstantially. She confessed to criminal behavior in her past. She shared her dark visions of bodies, water and death. On one Alpine Manor death, she placed her location in the nursing home in closer proximity to the victim.

The interviewer offered to investigate any lead she could provide to establish her innocence. She came up with none. More often than not, she seemed more satisfied just to have the company, to joke and laugh and share frustrations about her hot-and-cold relationships behind bars. She enrolled in a demanding apprenticeship in housepainting, sometimes showing up for interviews physically spent, her skin blushed from mineral spirits.

As an interview subject, she was easy to manipulate. She always protested probing areas concerning her parents, but it took little to break down her defense. "I don't want to hurt them," she would always say. She blamed no one but herself for her personality.

"I was stubborn and I wasn't like my sister and brother," she said one day. "I was a little monster. I *was*. I didn't want to be hugged and held and kissed and all that stuff. I didn't like it. And I don't know why, 'cause I love it now."

In time, two distinctly different personalities were evident. One drew cute pictures, wanted to cuddle little babies, wrote syrupy poems, called her lovers "pretty girl" and had the fears of a small child. The other drank Jack Daniel's whiskey, fought like a street hood, liked sadomasochistic sex and was oblivious to physical pain.

Her viewpoints of others also were riddled with contradictions. She could express two exactly opposite emotions about someone within the same session.

"Paul Lopez. Yeah, he's a good person, a friend, sure is."

Then, within minutes, "No, I don't like Paul. What he did to Robin just wasn't right."

She simply saw no conflict about such statements. It was little wonder a jury didn't believe her testimony.

With certain questions about her own psyche, usually involving her mother, she seemed to go very deep within herself. She became exceptionally silent. Her face turned red and her pupils dilated. Her features seemed gripped by a crushing mental oppression. She repeatedly expressed fear of being considered mentally ill, a "fruitcake" as she liked to call it.

"Do you think I'm a fruitcake?" she once asked.

"Do you?"

"Well, I wonder why I've done some of the fruity things I've done to myself. I do wonder, for real."

Gwen and the interviewer talked about her arms. "I did ten in one night, sure did." She said she was only speculating when she attributed the burns to her father during the trial.

"Because I really don't know why I did it," she said.

She said she felt numb, nonexistent, when she lit the cigarettes, she said. She only knew she "felt something" when the hot ash hit her skin.

Her interviewer asked her if she would allow herself to be tested by an independent forensic psychologist. He could evaluate her personality, maybe come up with some answers.

"Will it help my case?"

"Maybe," her interviewer said.

She agreed.

Before his evaluation of Gwen Graham, Dr. Michael Abramsky's work as a consultant in forensic psychology had involved him in some of Michigan's most notorious murder cases. He was popular among trial attorneys, not only for his twenty years' experience, but for his ability to communicate psychological concepts in a clear, simple manner to judges and juries.

Abramsky was already somewhat familiar with the Alpine Manor case. He had been contacted earlier about a possible evaluation of Cathy Wood when the prosecution and defense were still wrangling about psychological testing. Preparing for Gwen's evaluation, he studied the court transcript, the Palmatier polygraph video and other evidentiary materials. Then, in two afternoon sessions at Huron Valley, he interviewed Gwen and administered a series of standardized, objective and projective psychological tests.

Gwen shared some personal history in the interview. She said she often was called only "you" by her dad. She told Abramsky of threats by her father to flush her down the toilet, then of witnessing her dad pushing her mother's head into the commode. "They were just playing," she said. She talked about drains and her self-mutilation. She told the psychologist about her own sexual promiscuity and sexual play. She found it exciting, she said, when Cathy smothered her as they made love.

Her computer-scored objective tests, such as the Minnesota Multiphasic Personality Inventory, described a disturbed young woman. She was hostile, resentful and sullen, given to occasional violent outbursts. She was likely to have major problems in interpersonal relationships. She was likely to have poor judgement. She was attracted to danger and undaunted by punishment. She suffered from substance abuse. Outwardly, she might appear "aggressive, assertive, competitive and dominating." In fact, emotionally she was "dependent" and "passive dependent," her MMPI evaluation revealed.

Abramsky found her projective tests more enlightening. The first one he administered was the Rorschach, asking Gwen to comment on a series of inkblot images. She was slow and unspontaneous. She had difficulty seeing the people or faces or animals that most subjects will project during the test. Her only clear perception came when the psychologist produced a large color ink pattern.

"A pregnant monster!" she spouted. "It is!"

She giggled, almost euphorically. It was the kind of laughter Abramsky considered typical of someone who had broken through her own psychic defenses.

Next, they moved to the Thematic Apperception Test, or TAT. It was projective like the Rorschach. However, because it was less abstract than inkblot, personalities like Gwen's found it easier to articulate their visions and emotions, Abramsky would later explain. The test involved a series of nearly two dozen black and white drawings that pictured people in a variety of simple and complex situations. Gwen was asked to describe what was going on in each, what the people might be thinking and so forth.

Gwen struggled with some images.

A woman thinking, her chin in her hand: "She's thinking what she was doing as a little girl, but how old she is now. How she has to clean the house."

A woman with a younger girl: "She doesn't like what she's hearing. She's got to stop playing with dolls, but she doesn't want to."

The psychologist later noted, "Gwen has a tremendous block against any kind of mature activity whatsoever."

Drawings that pictured aggression also were revealing. One portrayed a man standing over the ravaged body of a woman prostrate on a bed. The man's head was in his hand, as though he was devastated by the discovery or devastated by the commission himself of some horrible act.

"Why should he be upset over a naked woman?" Gwen asked. "He has to go sit down. She's going to sleep."

Abramsky later said, "She doesn't see grief or guilt. She just doesn't see it at all. It's a joking type of thing for her. She doesn't see things at that level. Sophisticated emotions are simply not there."

Gwen reacted to pictures depicting what she thought might be immoral behavior. A boy who shot someone: "He's not going to mess with guns no more." A silhouette in a window: "A man breaking into a house. The lights are on. He'll get caught!"

The psychologist decided her sense of morality was what he called "primitive."

"Moral development covers a range as a person matures," he later explained. "In the earliest stage, something is wrong only because you will get punished for it. In the mature stage, you understand ethical principles and so forth.

"She is moral only in the lowest stages."

After the testing, Abramsky put together a complete psychological portrait of Gwen Graham. He also submitted his results to a private seminar of other consulting psychologists for input. They all agreed. She was a "low-functioning borderline personality."

The borderline personality, Abramsky explained, was one of several disorders that can develop in the first couple years of life and invariably continue through adulthood. "Low functioning" meant Gwen was of lower intelligence and sophistication, unlike "high functioning" borderlines who attain greater intellectual and social status.

However, their problem remains the same. Something very necessary to emotional development did not happen in Gwen's childhood, Abramsky predicted, something very early on.

"The mother-child bond is a very fundamental type of thing. The borderline's central problem is that a bonding relationship never occurs with the mother."

The psychologist was not talking about the more involved conflicts older children have with their parents. He meant lack of early, primitive bonding as a mother met *basic* emotional needs: A one-year-old cries; the mother does not pick it up to change, feed or comfort. A toddler is scared of the dark; the mother ignores its fears. A two-year-old is hit by a friend; the mother ignores the fight entirely.

"Either mother is too threatening to go to or count on in a reliable kind of way," Abramsky explained, "or mother cannot be there emotionally for the child at all."

If the bonding does not happen, the child's personality is stunted at that stage of emotional development, remaining "primitive" as the person grows into adulthood. The personality is hardly formed—on the borderline.

However, pathologically, borderline personalities continue to desperately seek the bond they never had.

"Their entire life is spent having these passionate attachments to people and then these constant tragic break-ups," Abramsky explained. "A kind of faulty bonding occurs. It's like a stunted plant. A real foundation for growth has never been established."

With that behavior comes the primitive trait of "splitting," such as Gwen's ability to like and dislike the same person with equal intensity. She was like a toddler gripped by the emotion of the moment, Abramsky said. Integrating two sets of feelings into an overall opinion was difficult, if not impossible.

The stunting extended beyond human relationships. Borderlines have very little sense of self.

"Their relationship to reality is somewhat tenuous. At times they experience a phenomena of not being real. A lot of times they will come apart when a bond with someone is broken, too. They can't handle the conflict, work it through logically. The burning phenomena, the self-mutilation, is a way for them to ground themselves in reality. The pain somehow makes them feel real. It's a contact with reality."

In fact, Gwen began burning herself after her bond with her father was broken because of the reported incest. While that alone may have been traumatic, Gwen already was in deep psychological trouble years before the event. She also slashed herself when Fran first tried to leave her. Abramsky pointed out other ways Gwen manifested the phenomenon.

"She's afraid of being washed down the drain. She has the feeling she's going to be sucked down. There's no sense of self, of solidity around her. The feeling that you can be sucked through those little holes in the bathtub is a childlike perception. It's appropriate for little kids because they don't have good, firm ego boundaries. That develops as you mature."

So does empathy. Gwen was incapable of understanding why the neighbors at Effie would be upset that she was shooting off a gun in the night.

"She understands right and wrong in the sense of someone saying 'This is right; this is wrong.' But when you talk about empathy, the ability to put ourselves in someone else's place, she lacks a lot of that."

Abramsky found that significant, considering her conviction.

"That could allow her to kill. She doesn't have a mature understanding of feelings, of guilt. Look at a child, a three-year-old who tears wings off a butterfly. What sense of guilt does she have? Even think about the concept of death for someone like this. Do you think three-year-olds really understand what death is?"

This lack of emotional development colored all her perceptions, influenced her behavior with others and made her sexually promiscuous, Abramsky said.

"Her behavior is asocial. Unlike a sociopath, who consciously breaks rules, she is essentially amoral. If you think of her functioning like a two-and-a-half-year-old kid, a lot of what she does, including those pictures she draws, make a great deal of sense. She's really never functioned beyond a particular level."

This was reflected in her own criminal defense, he added.

"Denial is the most primitive, simplest solution to all this."

The nature of the Alpine Manor murders, Abramsky believed, supported his analysis. However, it was quite unlike the way the case was portrayed in Grand Rapids.

"The whole thing of plotting, or spelling M-U-R-D-E-R, or so forth is not the way Gwen's mind works at all. This crime takes a certain conceptualization. It takes planning and timing. It takes someone who really plays chess . . . Cathy appears to be that kind of person. Bright. Manipulative.

"That's a higher kind of cognitive process than Gwen utilizes. Gwen expresses herself in very primitive kinds of ways. She goes out with Dawn and has fistfights with her. She can be a spiteful little girl, or violent. But she has an impulsive disorder. She's not a planner.

"I think Gwen could have easily killed the people, but the plot and the overall strategy is not her MO at all, not with all her problems. She's childlike dependant. Gwen is going to look at this like a little child. It was a game. There was a lot of play in it: Those little codes in the letters, the hiding under patient's beds. In Gwen's mind, this was an extension of that."

The Rorschach test figured into Abramsky's analysis.

"Primitive types tend to do poorly on Rorschach," he explained. "They get defensive about what they see and close down. She's terribly afraid of what's inside her."

However, Abramsky pointed out, the one image that did emerge from Gwen Graham's unconscious was extremely telling—the one she saw in the big colored ink blot. The "pregnant monster" symbolized the mother for whom she yearned, and the evil produced by their failure to bond.

The murders *were* a love bond, but not of a lesbian kind.

"The murders were a bonding behavior, a symbolic bonding," Abramsky said. "The two of them created their own little world, Gwen and her surrogate mother. She was the good little girl that did what Mom wanted, to win Mom's favor. And to Gwen the whole thing was simply play."

"Yes, the 'pregnant monster' is Gwen Graham's mother. But I also believe the pregnant monster is Cathy Wood."

Chapter 114

Gwen's mother Linda said there was a reason she didn't attend her daughter's trial. "We wanted to, but we didn't have the money or means to go."

She was the manager of a Tyler convenience store. Her second husband was a construction worker. They lived in a mobile home. The year of the trial, they brought home less than $12,000, she said.

Money wasn't any more plentiful in earlier years, she remembered. A woman of hardly five feet, by age twenty-two she had given birth to three children in three years. She recalled some advice she said came from her husband about child-rearing: "You don't hold children. It spoils them."

She recently changed her mind about that. She had just seen a TV program on child development.

"Now they say it doesn't spoil 'em to hold them," she said.

She wanted to contribute to people understanding her daughter. She was looking for answers herself, she said. With all the kids underfoot, she sometimes "lost my cool," she said.

"Would it help to know that I hit her with an electrical chord when she was about eighteen months? She was sitting there screaming, you know, how little babies do. I couldn't find out what was wrong with her. She wasn't hungry. She wasn't wet. She was screaming, and I lost it."

However, their conflicts she believed started in Gwen's teenage years.

"She was stubborn in a lot of areas. Her and I had some problems, but we worked all that out."

The most trouble Gwen had been in with the law before was traffic tickets. She had a bad habit of not paying her speeding tickets, she said.

After she moved in with Fran Shadden, Gwen told her that her father had made sexual advances, but she didn't know whether to believe her.

"I didn't know if that was a way of getting back at him or wanting to hurt me."

Gwen was a girl who needed a lot of discipline, "but not as much as she got," she said.

"I have looked back a lot and in wanting our kids to grow up right, maybe we overdone it," she said.

Later she said, "Believe me, I carry my own guilt."

Mack Graham had his own troubles in Heavner, Oklahoma, long after his daughter was put away for murder. His second wife had run off, leaving him with their preschool daughter. The girl suffered a seizure that blinded her and made her deaf. He had planned to take her trucking with him. Now, while she recovered, he had taken a year off from the road.

With his mustache and cowboy hat, Graham bore a striking resemblance to the Marlboro man, the advertising symbol of his daughter's brand. He spoke softly and slowly, with a hint of Southern drawl. He had visited Gwen once in Kent County jail. He hoped to head the way of Michigan again.

Mack never approved of Gwen's girlfriends.

"Gwen has always let others take advantage of her, use her," he said.

He knew about the trial and the story his daughter told. When it came to her allegations of incest, he chose not to deny or confirm.

"If I say one thing, it makes my daughter look bad. If I say the other, it makes me look bad. So I think I'll just leave it to her to tell it."

There had been mistakes, for sure, he said, things he should have done differently in the ways of child-rearing and such. He had tried to give his best, he said, but the bills and the cab in front of his eighteen wheeler had kept him away too much.

"That was expecting too much of my wife," he said. "She was young, twenty-one, with two kids and one on the way. It was expecting a lot, leaving her to do all that work."

Gwen and her mother got off to a real bad start when she was a baby, Mack said.

"When Gwen was real little, she never liked to be held. She'd always push away."

Gwen's mother didn't like this, he said. Before anything was resolved, Corey was born, eleven and a half months after Gwen.

Corey didn't push away. Corey took Gwen's place.

"Corey got held. Gwen didn't."

They battled for years, Gwen and her mom, Mack said.

For his part, he tried to raise her with "country psychology," teaching them about animals, the ways of caring and responsibility, the ways of life and death. Punishment came in the form of five licks with a belt, usually from her mother.

"Any time you feel you don't want a whipping from Mother," he told her once, "you can get one from me."

When she got older, the strap didn't seem to work. She would just bend over and silently take the punishment, her face turning bright red. He gave Gwen her last whipping at the age of eighteen.

Years earlier, he had tried to reason with her, give his daughter a little of his country psychology in a heart-to-heart chat.

"Honey, there are flowers and there are weeds," he told her. "You can neglect a flower, and it will turn into a weed. You can trim a weed, and turn it into a beautiful flower. Honey, I'm gonna make a flower out of you any way that I can—even if I have to trim you all the way back to the ground."

Mack Graham had no way of knowing she already was on the borderline. She had hardly broken through the earth.

Chapter 115

When people meet me, even the prosecutor, he thinks
I'm putting on some act. He says, 'Cathy you can't
be this sweet, and the part of you you're hiding from
me, I'm afraid of.' And I try to tell you, how can I
be putting on an act constantly, for over a year now?

—Cathy Wood, December 29, 1989.

Months after the trial, psychologists and others continued looking at the dynamics between Cathy Wood and Gwen Graham as more was learned about their behavior in and out of Alpine Manor.

They received no help from Cathy. After her sentencing, she became silent about the case.

"Mr. Schieber believed me, and the jury apparently believed me, and that's what I needed to do," she said, declining one of many requests for in-depth interviews. "I can't go over it anymore. It hurts me too much. I don't feel it. So, I can't."

In his contribution to the 1986 anthology *Unmasking the Psychopath,* leading psychologist Robert D. Hare proposed a twenty item check list for the psychopathic personality:

1. Glibness/superficial charm.
2. Grandiose sense of self-worth.
3. Need for stimulation/proneness to boredom.
4. Pathological lying.
5. Cunning/manipulative.
6. Lack of remorse or guilt.
7. Shallow affect.
8. Callous/lack of empathy.
9. Parasitic lifestyle.
10. Poor behavioral controls.
11. Promiscuous sexual behavior.

12. Early behavior problems.
13. Lack of realistic, long-term plans.
14. Impulsivity.
15. Irresponsibility.
16. Failure to accept responsibility for own actions.
17. Many short-term marital relationships.
18. Juvenile delinquency.
19. Revocation of conditional release.
20. Criminal versatility.

Psychopathy and its causes have been a source of study and mystery for years. Even the name of the disorder has changed three times: Psychopath. Sociopath. Antisocial personality. Some practitioners have simply written off the disorder as the embodiment of evil.

The impressions of those like Dave Schieber who saw a more "human" side of his star witness did not necessarily contradict the fact that Cathy Wood met much of Hare's criteria. The psychopath has always been known for a cunning ability to replicate and display the signs of conscience he or she, for all practical purposes, does not possess.

In his landmark work about psychopaths, *The Mask of Sanity*, psychiatrist Hervey Cleckley wrote:

> The observer finds verbal and facial expressions, tones of voice, and all the other signs we have come to regard as implying conviction and emotion and normal experiencing of life as we know it ourselves and as we assume it to be in others . . . Only very slowly and by a complex estimation or judgment based on multitudinous small impressions does the conviction come upon us that . . . we are dealing here not with a complete [person] at all but with something that suggests a subtly constructed reflex machine which can mimic the human personality perfectly.

Michael Abramsky, and earlier, John Hulsing, also believed that Cathy's behavior reflected the elements of the narcissistic personality disorder. The third edition of the American Psychiatric Association's *Diagnostic and Statistical Manual of Mental Disorders* lists nine criteria. Meeting five of them is indicative of the disorder.

1. Reacts to criticism with feelings of rage, shame, or humiliation (even if not expressed.)

2. Is interpersonally exploitative; takes advantages of others to achieve his or her own ends.
3. Has grandiose sense of self importance, e.g., exaggerates achievements and talents, expects to be noticed as "special" without appropriate achievement.
4. Believes that his or her problems are unique and can be understood only by other special people.
5. Is preoccupied with fantasies of unlimited success, power, brilliance, beauty or ideal love.
6. Has sense of entitlement: unreasonable expectation of especially favorable treatment, e.g., assumes that he or she does not have to wait in line when others must do so.
7. Requires constant attention and admiration, e.g., keeps fishing for compliments.
8. Lacks empathy; inability to recognize and experience how others feel . . .
9. Is preoccupied with feelings of envy.

In his book *The Narcissistic and Borderline Disorders,* psychiatrist James F. Masterson wrote that little was understood about why a child sometimes became stunted in an early stage of self-centeredness and remained that way into adulthood. As with the borderline disorder, however, mothers could have a powerful influence:

> Some of the mothers in the narcissistic personality disorders are basically emotionally cold and exploitative. They ignore their children's separation-individualization needs in order to mold them into objects that will justify their own perfectionistic, emotional needs.

Often, an individual will incorporate the characteristics of both disorders, Michael Abramsky said. A person can be a psychopath, while also displaying narcissistic tendencies. Both manipulate.

"High functioning psychopaths or narcissists are incredibly talented in that area," Abramsky said. "They have the ability to ascertain the needs of those around them and then exploit those needs for their own gratification or gain."

Those needs can be noble. They can range from a young man's need to help a teenager in trouble with her parents to a bright prosecutor's need to win a highly publicized murder trial.

A year after Graham's conviction, Michael Abramsky's finding of Gwen Graham as a borderline personality prompted Michigan State Police psychologist Gary Kaufmann to rethink his analysis of Cathy Wood. Cathy's breakdown at the end of the John Palmatier polygraph—the picture that had left him troubled—finally made sense.

As always, Cathy was crying for herself.

"It is extremely psychopathic that one would sacrifice themselves to bring another down," Kaufmann said. "The game of manipulation becomes more important than the outcome. That kind of risk-taking, in fact, is viewed as a form of thrill-seeking."

Cathy's role at the center of the case also took on new meaning for Kaufmann.

"The thing I've noticed over time with such self-defeating behavior by these kinds of people is that usually two things are accomplished with one act. She was able to manipulate, but she was also able to gratify her narcissism."

A new scenario of the Alpine Murder case was considered by Kaufmann, Abramsky and others familiar with the story. Made vulnerable after being turned in by her ex-husband, Cathy may have embarked on her ultimate high-stakes game. Controlling the early input, she appeared to have perfectly projected her own personality onto Gwen Graham. Among many who knew them both, Cathy's descriptions of her former lover to the police, judge and jury were more suited to herself than Gwen.

At times Cathy appeared to literally lay claim to Gwen's behavior. After Chambers' death, she said she drank Jack Daniel's, Graham's drink of choice. She said she felt sorry for Edith Cook, but long after Gwen said she killed her out of mercy. She said Gwen put a gun up her vagina, preempting Gwen's claim of the reverse to a jury.

"One reason I knew Cathy hadn't made up the murders was because Cathy only lied to make herself look better," Ken Wood once said. "Admitting to murder certainly didn't make her look good."

However, portraying Gwen as the manipulator, mastermind and sole executioner did. Switching the roles made more sense out of Cathy's own version of events. Setting up Angie Brozak to say outrageous things on the telephone was behavior typical of Cathy, not Gwen. Phone games also were played with patients' families. All the aides marked for death—Angie Brozak, Dawn Male, Robin

Fielder—were enemies of Cathy. They had something important in common. They were taking Gwen's attention away from Cathy Wood.

Besides the victims being mother figures, Cathy potentially had other motives to conceive and direct the series of killings. The shared secret offset the lure of Robin Fielder. Wood admitted she was a "child abuser" in a facility where residents were treated like kids. Aides who cared for half the victims were objects of her scorn. Outside Alpine Manor, Cathy Wood's life was in turmoil. Inside, she had power and control. The killings "were supposed to continue" not only after Gwen wrestled with Maurice Spanogle, but after Cathy Wood had a violent, disruptive fight with Ken. There also was evidence of attacks long after Gwen had left the nursing home.

"The ultimate power," said police psychologist Kaufmann, "is the control over life and death of an individual."

That Cathy Wood might have been able to manipulate Gwen Graham into the role of her personal executioner when they were lovers also was in step with conventional forensic psychology. Gwen not only had a history of parent figures prompting her to kill objects such as dogs and animals, she had the classic personality for the task.

In an article published in the April, 1990 issue of the *American Journal of Psychotherapy*, psychiatrist Theodore B. Feldmann and two forensic psychologists discussed "cofactors" in the commission of violent crimes.

> Forensic experience has led us to conclude that many violent
> crimes have a cofactor that precipitates the event. . . . The
> cofactor involved in these violent crimes is usually a person or
> persons influencing the perpetrator. It appears that most often
> individuals with severe borderline or narcissistic pathology are
> affected.

The often-quoted relief of "tension" was very likely more real than imagined. According to Dr. Feldmann, both borderline and narcissistic personalities, when stressed by forces beyond their control, have periods of traumatic "disintegration anxiety"—like

Gwen's fear of being sucked up—that violence seems to rectify, at least temporarily.

"In all the cases, the preoccupation with violence temporarily allows the traumatized self to restructure, providing temporary cohesion," Feldmann and his colleagues wrote.

"This appears to be the case, for example, in serial criminals."

Chapter 116

The Press stories—did it come out what happened to me when I was fourteen, that I was with this boy and we had sexual intercourse and I found out it was a girl? Are you interested back that far? It's a big factor. Oh my gosh! I'd have to tell you things like that?

—Cathy Wood, December 29, 1989.

The sounds of beating drums filled the chilled October air. The Comstock Park Marching Band was practicing on the high school football field, not a block down the street. Cathy Wood's mother Pat was outside raking leaves.

Over the two garage doors of the white New England-style farmhouse were signs. One for Cathy Wood's stepfather Chris, the other for her mother Pat. They read: "Pat's Pad" and "Chris's Dog House." A year after her daughter was imprisoned, the second garage door was closed. The couple were separated.

Inside the house, however, Cathy's mother had plenty of company. Her son, three dogs and five cats made the eighty-two-year-old farmhouse home. A frequent volunteer at the local Humane Society, Pat announced she had a special name for her pets.

"These are my kids," she told a visitor, inviting him inside. "I *adore* animals."

The interior was neat, but not obsessively so. Remnants of Cathy's life outside prison graced the house. There were her records, a couple dozen unicorns in brass and crystal and a bookcase of hardcover books. When Pat cleaned out the little house on Effie Place she found many more titles.

"She had a lot of paperback books. Boxes and boxes and boxes of paper books," she recalled. "Hundreds and hundreds and hundreds of books. I got rid of them. I told her, I'm not saving them."

Pat said she started reading to Cathy at a very young age, beginning with cloth books then moving into Golden Books. Later, her daughter's literary appetite made discipline difficult.

"Go to your room. That's the worst thing I ever did to her. She loved to be punished, because she loved to read."

She let out a gregarious laugh that filled the living room. The mother of Cathy Wood had the kind of large personality that left little doubt as to where she stood or what she felt.

She certainly did not approve of the portrait of a neglected and brutalized child that was painted by her sister-in-law to Judge Robert A. Benson.

"My ex-husband never really mistreated the children like the news media portrayed, as though they were beaten daily, not fed and got ridiculed. I was a working, normal housewife. I took care of the kids. The kids went roller-skating. They had their slumber parties."

She paused, looking her visitor in the eyes.

"I've always taught my children never to hurt anything. Respect. Courtesy. Maybe I stressed it too much. *I don't know.*"

She said the last three words emphatically, pausing dramatically between each.

"I did my *very* best. But obviously, I failed."

Sure, her kids dressed themselves, when they were older, she said.

"What's wrong with that?"

Yes, her first husband did drink too much and could be verbally abusive, she said. They met in high school, married while he was on leave from boot camp and had Cathy and Barbara in Soap Lake, Washington. Cathy was born near the Air Force base where he was stationed. Assigned to a canine unit, he went to Vietnam. He came back from combat changed, she said.

"My first husband was an asshole," she said. "There's no doubt about that."

The kids saw little of him, however. He slept days and worked midnights, she said. She worked in an office all day, but was home by five—for them. The mouth-stuffing incident reported by her sister-in-law in her letter to the judge was inaccurate. She called Cathy's aunt and let her know that herself.

"I was *not* there. It was at a lunch. I would not allow that, and John would never pull that if I was there. You *have* to be proper. You can't make displays, and you cannot ridicule children. You *cannot* . . . that is not allowed."

She admitted he might have "pulled some stuff" while she was working.

"But never when I was there. Because then, he would have to answer to *me*. My first husband loved me. He still loves me. I don't know why. But he hated me for my strength. He *hated* me for my strength."

An earlier newspaper profile of Cathy indicated she had been teased as a child by neighborhood kids for her weight. Hogwash, Pat said.

"Nobody teased her. No. No . . . She felt insecure, but no one teased her. Who would tease her? Cathy was too big. She would pound them to death."

A few days earlier, Pat had seen the videotape of Cathy's polygraph with John Palmatier. She appeared to react calmly to Cathy's scathing portrayal of her as a mother who wouldn't let her have cookies when she wanted them.

"You know you always hurt the ones you love. She was hurt and she was angry and she came out with the last cookie in the jar."

Yes, she said, she liked to play with the kids, as Cathy said in the video, but that didn't mean she was nuts.

"When they played jacks, I got right down with them and played jacks. I always had a lot of fun. When they went to other people's houses their mothers never did that. I can rake leaves and jump right in the leaves with them.

"I'm me. I cannot change me. I'm sorry. I can be very stuffy. I can be very high and mighty and I can just have a lot of fun. With children, why should you be stuffy? I thought I was putting them at ease. I guess not."

She was sensitive to the differences between Cathy and Barbara. Cathy had three friends, Barbara had thirty. The phone "rang and rang and rang" for Barbara. Cathy "sat alone in a corner" and learned to play chess.

The David/Debbie incident was disturbing.

"I'm yelling and ranting and raving, what's going on? I probably shouldn't have yelled at her. I ranted and raved and yelled at Catherine . . . I don't think I did anything different than anybody else would have."

Did she threaten to put Cathy in a mental institution?

"Now why would I do that?"

When Cathy married Ken she was disturbed.

"I was disappointed. I was angry. I was hurt."

At first he seemed decent. It was a requirement, she said.

"They had to come to the door. And they had to be a gentleman. And they had to be nice. And they couldn't use filthy language. That wasn't *allowed.* I was a typical mother."

But Ken sequestered Cathy, she said. She had been told by her daughter that when she tried to diet, Ken filled the house with junk food.

"He was very possessive of Cathy. He wanted Cathy to himself."

She had little use for him now, and she knew he had little use for her. She called most of his stories about her "ridiculous."

"I'm a bad person, a very bad person. That's all right. He can think that, 'cause he's going to anyway."

Ken was blackmailing Cathy about the murders, her daughter told her.

"He wanted money, for a year. When she didn't have the money, and couldn't come through, he turned her in."

Yes, Pat had done her share of fighting her daughter's battles. She took on Ken several times. She pried Cathy's vacation pay from Alpine Manor. When Gwen Graham was sent to Huron Valley she lambasted prison officials.

"I was making waves at the prison. What are they going to do with me, lock *me* up?"

Her daughter's prosecution and conviction was a sham, she said.

"They treated her unfairly, all the way down the line."

On the other hand, Pat said she should have made her daughter face up to her own responsibilities earlier than she did. She remembered when she asked her to start paying rent on the little house on Effie, one of her rental properties. Cathy hadn't paid rent in two years.

"Mother, you can't make me move out," Cathy told her. "This is my house. *You* get out."

"I served papers on her," she recalled. "I will not have her talk to me that way. She was angry how I evicted her. One day she came in the yard. I was taking the trash out. And she comes in, 'Hi mom.'

"I said, 'Get off my property. I can't *afford* you.'

"Her smile faded, 'cause she thought all had been forgotten."

Pat laughed, deeply, at the memory. She was still chuckling as she continued.

"One of my other renters was there paying me the money, and she had never seen that side of me . . ."

Later, the mother of Catherine May Wood pulled out two picture albums, stuffed with portraits of the past. Cathy was born with a birthmark on her forehead, but it faded in a year. There was a picture of a pretty toddler in a smart dress and stitched leather shoes. There was a photo of Cathy in a fluffy petticoat, and another in a duck hat, standing next to her dad. At ten she was standing next to a Christmas tree. She was straddling a big war cannon as a teen.

"There she is at her wedding," Pat said, turning a page. "Happy bride? Is that a happy marriage? Now, look how pretty she is here. Here, she's at home."

When she was done with those two books, she stood up.

"Now," she said, "I've got something else to show you."

She had another photo album for her visitor before he left. She was smiling broadly, holding it in front of her in her upturned palms.

"*This,* is the neatest one, here," she said, placing it in his lap.

Inside, were pictures of all her dogs.

Grand Rapids Press reporter Ken Kolker had scored one exclusive after another in his coverage of the Alpine Manor murder case. After both defendants were imprisoned, he pulled as much as he could together in a final story called "Fatal Friendship" for a Sunday edition in early 1990.

Kolker was relaxing at home when he received the phone call. Again he had a first, but with the trial over with, he had no news event to peg the information into a story.

"This is *David/Debbie,*" the voice on the other end said.

The caller's voice was filled with contempt. She had read all about Cathy's version of their relationship in Kolker's story—and she was fuming.

Yes, she knew Cathy Wood.

However, she said, everyone was missing some very important facts. She never had a romantic relationship with Cathy. In fact, she was the girlfriend of one of Cathy's friends. She and Cathy were only acquaintances. She wanted the reporter to know one more thing. Cathy knew she wasn't a boy. She had always made that very clear.

"The way she described it, the whole David/Debbie thing wasn't a total fabrication," Kolker later said. "It was a spinoff."

David/Debbie appeared to be another one of Cathy Wood's perfectly executed half-truths.

Chapter 117

> *I'll always love you most, Cathy, and I'll make right this wrong I've done to you.*
>
> —Gwen Graham, September 8, 1987, in a letter from Tyler, Texas.

Stephanie Engman flung the Sunday newspaper into the wall. In seconds she was hurling or smashing anything she could get her hands on in the dormitory room.

When she came to her senses, the *Grand Rapids Press* lay on the floor, the pictures of Gwen Graham and Cathy Wood staring up at her from an article headlined "Fatal Friendship." The stories about the pathetic, insecure fat girl had her in tears.

They were not tears of sympathy.

"Everybody was feeling sorry for the woman who helped put washcloths over my grandmother's face," she later told a friend. "Feeling *sorry*—when it was nothing but a big joke, for fun and for power."

Nanna used to always say, "Well, fiddley dee, we'll have to change that won't we." Stephanie's first impulse was to write the newspaper. Then she thought about another mob of reporters at her door.

Yes, there were things she had to change. Not long after the article, she left Hope College. She needed to find a way to live with herself and others. Wood and Graham had not only taken her grandmother, they had taken away her ability to trust anyone or anything again.

"I have to find a way to forgive them, but not forget."

She had to find a way.

"Hating isn't fun and it makes you very tired," she told a friend.

Her father, John Engman, the lawyer, made up contracts for the family to sign. It called for any family member, no matter where their location, to attend any parole or pardon hearing for Wood and Graham.

Engman had no doubt his mother-in-law was a murder victim. The testimony about the souvenir from Mae Mason was alone convincing. He remembered the little house with the swinging door that Cathy had described. It was one of Maisy's key chain charms. The kids used to play with it on the floor as toddlers.

Soon, more lawyers were involved in the Alpine Manor matter. First Nancy Hahn, then the Engmans and the Hundermans decided to file suit. Early on, Hahn's Grand Rapids attorney J. Clarke Nims received a phone call from another lawyer. Her name was Nancy Gage. She suggested he quickly videotape a deposition. She had a client, a former Alpine supervisor, who was very sick with a bad heart. She wanted to talk about short staffing and the complaints no one would listen to about Gwen Graham and Cathy Wood. Her name was Tish Prescott.

At first, John Engman was reluctant to sue. Then he saw the former supervisor's deposition.

"I can't express how angry it has made me," Engman said. "This is your worst nightmare because you have the guilt. I have spent a lot of time with that. And it has bothered me, because I *swore* I would never put anybody in a nursing home. I will live with that for the rest of my life."

One day, the Engman's daughter Sari noticed a pattern when

her eighty-nine-year-old grandfather visited for dinner. People around the table often were cutting him off, simply because he was slower, simply because he was older. Maybe that's why he doesn't talk so much, she told her mother. He knows nobody will listen.

"Look at me, Grandpa, I'll listen," she decided to tell him one day.

The Hundermans listened to their minister, before they made their decision. A good day's pay, for a good day's work. That was the way of their church.

"Suing is not the Christian Reformed way," the minister told them. "But if this is the way you feel, you must do what you have to do."

Jan had received flowers from Alpine Manor owner Ron Westman. A bouquet arrived for Thanksgiving, then one for Christmas. Then, the flowers stopped.

"Emotionally, the lawsuit won't accomplish a thing," Jan told a friend. "But I think it's going to make a point to a lot of nursing homes."

Some just needed to simply find the truth for themselves. Al Van Dyke didn't come to grips with his mother's demise until a year after her death, when the former homicide cop walked into Walker PD and had a good talk with Tom Freeman—cop to cop.

Other families felt the nursing home was a victim among the rest. Ted and Maxine Luce were out to dinner one night when a friend approached them at the salad bar.

"I'd sue them people, I would," the friend said loudly.

"No, I don't think I'll do that," Ted said. "My mother had real good care there."

A couple of minutes later Ronald Westman walked over to their table. He had apparently heard the exchange.

"I'm glad you feel that way, not bitter," he said.

A year after the trial, Westman sold the nursing home to a hospital group. It was renamed St. Mary's Living Center. The new administration changed the residents' birthday board. They stripped the walls of the material geared for the mentality of children. They put newspapers and magazines in the day rooms. They dressed the nurse's aides in regulation uniforms.

The worst of the emotional aftermath never found its way into court depositions. It eluded description in the cold, precise language of the law.

Linda Engman's pain was very private. She was never one to put her head on her husband's shoulder and bawl. Often, she simply found herself wide awake well after midnight, when her big glassy house was very still. Invariably, she went downstairs, drawn to the wood stove that kept the house warm in winter months. She would light a cigarette there and begin thinking. Sometimes she pondered washcloths and pastel walls and fluorescent lights and other terrible things.

"You start opening that door in your mind a bit," she told a friend. "You open it, and then you have to shut it quickly. You have to shut it for sanity's sake."

Often, she found herself sitting on the floor, staring out through the tall walls of glass. The room blackened, she could see the brown river running by swiftly outside in the night.

Time brought sobriety, recovery and a new attitude for Dawn Male, and a new perspective on the whole Alpine Manor affair. Cathy Wood was able to captivate us all, she thought, simply because we had no respect for ourselves.

"I'm sorry it had to happen to Gwen. My life as a kid may not have been as severe as Gwen, but I got a lot of physical and emotional abuse. I'm glad it wasn't me. I think it could have easily been me. I was just as vulnerable as Gwen, at that time. Now, I *see* Cathy."

Dawn couldn't foresee something like that ever happening to her again. She still was in Lakeview, but the little town had new horizons. She went to work in a nursing home again, but also took an entrance exam in law enforcement at Grand Rapids Junior College. Dawn wanted to be a conservation officer. Dawn Male might even consider being a cop.

A year after the court case, Dawn still doubted the murders had occurred. She suspected Gwen Graham had been framed. So did Angie Brozak, Ladonna Sterns, Tony Kubiak and many others. They couldn't square the story with the pathological lying of Cathy Wood and her profile of the Gwen Graham they knew.

"You have to ask this question," Dawn told a friend. "Why would Cathy jeopardize years of her life in prison? My answer is this: Either the game isn't done, and there's a subplot I'm not figuring out, or the game *is* done, but she made an error somewhere in the game, and now she's stuck."

They all wondered if Cathy was simply waiting to make another move.

Ken Wood found some freedom nearly a year and a half after his ex-wife was imprisoned. He was working in a convenience store, raising Jamie and getting a few laughs as a new member of a comedy troupe putting on a show for local cable TV. One night Cathy called from prison. Mysteriously, she seemed to know about his new avocation.

"So, are you having fun with your comedy friends?" she said, playing coy.

"Cathy," he said. "Whatya want. I'm busy. I don't have time anymore for all this crap."

For the first time, Ken Wood really just didn't give a damn. He found the feeling joyous.

A couple of weeks later, Ken received some terrible news. The grandmother he dearly loved had a stroke. When Ken's father admitted her to a nursing home, a friend who didn't know the family's connection with the Alpine Manor case, asked his dad:

"Now, do you feel comfortable with her in a nursing home? Remember those two girls?"

Ken was overwhelmed when he walked into his grandmother's nursing home for his first visit. He kept looking at all the aides. He thought, who are these people? Are they answering my grandmother's buzzer? When she complains about a headache, does anyone really care?

He couldn't shake the feeling that everyone was looking at him. He wanted to make sure his grandmother got the best of care.

Robin Fielder tried nursing home work again, but quit days after she took another job as an aide. She was bathing a naked patient when another worker, a woman in her thirties with heavy, caked makeup, walked into the room.

"I know who you are," she said, glaring. "I was at the trial. You are as guilty as they are. Either you quit, or everybody around here is going to know who you are and what you did."

Robin was shaking when she told the supervisor she quit.

"It's not fair," she said. "I'm not guilty."

Later, she gave up on the medical field, writing off her two years of schooling. She began studies in computer sciences, trying to forget her outrage over the sentencing of Cathy Wood.

"To know that she was the cause of all this, I was real mad," she told a friend. "She hurt me. She hurt my family. She hurt the patients. She hurt the patient's families. She hurt Gwen's family. She hurt her own family. They both should have had the same sentence. She was as guilty as Gwen."

Robin was troubled by other memories. All her pictures from childhood to her teenage years as a cheerleader were in albums left in Texas. Gwen's family had them. Gwen was pleading with Robin to come to the prison herself and ask for them in person. Robin knew Gwen might try anything to see her again. But it was a trip she was incapable of making.

Someday, Robin Fielder, hoped to get the rest of her life back.

Guilt and punishment were discussed around the Walker Police Department. Roger Kaliniak and others did not find the kind of satisfaction that usually followed the conclusion of a case of this magnitude.

"I don't think Tom is one hundred percent satisfied either, from my own gut feeling," he said.

Tom Freeman wanted to know more about Gwen Graham.

"God damn, I wish she would talk to me," he told another investigator. "I wish she would cop to this thing. I'd like to know if there are other bodies."

One day, Freeman received a letter from Cathy Wood.

"I've figured out now how police work a little bit," she wrote. "I hope some of the things you told me were sincere."

She added a postscript: "Someday you'll have to let me beat you at a game of pool."

David Schieber was also getting letters from Cathy Wood in prison. One belittled the Walker detective whose tenacity broke open the Alpine Murder case.

Cathy wrote: "The definition of 'policeman' sure doesn't say: 'see Freeman.' "

Cathy sang the praises of being in a federal prison to the assistant prosecutor. "Bonjour Monsieur Schieber." She had a French roommate. She was taking a course in existentialism.

"The difference in prisons is amazing," she wrote. "We're never locked in our rooms and I'm treated just like everyone else. Even all the people have been good for me. It's helping me be a little more assertive in getting what I want."

The assistant prosecutor wrote her back, telling her about his cases and heavy workload. Soon, they had a regular correspondence going.

"I wish I would have had a father like you," Cathy wrote in one letter.

In another, "I got a lot of my confidence from watching you. Sixteen years is quite a slice of time, but maybe I need it to get myself together. So when you're a famous judge, I may have to sneak in and watch you."

Later, one bright morning, Walker Deputy Chief Bill Brown wondered over coffee whether justice had been served.

"Most people get hung up on the fact that the person who is the trigger man, the killer, is the worst," he told a companion. "Gwen is the hands-on murderer. But without Cathy, it never would have happened. Who should be dealt with the harshest? Then, again, you have no choice. There's the old theory that the first one to the window gets the deal. That's the way the game is played."

Gwen Graham came to the attorney's visiting area wearing a prison ensemble—shirt and pants in bright white. They were state issue for a prisoner in solitary confinement. The soft cotton material was blemished by serial numbers in faded black dye.

She asked about Robin Fielder.

"How's she doing? Okay?"

Her interviewer nodded.

She frequently asked about Robin, sometimes tearfully. She never provided a detailed rebuttal to Robin's accusations at the trial.

"I will never say anything bad about Robin," she said. "I just never will."

However, her blanket denial continued.

"I didn't kill anybody. No. No. No. I didn't kill anybody. I didn't watch anybody kill anybody. No. No. No."

The interviewer asked her to speculate, about someone else who might find himself in her situation.

"Would that someone ever tell if they did really kill these people?" the interviewer asked.

"Why wouldn't they?"

"Well, then it would take away her last option. Then someone else would be in total control of her life."

"Cathy has already taken away my life. By me being here, Cathy already has me under her total control."

"But would another person ever tell?"

She thought about it hard, then answered.

"No, you wouldn't tell. Sure wouldn't, for real."

Earlier, she had wondered about her appeal. It had been nearly a year since it was filed. Still there was no word from the court. The appellate issues ranged from the relevancy of Cathy Wood's testimony about her "lesbian life-style" to the court's failure to grant psychological evaluations.

If Gwen received a new trial, might she try to plea to a lesser charge?

"No way. If I was on the parole board, and somebody said I killed six helpless people, I'd say 'No way.' "

Six helpless people. Marguerite Chambers. Myrtle Luce. Mae Mason. Belle Burkhard. Ruth Van Dyke. Edith Cook. Six people died on five days in 1987.

There was the very real possibility her appeal would be denied, her interviewer pointed out. As Gwen considered that her shoulders slumped. She stared at a wall of cement block in front of her.

She looked hurt, confused.

"Then, what's going to happen to me?" asked Gwen Graham. "Am I going to be here forever?"

No, five mandatory lifetimes, if she had that many to give.

It was as far beyond forever as any mortal would ever get.